William Stuart Gould, M.D.

A HEART WIND FROM THE DESERT

A NOVEL

ALSO BY BILL GOULD

At Yonah Mountain

Captain Iron Mustache

In Black Granite

C.O.L.A.

Raphael's Blanket

Lincoln Friday

Sabrina's Suit

Sass

William Stuart Gould, M.D.

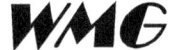

WMG Ltd. Publishers
288 Lexington Avenue
Suite 6-F
New York, New York
10016
wmg.ltd.publishing@gmail.com

This book is a work of fiction. Names, characters, places, and incidents are either products of the author's imagination or are used fictitiously. Any resemblance to actual events, locales, or persons, living or dead, is entirely coincidental.

For information about WMG Ltd.'s Speakers Bureau or discounts for bulk purchases, please email: wmg.ltd.publishing@gmail.com

ISBN: 978-0-9912237-4-9 (e-book)
ISBN: 978-0-9979804-2-4 (pbk)

To my parents

PROLOGUE

Mid 2002
Charles De Gaulle Airport
Paris, France

*A*n *American in Paris* was playing softly in the background as Dr. Solomon Forte shuffled, head down, toward check in. His right hand towed a dirty suitcase, lashed to which was a six-foot spear. His left hand, heavily bandaged, clutched the sides of a tattered cardboard box marked with the faded words:

**USAID
A GIFT FROM THE PEOPLE OF THE
UNITED STATES OF AMERICA**

The music only further depressed him, for it culled memories of his mother and father, poor immigrants who had so loved Gershwin. And Michaela and Dana had loved *Rhapsody in Blue*, and *Porgy and Bess*, and now they were gone. Everything was gone.

He checked in and left the suitcase and spear as baggage but asked to keep the cardboard box with him. As he passed through immigration and security, officials in both areas had him open and reseal the carton several times. Finally cleared, he entered the departure lounge, catching his reflection in a mirrored partition, barely recognizing the bearded, gaunt man staring back. He was nearing forty. The hair that had been jet-black and neatly cropped just months before, when he left his damaged medical practice in Whitaker, was now streaked with gray and unkempt. As he rounded a corner in the lounge, he exhaled as he caught sight of Gate M-49.

BRITISH AIRWAYS—WHITAKER NON-STOP

His eyes locked rigidly on the symbol of the last sector of his journey. He was not surprised that the notion of soon being home was so devoid of warmth. The single ember left in him was the fragile promise of coming back to Europe to be with her, to test their passion, to see if it would survive the real world.

Though his lips turned down at the sight of the word "Whitaker," he accepted that there was no choice but to return to the U.S., to salvage what might be left of his career. Was that first, or was she? He shook his head, wondering, but quickened his pace, hungry to find a seat at the gate and nap for the hour before boarding. Maybe it would calm the buzzing in his ears and the strange nausea from weeks, or was it months, without sleep.

He was oblivious to the glare of a security gendarme until the officer poked his index finger at Sol several times and bellowed a second time, "*Hein, Monsieur, venez ici. Qu'est ce que c'est, celui-là?*"

Sol's shoulders tensed, startled by the raised voice, and his head jerked left and right, eyes darting, searching warily for the threat, but seeing not a single rock flying at him, nor a crazed face brandishing a Russian assault rifle, he walked on, unaware that it was he who was the target of the shrill policeman's attention. The guard, puffed his chest and commanded in nearly unintelligible English, "You, Meester, you came 'ere."

Sol stopped in his tracks, surprised, though not intimidated, for he had been through the drill countless times since escaping Whitaker, stomaching brigades of self-consumed bureaucrats across the world. He shook his head skeptically and walked to the gendarme's counter, smiling stiffly as he placed the box on the floor.

"No, no, you put 'im 'ere for ze inspection." The man tapped the counter indignantly.

Poker-faced, Sol lifted the box onto the kiosk and mumbled, "Your pals at security already looked at it twice. It's a paper truck. Just a toy."

"*Mais oui*, ze paper truck." The gendarme shot air from his cheeks as if confronted with a lunatic. He pointed to the box. "*Ouvres cette boîte.*" He flapped his hands in the air over the carton.

Sol, spirit worn thin by government-generated calamity over so many nations, the endless days of travel, the loss of nearly forty pounds, and the poison of having tried so hard to do right, and having nearly been murdered for his pains, all of it, at that instant, climaxed. As if one of the mad schizophrenics he'd studied in medical school, he took notice of a hallucination crowing deep within his head. He recognized the voice, though, of his dear André, grunting, "*Ça suffit*, it is enough, Soli. You must not listen to zis bastard."

So Sol snapped back at the policeman, "It's enough already. It's a pain to open. I just got done rewrapping it for the nth time. I'm done with your crap."

He took a step away from the security official, but the man shrieked, "You, Meester, you come 'ere. You open ze box! It is my order." He jumped forward and seized Sol's arm.

Sol pulled away forcefully, but the gendarme managed to grasp a handful of Sol's faded shirt, which sent two buttons skittering along the floor. When Sol's eyes dropped to watch them spinning away, the officer reached around and snatched the box, slamming it onto the counter. Sol braced, lips curled down as his hands shot forward to grasp the policeman's wrists. The gendarme gulped nervously and leapt rearward, but the escape was thwarted when his back hit a wall. He groped for his whistle, put the wrong end in his mouth, and blew over and over. With but nothing but a hiss, he pulled the whistle free, and screeched, "*Urgence, urgence*," so loud a tense hush descended over the entire departure lounge.

But one officer responded, a gendarme who approached indifferently, sidling up to his compatriot, hiding a smile. "What is eet now, Marcelle?" he croaked in English, turned more to Sol than his compatriot.

"Zis man, 'ee disobeys me. I tell 'im open ze box for ze inspection. 'Ee run away."

The second officer nodded perfunctorily and spoke quietly. "But 'ee is still 'ere. Where did 'ee run?" Turning to Sol, he asked gently, "Please *Monsieur*, allow ze officer inspect ze package. We must, *Monsieur*. It is our law. Please understand."

Sol's shoulder's relaxed, and he undid the twine carefully, though not fast enough for Marcelle, who grumbled impatiently and pawed at the cardboard flaps, ripping one.

The second official shook his head and took Marcelle by the tunic to a corner. They spoke in hushed, angry tones, though Sol had to roll his eyes and snort a laugh when Marcelle's voice rose to hiss the word e*xplosif,* loud enough to be heard throughout the lounge. The two men took deep breaths and stepped back to the counter. Marcelle lifted his chin bravely, thrusting a hand inside the cardboard box as if it might be the last act of patriotism he would ever execute for his beloved France. But all he extracted were scraps of dirty, sewn-together cardboard shaping a foot-long model of a British Land Rover, the axels fashioned from tree twigs, red bottle caps shaped into headlights and wheels. A frayed length of tattered nylon filament had been tied to the front, allowing it to be pulled along—a child's toy.

Sol snarled, "Please be gentle with it," but the gendarme twisted the curio in all planes, searching for contraband. When he poked his fingers inside, he managed to crack the "windshield" which had been created from a discarded glass microscope slide. Sol raised his hand again, but Marcelle jammed the toy quickly into the carton, crushing a corner. He brushed the box aside with a sweep of his forearm, summoning another passenger. Sol began to protest, but the policeman fluttered the back of his hand disinterestedly, dismissing Sol. When Sol continued to glare at him, the policeman barked, "You, Meester, you know what is Nine-Eleven?" He shook his index finger indignantly. "You want im in ze States, okay wis me. *Mais* we do not allow 'im from 'ere."

Sol braced and his fists tightened, but the second gendarme took a step toward the desk, placing himself between Sol and Marcelle. He patted both of Sol's arms gently and shook his index finger no, then asked, "*Monsieur*, it is okay to look at 'im, *s'il vous plait*?"

Sol heaved a cheerless sigh, pulled the truck from the box, and handed it to the man, who also inspected it closely, but tenderly. He appeared astonished by the resourcefulness that had gone into its creation. *"C'est incroyable, non?"* He spent a moment unbending the wrinkle in the dusty cardboard, but Sol smiled, looked at his watch, and then at the gate. "A gift from the children." Sol pointed to the stamp in his passport. The officer nodded approvingly as Sol placed the toy back in the box, holding the torn flaps in place as Sol wound the string about the carton. He added as Forte started toward the gate, *"C'est un camion en papier. C'est intéressant.* I sink you say, 'paper truck.' So interesting. *Bon voyage, Monsieur. Et merci.* Our nation sank you."

On board the 747, Sol was directed left, then upstairs. At the first-class compartment, a flight attendant looked at him closely and nodded with a smile. "Ah, so you're the one. We've been waiting for you, Doctor. We'll take good care of your kit.

She placed the cardboard box carefully into the luggage rack directly above Sol as he flopped, exhausted, into his seat. Another flight attendant stopped by Sol's elbow. She tipped a bottle of Moet & Chandon toward him. "Would you like champagne, sir?"

"Do you have ice water, ma'am?"

"Yes, but how about a soft drink, Doctor? We've got…"

"No, no, just ice water, please." Sol considered explaining himself, justifying why a man so weary would turn down champagne for water, but his eyes dropped and he looked away.

The woman answered softly, "Yes, of course, sir," She brought a goblet of perfectly clear ice water, a twist of lime curled over the edge. "We're privileged to have you aboard, Doctor."

Sol nodded and smiled faintly, then sipped the water and let his gaze drift out the window. He, though, perceived nothing then, nor when the plane lifted off and circled toward the west, unlocking a broad vista of Paris, the Eiffel Tower reflecting in the cut crystal of his glass. As the magnificent city faded, his mind remained mired in a buzzing silence, as if his heart had stopped.

CHAPTER ONE

Earlier 2002
On the Bus
Making for Umm Balla Village
Western Darfur Province
The Sudan

Solomon Forte, looking far younger than his nearly forty years, muscular, clean-shaven, with close-cropped ebony hair and twinkling deep, deep blue eyes, sat sweating profusely, clasping a chipped, scratched glass of sloshing, murky brown water. His eyes drifted closed, his consciousness spinning into a trance in which he sat camped beside a wintry river in the mountains outside Whitaker. The rattle of his hands in the dream was not a product of the vicious jolting of the bus he had boarded so many hours before, but of shivering. Then a nuclear thud jarred him, and his eyes opened as wide as the flat, reed baskets on the women's heads in the last hamlet. He thought of jumping free and taking his chances on foot for the final hundred miles, but the bus settled back onto the hardened sands of the sub-Sahara, decades-old tires regaining purchase, the desert ship resuming its cruise westward.

Staring at the larger particles of mud in the bottom of his water glass, he became hypnotized, again unable to keep his eyes open, his last thoughts before sleep those of petitioning God to make the pebbles in his water glass pure nuggets of gold, pretending the rumbling of his arms was now him panning for precious metals. But he could not keep the deception alive, and every few seconds another crash woke him, forcing his eyes open, reminding him that he was stuffed into the bed of an ancient, ten-by-twenty-foot freight truck, one converted decades before into a fourth or fifth world, long distance coach by the African counterpart of Carl Eric Wickman, the father of Greyhound.

Sixty-two fellow travelers bounced on mopane planks, the precious African hardwood into which had been worn smooth concavities, a memorial to the decades of forgotten souls who had squeezed, six and seven abreast, aboard that vessel to cross the Sahel. Sol sat dead center, only infrequently able to make out the ten or twelve pairs of emaciated black legs hanging over the open sides of the bus. The bucking limbs were somewhere attached to the voyagers of lesser means, the destitute consigned to the roof. The disenfranchised were fated to spend the morning and early afternoon broiling in the angry sun, holding on for dear life to what they could grab of the pitching bus, and then endure hour after hour of the afternoon battered by heat *and* the daily *haboob*. He had read about the bone-dry hurricanes that took greater and greater bites of the Sudan each year, the intensity and frequency of the wind escalating by the month, as the Sahara inexorably consumed Africa. He could not, though, have imagined the passion of its winds and the pain of the sand blasting in his face at eighty miles per hour.

From his sheltered seat, Sol could hardly make out the passengers, those of even tighter pockets than the upper level wayfarers, who clung to the sides of the bus, their faces and bodies twisted away from the swirling sand that enveloped the truck even when it was stopped. And stop it did, every few minutes, three dusty twelve-year-old boys ordered to jump down from the roof to change tires or dig wheels out of hidden desert pits. They slogged on like dogs, hissing "*Al hum de ley la*," praise be to God, over and over as the driver stood above them, stick in hand, flicking it menacingly as he yapped at them to work faster.

It did not take long for Sol to appreciate that his fellow travelers had not bathed in many months—some, not for years, a fair percentage, never. On the southern edge of the Sahara, in the Sahel, the precarious band of semi-desert, semi-habitable land that stretched across Africa from the Atlantic to the Indian Ocean, water was for life, not luxury. And though Sol had showered at the guesthouse in El Fasher the night before, or had it been two nights, his own odor had already begun wafting into his face, a spoor far more fetid than that of his neighbors. Somehow, theirs was neutral, not unpleasant, a sweetish aroma, one he had never before encountered.

But the foreign scent only added to his loneliness, and when the sting of the yellow silt swirling through the bus waned for a moment, he opened his eyes wide, realizing he was but a solitary white dot in a sea of dark, dark black, lurching across a desert at the entrails of the Earth in a death trap. He wanted to ask his neighbors why the driver insisted upon coursing such a parabolic itinerary along the very edge of the thirty-foot-deep, dry riverbeds, but he was sure he could not commune with a single soul. He wondered what would happen if the vehicle lost its balance and rolled into the river bed, if they would all die. Would there be a record of the tragedy, or would all the evidence be consumed by the flock of vultures that had been circling the bus for days? And what would become of his bones, how far away would they be scattered by the incessant *haboob*? Would they be distinguishable from those of his companions?

Surely these people had families. Someone would ponder what had become of the family patriarch. He shook his head and wondered if his own passing would be noticed in Africa, or even at home. He had lost everyone and everything. Maybe those who did remember him would just assume he had carved a new life for himself and never ask, "Hey, whatever became of Solomon Forte?" But another frightful bounce snatched him from his weepy musings, his mind now concerned more with the sliver of tooth that had just sheared off an incisor. So, that was why most of the passengers had clamped between their teeth a twig the girth of a chopstick, a desert mouth guard.

Though he was a medical doctor, trained to intervene boldly and save lives, he found himself powerless to stop the abuse. They were all at the mercy of a driver most adept at causing the bus he piloted to slam in three disparate directions at once. They could do nothing but sit and await their fate.

While the mass vibrated, mumbling prayers to their God, Sol reminded himself yet again that he was a scientist, conditioned to tap rational thought, not totems. He considered ways to soften the vagrant, tortured course through the desert, eventually deducing that the expedition had to have been purposefully designed, the heaving of the vehicle an unpleasant, though necessary, facet of life in the Sahel. The gnarled man at the wheel could not reasonably be considered suicidal and have lived into his late thirties, a venerable age in Africa. It followed logically that the violence of the journey must have been an adaptive measure, a skill perfected over many years and thousands of journeys through the sub-Sahara.

This was a course that hugged *masars*, the tacit borders through the sands that defined ancient, nomadic routes, separating murderous rival clans. He'd read about them on the plane over, and now understood that if the driver wished to save his own skin, he really had no choice but follow the unseen lines deftly to circumvent whatever ambush the desert might hurl. That could be, he assured himself, the only coherent explanation for the sadism of the voyage. The driver, he concluded in the end, had to be a savvy professional, though Sol tried hard not to think about the tattered, dirt-caked, brown *jellabiya*, desert gown, and once-white *immah*, turban headdress, in which the man was clothed. It was just his work clothes, Sol nodded weakly, not the index of his proficiency.

In fact, Sol could not really tell what was happening in the cab, or for that matter, two rows ahead. He was totally encased in the blowing *jellabiyas* and *immahs* of his new comrades, and even if they had been stripped down to the underclothes most didn't wear, he was so far ensconced into the center of the vehicle, he was barely able to discern if it was still light outside.

His mood had been quite temperate initially, when the bus first departed El Fasher on the several hundred-mile excursion. He noted that the other passengers sat calmly, speaking in whispers with their neighbors, and he assumed they knew what they were doing, that they, too, wished to survive. But after Nyala, the bus left the relatively paved road down from El Fasher, now forced to navigate the *masars*. When the serious bucking began, he soothed himself by repeating in a hiss that this ritual had been played out across Africa safely millions and millions of times over the past century, though as they entered the actual desert, and the life-threatening cuffing began, even his most stoic neighbors were yelping. Several of the men mumbled over their prayer beads that it would surely take all of Allah's power to grant them continued life until the end of the journey at Umm Balla.

Dozens of Sol's acquaintances apologized for the wretchedness of the trek across their country; some even dug into the pockets of their *jellabiyas* and offered their pale guest tiny crystals of sugar in reparation. He laughed to himself sourly how different it would have been for a lone black man on so ill-fated a journey in the United States. Sol tasted no anger, saw no fearful stares. Not a single soul on that bus leaned away from him to avoid grazing the strangely colorless creature. His fellow passengers had even huddled at the bus station in El Fasher to discuss the extraordinary presence of the ashen visitor, and they came away in one voice, insisting that Sol be given the seat of honor at the core of the mass to screen him from the *haboob*.

As the heat bore down on the lurching vessel, the travelers came up with an extra water glass. They passed it to the rickety vehicle's side walls, three-foot-high panels of once-painted tin. Before jumping aboard, Sol had jiggled the metal sheets, forcing himself to ignore that they were not much thicker than aluminum foil.

A bearded, grizzled, very black, old man in a threadbare *jellabiya* sat at the far end of the middle row, squashed against the side panels. He tended a water-filled, cowhide bladder that hung outside the bus. Suspended from the luggage rack topside by a single tether of rawhide, the bag pendulated freely, most of the time out of sync with the old man's grabbing. Occasionally, his hand would coincide with the bag's arc so he could draw off a pint of water through a small nipple in the leather then pour it carefully over the outside of the cask until the skin dripped. That did wash away the tarnish of stuck-on sand, but no matter how often he went through the drill, seconds later, the skin was again encrusted in a thick patina of yellow, desert silt.

Sol laughed aloud, satisfied he was the only speaker of English within a thousand square miles. "Waste of time, my man. Water inside that thing's dirtier than the outside of your bag."

A woman's soft voice several rows behind caught Sol's attention. It took a moment for him to realize that she was speaking to him, and in English, the first he'd heard in days. "You see, sir, when the water on the outside evaporates, it cools the liquid inside. It is primitive, but it is the best these people have."

Sol tried to turn and look at the source of the faraway murmur, but he could not rotate his shoulders more than a few degrees before his face was covered with the tail of a neighbor's blowing *immah*. He worked to thread his arm between his closest six neighbors and raised it to wave, "Thank you, ma'am." The sudden spoor of his own body stunned him, and his involuntary breath of blistering air scalded his nose and throat. He thrust the glass back to his neighbor, begging with his eyes to send it along for a refill. It was true; each time he passed his cup for a recharge, it came back cool.

Sol also noticed that everyone else handed over a tiny coin for their water, though the metal was so light, even a wisp of breeze blew it overboard. Then there were shouts for the driver to stop so the old man could dismount and recover his capital, but after the third time, the driver yelled back, "Too damn bad. Be more careful."

That set the old man grumbling, his irritation intensifying each time Sol's glass arrived without the requisite fraction of a Sudanese penny. But the other passengers barked back at the man to just fill the cup and be hospitable.

Hours later, the truck pulled into one of the lone, ageless hamlets strung out along the Sahel. It lay between the city of Nyala, which they had left many, many hours before, and the prehistoric settlement of his destination, Umm Balla, many, many hours in front of them. The bus shuddered to a stop at an open area surrounded by a collection of several dozen thatched-roofed, mud huts. Sol stood and waited his turn to make his way to the tailgate. He jumped from the van, stiffly moving across the primitive town square, ignoring the disbelieving stares. He stopped at a twelve-foot-by-twelve-foot paddock barely framed by four short walls of rotting grass mats. The sides were suspended by vines from a scraggly baobab tree, the delicate leaves barely screening the occupants from the scorching sun.

He pretended to walk away but hid behind a tree and stared around the knobby trunk into the enclosure. It was a *madrasah*, an Islamic school. A dozen young boys swayed in prayer as the *mualim* swatted the less attentive in the back of the head with a stick.

The woman from the bus who had spoken to him in English approached and asked if he understood what he was seeing. Sol shook his head no, and she whispered a translation of the *mualim*'s rantings.

The man kept pointing his cane south, warning that nothing sat between them and Mecca, so the boys better accept that Allah was watching them very closely.

He droned menacingly, "You will submit your will to Allah. You have no right to desire anything, nothing. Your only desire shall be to become better at submitting your disgusting desires to the will of Allah, as commanded in the Quran. If you fail, you are doomed to suffer the fire of hell for eternity. Death is no escape. Let me warn you, lest you think that if you die, it will all be over. No, *No*, **NO**! If you do not submit to Allah's will in this life, death is only the beginning of the pain for those who do not learn that you ask for nothing other than to give your filthy cravings away to Allah. That is the only way to avoid the pain. If you do not, you will dwell with the devils, the Jews. Submit or suffer for eternity next to a Jew."

When the man ceased, nearly breathless, Sol mused, "Sounds about like the curriculum at St. Mary's Academy."

Sol noted that the children's faces were, as they rhythmically echoed the platitudes without expression, far darker than the kids in Khartoum, the features even more African. He remarked to the woman, "This really is Africa, isn't it?"

She smiled and walked off, calling over her shoulder, "Sir, please be careful."

He watched that class end and, without a recess, the boys took up twigs to copy Koranic verses in the dirt. The *mualim* stopped to stand over each of his students, breathing fire and brimstone, occasionally snapping the boy in the back of the head until the correct words were scratched in the sand. With the master calmed, there came an angry growl and one step to the left to swat the next child. A few of the students clutched slates on which they penned stanzas with sharpened sticks dipped in water. The *mualim* did not hit the moneyed boys nearly as briskly as he did those who scratched in the dirt.

At first, Sol was angered and turned away, but his eyes drifted down to his own knuckles. He wondered if he could make out little scars where the nuns had bloodied him with rulers at St. Mary's, retribution for using his left hand to write out catechism and throw dodge balls during recess.

Sol drifted back to the northern border of the square, nearing the bus, where camels were parked willy-nilly. The colossal beasts, the largest, strongest dromedaries on Earth, grunted and carped in a cacophony that rivaled the prattle of spectators at the stock car races back in Whitaker. Several of the animals, the trusted few, were permitted to move freely, to graze arrogantly. They refused to eye the unwashed masses, the lesser caste, those hunkered, one front leg flexed a hundred-and-eighty degrees at the elbow, the upper and lower bones painfully lashed together with slips of desert vine.

The creatures were seemingly unconcerned with the layers of kidney bean-sized flies, waves of which colonized yawning sores, bleeding patches rubbed open where they had been laden nearly every hour of every day of their lives. The *jamali*, camel drivers, often loaded the animals with five and six hundred, and if need be, nine hundred pounds of cargo, far more than the three hundred that should have saddled their most important link with survival, and into whom they had poured their entire life savings.

The camels brayed and spit wads of stinking, half-chewed cud at each other, some crawling painfully, rubbing hobbled forelegs along the ground, squandering their vitality to nip at their neighbors' lesion-covered hides. They seemed more interested in wounding a brother next door than breaking their motley bonds and fleeing into the desert.

There were also burros, dozens of them. They appeared in and out of the wilderness, elfin creatures compared to the donkeys Sol had seen at home. Men fully robed in thick *jellabiyas* straddled the filthy creatures, the riders' knees bent high to keep their one and only pair of ragged sandals from scraping the rocky earth. A clutch of chattering women followed on foot, their heads balancing five-foot-wide flat baskets of wilted produce.

While the camels had had holes burned in their noses to attach rotten string for steering, the burros had been spared that torture. As Sol watched the burros come and go, he realized that guiding an ass was less intricate than maneuvering a camel. Donkey riders journeyed bareback through the wastelands wielding two-foot tree limbs, clubs, with which they swatted the burro in the head on the opposite side they wanted it to turn. The beast, whose head shuddered as if surprised at the millionth iteration of the insult, veered away from the blow and found its eyes now pointed in a new direction. And that is where it headed, Sol laughed, like the kids in the *madrasah*, or, after he gave it a bit of thought, like the students at St. Mary's Academy in Manhattan. His concern for the welfare of the donkeys suddenly vaporized in the heat, though, for it struck him, a burro born in the Sahel was just the reincarnation of a Nazi death camp sergeant.

He turned his attention to the eight-foot-wide dust path running through the settlement. There lolled the fortunate burro or two, creatures only recently departed to their final reward, stiff carcasses reposing exactly where they had dropped, legs locked straight up into the uncaring yellow sky. What was left of them sat encrusted in a veneer of flies so impenetrable, the scraggly, ill-tempered dogs, and even the orbiting vultures, snubbed the carrion.

Gaggles of very dark people milled about the center of the square, for it was Wednesday, the cusp in the week when desert dwellers, both two and four-legged, came together over all of central Africa to trade wares at the *suq*. The arriving women skulked to tiny patches of dirt in the square, hunkering to spread their produce on the sand. The men repaired to shady corners to fuddle, drink tea, and smoke cigarettes pulled from red and white packs stamped "LIFE".

There were also dozens of nomads striding about, cocks of the walk. The squatting women, pastoralists, scrub farmers, lowered their eyes, shushing each other as the burly men tramped past. These incredibly thin ladies, delicate twigs compared to the tree trunk nomads, hawked tiny species of flaccid vegetables Sol had never before seen or imagined. The women had, by and large, set up shop next to their friends so they could while away the torpid afternoon chattering. They wore identical *tobs*, wrap-around gowns, the traditional dress of desert women since long before *The Bible* had been scripted. The frocks in which these voluble merchants sheathed themselves were tattered and sun-faded, frequently falling open at the midriff. Every few minutes the ladies would spring to their feet, turn away from the crowd, and ever so carefully rewrap the material, ignoring customers, even those with their hands out proffering wrinkled bills.

A different clique, businesswomen who spent less time jabbering with neighbors, tended larger, less-wilted inventories. Each sat in a parallel series of roofless, two-foot-wide, four-foot-long, two-foot-high, mud-walled stalls. These vendors sporadically ceased nattering long enough to reorganize their wares and shoo away flies with spade-shaped reed fans. Occasionally, one of the women exchanged a word or two with the nomads, but never locked their eyes. Spread before these merchants were quarter-filled straw baskets of sorghum, *durra*, the raw grain upon which the Sahel subsisted. To Sol, it looked like kasha, the traditional staple his Jewish medical school friends served when he visited them on religious holidays.

A few entrepreneurs tended dried mud bowls of wrinkled green coffee beans, and some presided over banana leaves piled with stunted, though less wilted, vegetables than those pushed by the chatterers. These ladies wore bits of gold in their ears and donned *tobs* a trace more vibrant in their reds and yellows, though they, too, frittered away much of the afternoon redoing gowns, a duty that came before cultivating customers.

Finally, in a wind-protected corner of the square, under the shade of scraps of woven grass, sat the ladies who sold cloth for *jellabiyas* and *tobs*. Their wrists were ornamented with a very thin bracelet or two of precious metal, and several had capped their front teeth in the deep orange gold of the third world. These women would not have to worry about where their nest eggs were hidden when it came time to run from the next horror. Behind each of these noblewomen sat eight-foot-wide mud huts shielded from the sun, tiny enclosures freshened by the desert breeze. Here labored the tailors, all men, artisans driving the treadles of hundred-year-old Singer sewing machines.

Sol stood behind a mound of garbage and considered the process. Customers haggled with the bejeweled ladies out front for a meter of red and yellow flowered cloth. With the price settled, a piece of material was cut with rusted, antediluvian scissors and handed to the shopper, who took it three paces into the tailor shop. As a man dared not touch a woman publicly, the clothier looked his customer up and down, reckoned the measurements, and a new *tob* was ready before the client had time to buy a stalk or two of the bizarre vegetables.

In the furthest corner of the square, a serious old man stood in the open tending a tripod of tree branches from which hung emaciated sides of rank, fly-encrusted mutton. Next to his shop sat another merchant, AK-47 assault rifle slung over his shoulder. He groggily guarded a raw-wood table swanking the severed heads of his neighbor's dispatched sheep, the inventory facing outward, dress-right-dress, tongues hanging in the same direction, dust-coated gray eyes propped open with twigs to stare straight out at would-be purchasers. Sol noted that the legs of the table, though only tree branches, were interestingly tooled, but as he took a step closer, he realized it was just years of dried blood that had drooled into spirals and twists.

Sol looked back to the bus to witness the last dozen or so of his fellows, the penniless, creaking tiredly over to the *suq* to rummage for scraps. Some of the passengers did not even bother wasting the calories on so futile a quest, satisfied to remain behind in the shade of the bus and kneel on tiny patches of ground to offer afternoon prayers. They rolled open half-bath-towel-sized prayer rugs. Sol could see that at one time they had been colorful and finely woven, but now were dirty and moth-eaten. The faithful washed their feet with water trickled from undersized brass teapots hidden beneath the folds of their robes then faced south toward Mecca. This was the fifth time since the journey commenced that prayers were offered, but the first time in a village. The other sessions had been far out in the blowing sands, where Sol had remained aboard the coach to avoid the winds that thrashed the kneeling disciples.

Sol sauntered back into the *suq* to comb for something edible. He considered buying food for the religious travelers, and walked until he came to a line of young ladies hawking small cylindrical bundles of the twigs his fellow passengers used to protect their teeth from the mad jolting. His tongue ran over his chipped tooth, and he asked with hand signals if he could inspect the product. With the good-natured laughter, he picked up the packet and shrugged his shoulders. One of the teens jumped up, redid her *tob*, and pulled a twig from the pack. She rubbed one end on a rock until the fibers frayed, placed it in her mouth, and buffed each tooth carefully, starting with the molars, moving methodically around the dentition, and finishing off with a flourished polishing of the incisors. When she was done, she rewrapped her *tob*, smiled broadly, pulled her lips back, and flashed a perfect set of burnished teeth.

There was more laughter when Sol mimicked the process, surprised that the wood of the toothbrush tree had a medicinal, refreshing tang. He reached into his pocket to pay for the bundle, but found only a US dollar. The woman gasped and pushed it back into his hand, so he took a few steps away and left the dollar under a stone. He pointed to it and then to the semicircle of ladies.

A few yards away, he approached an ancient, toothless woman, perhaps forty years old, hawking a tattered grass dinner plate of what appeared to be brown marbles caked with straw, mud, and pea-green pustules. When he did not stop, she scowled. He looked away, but when his trailing leg passed her, she thrust the basket forward. Though he saw the edge of the basket out of the corner of his eye and spun to avoid it, and though he never actually touched the wicker, the contents launched into the air. He watched, tensed, as the marbles hurtled a foot or two off the basket only to coast in a parabolic, slow-motion back to Earth. He was struck for an instant that even here, the laws of physics prevailed. There was barely a tinkle as the marbles succumbed to gravity's clench, a sound much softer than the woman's screams.

The volume of her rage only amplified as she lifted her wasted buttocks off the three-inch-high, worn wooden stool upon which she had been perched for most of the afternoon, if not most of her life. She redid her *tob* and squatted to gather the remains of her livelihood, jamming the yellow-brown goo of mud and mucus menacingly up toward Sol's eyes. He stood speechless as the old lady spun away, apoplectic, gesturing wildly toward the men hunkered in the shade, gangs of them still drinking steaming tea and sucking on their LIFE cigarettes. The timbre of her ire deepened as she sang out a string of Arabic epithets, not one word of which he could echo, but every single syllable of which he absorbed. He stuck his hands into the pockets of his scrub pants, but the money was gone, his dollar in the hands of the young ladies selling toothbrushes.

A bearded nomad encased in a grimy brown *jellabiya*, an AK-47 assault rifle gripped tightly, abandoned his tea-drinking to march forward. Roughly, he pushed aside a throng of farmers and stood above the woman. She offered up in her palm for his perusal tiny, nearly colorless yolks, then pointed at Sol and pleaded for the nomad's help.

The man grimaced, raised the AK, took a faded bill from a pocket inside his robe, shook it angrily in Sol's face, and motioned for Sol to compensate the woman.

Sol looked up into the black eyes of the sizeable man and started to back away. But he stopped and spread his feet apart, making the split-second decision not to run, but to establish his territory. He remembered the yellowed pages of a book written by an Englishman who had travelled the Sudan in the early 1900s—to show weakness in the Nubian Desert was tantamount to committing suicide. On the other hand, though, he reminded himself that he had been sent to Darfur as an ambassador of peace, or so he'd been tutored by the directors of Please Help the Children in offices on three continents. He nodded gently, smiled, and mumbled softly, "I am very sorry, sir. I will pay for the eggs." He reached into his pockets and turned them inside out, revealing the absence of cash. He pointed to the bus and then to his waist, mimicking a fanny pack. The large man's dark eyes glazed over, and Sol sputtered, "I'll be right back."

Sol started to shift off, taking perhaps three steps before his egress was barred by a half dozen of the brown robes. As their jeering deepened, another squad of nomads materialized behind him, obstructing any chance of escaping to the *madrasah*, to seek asylum in a house of worship and appeal to the *mualim*. He stopped and took a deep breath, organizing his thoughts, conjuring a plan to draw upon his years of experience dealing with people *in extremis*. However, what the patients to whom he had offered his healing services in America did not wield, aside from one unhappy man who had come at him with broken bottle of Jack Daniels when Sol would not fill his prescription for narcotics, were assault rifles. In the village of Boranga, every male over the age of five brandished an abused rifle, mostly AK-47s, their wooden stocks etched over the decades with the initials of soldiers who had toted that weapon in uprisings from Russia to China to North Korea to Viet Nam, back to Russia to Laos to Cambodia to Nicaragua to Sri Lanka, and finally to their last stop on Earth, central Africa. While most of the men held their weapons at the ready in two hands, a few of the particularly well-armed slung their AK-47s over shoulders, resting their palms on long-barreled, Old West six shooters stuffed into the belts of their grimy robes.

Sol wiped away the sweat that had begun to drip in streams from his face. He croaked as he pointed an index finger toward the bus, "I told you, sir, the money's over there."

When no one budged, he pointed to his pockets and let his hands drift toward them very slowly to reassure his audience he was not reaching for a gun. It was a gesture he'd honed during his residency in the South Bronx. He would reason with these men, and they would allow him into the bus to make right his misdemeanor.

But before his hands reached the flapping pockets, a woman's soft voice called from behind. "No, sir. Do not touch your money." He turned. It was the woman from the bus. He looked at her this time. Her complexion was *café au lait*, flawless, her features aquiline, her gown bright, trimmed in silver tread. Her facial features were an exotic fusion of European and African virtues, far from Sudanese or Kenyan. Dangling from a gold chain about her neck was an ornate crucifix, quite dissimilar to the one propped on the altar of his church in Little Italy. She was a Coptic Christian, Egyptian or Ethiopian, a follower of the Gospel of Mark.

The woman moved closer and whispered, as if the onlookers could have understood, "Sir, these men are Bedou. I think you call them Bedouins. To them, you are not a human. The rules of their society do not apply to you, and barely to me. If they see that you have money, they will kill you for it. Let me drop a three-cent note on the ground in front of the old lady. You walk back to the bus and take your seat. You may repay me in Umm Balla."

The woman turned to the burgeoning crowd and spoke in Arabic, Sol recognizing only the words *Doctori* and *la dollars* repeated over and over. She turned and spoke to Sol again. "I told them you were a volunteer doctor working in their country for free, and that you had spent your last money on a toothbrush. I told them you had no more dollars, and that I had had to buy your ticket for the trip into the desert. You must go to the bus now and wait. Do not turn back and look at these men."

She pulled a faded, torn bill out of her pocket and placed it under a stone in front of the old woman. Though the ancient storekeeper reached for it, a strapping Bedouin pushed his way forward, scooped it up, scowled when he realized it was only three cents, and took a half-penny from his *jellabiya* and dropped it in front of the old lady. Though the coin blew away before it hit the ground, the cachectic woman waited, hunkered, eyes down, until the nomad stalked off. When he was many paces away, she scampered after the money.

Sol, aware from his readings of desert society that he had lost face by allowing a woman to fight his battle, considered turning toward the men to make a final defiant gesture with his middle finger, but he surveyed the territory beyond the bus, the barren moonscape that was to be home for the next half year, if he was still alive in five minutes. There was nowhere to hide for the next hundred miles, and even if he jumped into the cab and hijacked the bus, the nomads would just follow, plodding across the desert on their camels at three miles-an-hour. There was no hurry. Eventually, they would track him down in Umm Balla to extract whatever justice they deemed fitting.

He started toward the bus, swaggering, until the New York City inside him gnawed so potently, he could not stop himself from turning back and snapping his fingers up against his chin. He spun around and strode even more arrogantly toward the bus.

Sol had been one of the first passengers to board in El Fasher, before the luggage rack and top of the cab had been loaded, and before the bus had made a dozen stops in the desert to add passengers, lone souls who appeared out of the dunes. He had been unaware that the roof was now packed five feet high with tattered cloth bags, most not much bigger than basketballs, the entire personal belongings of the majority of the passengers. There were also a few chicken coops fashioned from lashed twigs. Each was loaded with guano-encrusted, wilted fowl squeezed together even more snugly than the human customers below. He wasn't sure what species of bird was native to the desert, but he could make out very small bodies and diminutive combs as anemic as the women's *tobs*. Sol imagined them to be exotic desert capons, but one escaped and ran several revolutions around the bus until its owner fell on it. He realized it was just a chicken, another stunted desert creature, as were the grand majority of the living things he had encountered over the past days, aside from the nomad men and their camels.

A few old cardboard suitcases sat out in stark contrast to the bulk of the decaying gear. Most striking, however, were the people frying on top who had not been able to come up with the twenty-five-cent fare for the accommodations below. Over the rusting cab dangled legs which covered much of the small piece of glass that remained of the windshield.

Sol grabbed the camera out of his fanny pack, but as soon as the device rose above the tin foil side panels, a cluster of Bedouins sprinted over, pointing at themselves wildly, demanding their pictures be taken. Though Sol recognized them as the same group that had been so angered thirty seconds before, they were now smiling, striking poses for the camera, some with AK-47s pointed ominously at Sol, some with AKs pointed at the heads of fellow tribesmen. Sol turned to start snapping shots and got one off before the Coptic woman lifted herself aboard and gently pushed the camera down.

Sol was quite surprised, first that she had touched him, and more so when she placed her face near his ear and whispered, "Now they're going to demand money for having taken their photograph. *Doctori*, you should really sit down in your seat and read a book."

Her scent was curiously pleasant, even arousing, and he furtively drew in a deep breath through his nose. He turned to look at her again, the regal features, her elegant hands, and did not pull away as quickly as he might have. He was not sure, but thought she also hesitated for a moment. Then he caught another whiff of himself, and so must have the alluring woman, for she turned and was gone.

Though Sol calmed himself, he tried hard not to exhale so vigorously that he would disperse her scent. His musings ended when the growling outside the bus escalated into yapping, and he looked into the souring expressions of the locals whose heads reached over the sides of the coach. The man toward whom Sol's camera had been directly pointed yelled something about money and hoisted himself onto the tailgate, but the exotic woman rushed to the back of the bus, took out another three-cent bill, scowled, and dropped it behind the man. It caught the wind and the nomad dismounted, *jellabiya* flapping as he chased the note across the square.

When the lady was sure he was gone, she stepped over several benches to take a seat next to Sol. With her nose pointed away, she spoke softly. "*Doctori*, you must understand, these people have nothing, including manners the way you have been taught. Their lives are short and painful, but they have a strict code of honor amongst themselves, rules of life you and I would have difficulty living up to. Mostly, *Doctori*, they worry where the next meal will come from and how to stop the farmers from taking more land that has been theirs for thousands of years. They do not read or write. They have never seen a book, even the Quran. They know nothing of the world outside this scrap of sand."

"But, ma'am, excuse me, there's a school right over there. The kids are learning to read and write."

She sighed but tightened her jaw. "Excuse me, sir, but you do not understand. The boys in the *madrasah* are from farming families. The farmers and the nomads are as different as you and I. The Khartoum government arms the Arabs, that is the nomads, and pays them to massacre the farmers. The peasants run, and the government designates the land as abandoned. They claim it for themselves so they can seize the oil and water rights. The nomads are just waiting for word to start the killings. Soon it will lead to a war throughout the Sudan. Do not interact with these people. Please."

She raised a graceful finger and pointed majestically at the mob of camels still spitting and nipping. "The nomads are born on the camel, they marry on the camel, they live for thirty years, the strong ones perhaps to forty, on the camel, and one day get off or fall off their camel and lie there until they die. The tribe will stop at that spot just long enough to bury them, but there will be no marker, no heaven, just the next day's fight to find a mouthful. So, you must forgive them, but you must also be careful. Here, there is only one code, and it is of the nomads for the nomads. There is no law protecting you. Their system is strict, brilliant, and time-tested. It enables them to survive on nothing. It has to be that way.

"And you, *Doctori*, are not Bedou, so to them, you are not a person. If they were to kill another Bedouin, they would be executed, and very painfully, for they had committed a crime against Allah, one that caused harm to the clan. But if they kill you, there is no punishment, for your death does not matter. It will have no effect on their world, on their lives, or on their ability to find food tomorrow to feed their children. I know you mean well, but that will not help you here. You must be careful."

Sol thought for a moment, taking in what she had advised, but shook his head slightly, adding serenely, "Thank you, ma'am, again, but I have to tell you I did my residency in the bowels of New York City. I got along with everyone very well. Never once had a problem, and those were tough, dispossessed folk. People are people. If you treat them with respect, that's what you get back."

Her face hardened. "If you believe you understand life here, you will not survive. In Darfur Province, outside the clan, there is no law, there is only the gun. In the old days, there was sort of an uneasy peace. If a farmer killed a nomad, his own people punished him. They made him pay a grain levy to the nomad's family. And the nomad's family would wait until a famine year to collect the debt. Are you that clever?

"But now, it is war between them, the Arab and the non-Arab. Can you tell them apart?"

"I thought all these people are Arabs."

"You see, *Doctori*, they look the same to you. Both sides. They speak the same language, or so it seems to outsiders, but their clans are different, and their hearts are different. With these people, you can't tell who is going to shoot you if you say the wrong word. For one tribe, what you say kiddingly will bring laughter, for the other, execution."

"Is it going to be the same with the refugees in the camps? Are you saying there isn't any law in the camps? That's not what my organization told me."

"I am afraid there is no law anywhere in Darfur, or really even in Khartoum, the capital. The rules now are in the hands of the monsters in Bashir's government who are killing the refugees you came here to serve. But the people in the camps are farmers, victims of the Arabs. It will be somewhat easier with the farmers, but the workers in the camps, the ones they call checkers, the ones who will do all the work for you, they are Arabs, so everything you say and do must be measured. Some of them are good men, some are not. It is hard for an outsider, or even for me, to tell the difference. Please never let down your guard. This is a very harsh land. And now with the genocide, these people have nothing but fear and hunger to drive them, both sides. A penny here, a penny there, it's worth a mouthful of *durra*. That is all that matters."

Sol's head drooped, and he mumbled, "How did you know I was a doctor?"

"Everyone knows. These people do not have telephones, but their news travels faster than it does in your country, or mine."

Sol asked, "Where are you from? I see you are a Coptic Christian, but you speak Arabic so fluently, so I don't think you are from Ethiopia."

"You know I am Coptic? Very observant. I am Egyptian, from Alexandria. I am a professor of obstetrics."

"You're a *doctor*!"

"Is that so surprising?"

"Of course not, but are you practicing here?"

"I am on my sabbatical, one year to work for the UN in El Fasher. I am going to Umm Balla to teach the women prenatal techniques."

"Then we will be working together!"

"Not really. Two different worlds. There is the local population, and there are the refugees, though both are being decimated by the government. You will be caring for refugees. Those people lived in the country of Chad. The border is not far from Umm Balla. And, please, stay away from the frontier. One side or the other will kill you if you get lost and cross the line in the sand by one meter.

"The Chadians have been driven out of their country by a government as murderous as the one in Khartoum. The people I teach about safe pregnancy and infant care are Furs, the indigenous population. They are the people of the village of Umm Balla and all the villages in this province."

Sol was bemused. "Furs. I don't know about that."

"They are the tribe that has lived here for many centuries. *Dar* just means, 'the place where,' so Darfur means the land of the Fur people." She waited until Sol nodded, then asked, "Have you been to Egypt?"

"I have. To visit a close friend and his family. I plan to visit Alexandria on my way home, *if* I make it." He smiled.

She smiled back, "You will be fine. And you must visit Alexandria. It is the cultural center of the Arabic world. My university is there. It is spectacular, not what you think. Maybe when you are done here, you may even want to learn Arabic. Then you can read so much wonderful literature about these people.

"But back to you. The police in El Fasher were watching you, to see if you had contraband, maybe illegal drugs or alcohol. Or maybe they thought you could be a spy for your government to search for terrorist bases. The last white man who got his permit in El Fasher to travel to Umm Balla worked for UNICEF. He had two bottles of Ethiopian whiskey hidden in sealed water bottles. They caught him and sentenced him to ten lashes—immediately. It almost killed him. He spent weeks in the hospital in El Fasher before he was recovered enough to fly home to Holland. This white man had to share his bed with a Sudanese man who just lay there waiting to die of TB. Each man hated that he was going to die next to an infidel. We had to bring both of them food and medicine. There were a hundred people in the ward with one toilet that didn't work. You would think the UN would have supported him, but they didn't care, too fearful of offending the local imam, so the boy's family had to pay $20,000 for his hospital bill before the government granted him an exit visa.

"Really, *Doctori*, he was lucky. The usual punishment is twenty lashes for alcohol, but because he was a foreigner and the government was alleging to the world that they were compassionate, they ordered he be treated with mercy. And you must be careful, *Doctori*, the sentence for adultery is one hundred lashes, even if it is with one of your own.

"When you went to have your permit to work in the Umm Balla Camp approved by our UN staff, they charged you one hundred dollars for the license..."

Sol's face tightened as he interrupted. "I know. That's more than it costs at home."

"You see, sir, the reason is the UN has to pay *baksheesh* to the police, or you would have been sent back thousands of kilometers to Khartoum and made to go through the whole process again and then again until you paid. And we will be stopping in more towns, and you will have to pay them as well. The authorities will arrange for you to have very little money left when you get to the Umm Balla Camp."

"You mean I have to register again?"

"Yes, in every town that has a police department. If you do not pay, they will put you in a little room with just a chair to wait for the next bus back to Nyala, then one back to El Fasher, then to Khartoum. That could be two or three weeks on the road. All you will get is weak tea, which you will have to pay for. *Doctori,* how long do you plan to be in the Sudan?"

"Six months, but I've already wasted nearly a month in Khartoum just convincing them I'm really a doctor. I had my degrees copied and notarized before I left the U.S., but those people in Khartoum tried to get me to pay like five hundred dollars to get the three degrees translated into Arabic, and a hundred more to get them re-notarized by the same guy who translated them. Then I had to get a physical for two hundred US. A man in a dirty white coat walked into the room, glared at me, and left. Every day they harass me is a day less I've got to treat patients in the Umm Balla Camp."

"That is the whole point, *Doctori.*"

As they spoke, the passengers began to filter back to their seats, and the woman stood to return to hers. As she turned she added, "Oh, you will have much time in Umm Balla to treat refugees. More than you want. In a few weeks, you will be dreaming of home more than anything in the world. I have seen it many times. In three months, you will be looking for reasons to leave. Umm Balla is a very brutish place."

With the bus repacked, the driver spit on the ground, lit an oblong cigarette, and climbed aboard. He barely managed to start the engine before a commotion arose at the rear of the vehicle, and he shut off the engine with a groused "*Al hum de le la*" then another, more piercing, "*Al hum de le la*" as he bristled to the tailgate, lips curled down. Several passengers at the rear of the truck were pointing at a man in Bedouin robes, who had squeezed into the bus, making his way toward Sol. The driver leaned his head into a gap in the last row of passengers and grumbled at the interloper to get off unless he paid for a ticket. When the mendicant did not listen, the driver went to the front to fetch his rifle, a bolt action .22 as old and rusted as the bus.

A sub-clan of the Bedouin men, who had been but laughing spectators at both the egg and photography skirmishes, now trotted to crowd the area behind the bus. The Bedouin women, though, dared not approach within twenty paces of the men, and formed their own half-moon behind them. The farmers fell into a sloppy crescent behind the nomad women, and *their* women a final semi-loop even further back. The focal point of the four concentric arcs was the blue-eyed, Caucasian man climbing madly over benches toward the front of the bus, just steps ahead of the arm-waving wanderer.

The UN doctor placed herself, once again, between Sol and an enemy. The man, grunting like a wild hog, came to an abrupt halt, pulled the three-cent note from his *jellabiya*, and reached around the woman's shoulder to shake the bill menacingly at Sol. With each flip of the bill, his snorting loudened. When the UN lady told him for the fifth or sixth time that the white visitor had no money, the nomad put his hand on the slide of his AK-47 and tightened his fingers, preparing to chamber a round. The other passengers pushed past Sol to leap from the vehicle, some landing on their faces in the sharp sand.

The woman, Sol, and the agitated Bedouin soon had the entire truck bed to themselves. Though the driver had started up into the back of the vehicle, when he saw that the antagonist was not one of his patrons, but an agitated, armed Bedouin, he slithered away to hide behind the rear arc of farmer women.

For a moment, not a single sound ejaculated from the one hundred or so members of the family of man gathered in the middle of the sub-Sahara. Though the camels, donkeys, sheep, and chickens persisted in their strident discord, Sol perceived nothing but a hum of static and the image of the assault rifle muzzle hovering inches from his face. It seemed very peculiar that his own sweating had ceased, and he found his thoughts drifting to the endless lectures in medical school about the sympathetic nervous system, and the fight or flight mechanism that saved people's lives, but were about, he feared, to fail him. For a moment, he wished he had paid better attention to those lectures so many years before, reasoning that if he knew more physiology, he'd be able to cull that science to save himself. But the strident clack of the Arab charging his AK-47, a ten- pound assault rifle with eleven parts, drew Solomon Forte from his musings. There was nothing left to do but put on his nastiest Bronx game face.

Whether it worked or not, Sol and his audience would never know, for as the weapon's slide went forward to chamber a round, a piece of the mechanism snapped off and sprang upward, arched, and landed with a feeble clank at the doctor's feet. Sol picked it up, noting that the metal was so rusted it had broken off, never again to be part of any serious firearm. Sol approached the man slowly and handed him the fragment. Several of the Bedouins broke out in gasps of laughter, and one lifted his rifle, pretending to offer it to the red-faced black man, but at the last moment, pulled it away, chuckling that he didn't want old Ahmed to break his gun as well.

Each semicircle waited for the one in front to start howling before they took leave to enjoy themselves. Even the driver snickered. The only souls in Darfur Province not amused were the three on the bus. Sol was now so close to his adversary, he could not miss the fungating ulcer that broadened along the Bedouin's jaw, dove down precipitously onto the neck, and finally disappeared under the *jellabiya*. At first, Sol thought it was a basil cell cancer, a curable lesion, one even he could treat. But as he leaned closer to inspect it more carefully, it was clear the cancer had penetrated the hidden tissues deep under the skin. It was probable that bits of the tumor had already broken free, travelled via the blood stream, and were now growing freely all over the man's body, even in the brain. Sol shook his head and accepted that is was too late, that there was nothing to be done in the futility that was the Sahel, or for that matter in the U.S., even at the finest of cancer hospitals.

He took a last look at the lesion, knowing in the real world he would likely never again see a malignancy so advanced. He wanted badly to take a picture, but instead focused on the surface of the tumor, committing the wound to memory, perhaps someday to write about it in a medical journal. When he noticed the surrounding skin lined with angry, red tissue, he followed the slender scarlet streaks that radiated from the cancer like roads on a travel map in a far-off world that actually had roads and maps.

Sol pointed to the wound and asked the UN woman to query how long the lesion had been there.

"One week," the man grumbled in guttural Arabic, his eyes suddenly lowering.

Sol's face tightened in disbelief. "Uh huh. How 'bout a couple three years?" But he smiled thinly, nodding, willing to accept whatever he was told by a patient until proven otherwise, the rule of law set for his medical school class by its mentors. Maybe it was as he had read in his hundred-year-old book of tales about the Nubian desert, that the perception of time amongst the nomads was not as it was in the West, and he pretended Einstein's Special Theory of Relativity was playing out before his eyes.

But the nomad grunted and lifted his head for the doctor to get a better look, dragging Sol back into the Bedouin's frame of reference. Sol asked the UN physician, "Ma'am, do you have any suggestions?"

She shook her head. "I deliver babies. You know far more about this than do I."

A few seconds passed while Forte pondered his therapeutic options, finally raising his extended index finger in doctoral exclamation. He nodded confidently and pushed past the stunned man. Sol climbed onto the roof of the bus to dig through the mountain of baggage until he found his myriad duffle bags. He opened the sacks, searching in each as the audience stood stupefied, never dreaming one man, even the devil, could own so much. He called over his shoulder that he would treat the man as soon as he came to the right medicine. The UN lady translated.

In bag number five, he found several little cardboard boxes, dropped back down onto the tailgate, and asked the UN woman to translate. "You must take the pills three times a day, at eight, twelve, and say six in the afternoon, and this salve goes on the sore once or twice a day."

She nodded gently to Sol then turned to the man and commanded brusquely, "Take one when the sun is on the ground in the desert after you get up, one more when the sun is overhead, and the last when the sun is on the floor of the desert again. Take them until seven suns have come and gone." She grasped the five fingers of his right hand, then pointed to the thumb and index finger of his left hand. "And put some of this medicine on your neck when the sun is directly overhead."

"Do you understand, sir?" Sol queried.

The woman translated, and the man snorted. She muttered, "I guess that means he does. You can never tell with these people."

Sol handed the boxes to the man, who snatched them without a word. Had Sol not been looking at the breech of the broken gun, wanting to see the bullet that had been intended for him, he might have perceived the subtlest nod from the nomad as he turned to leave. But Sol was not concerned with the ritual of gratitude on the edge of the Sahara in the midst of a terrible famine and a worse civil war. For a purpose he could not fathom, all he wanted was to remember what the bullet looked like, perhaps believing that someday the vision of something so small ending a life would help him master another pointless catastrophe or meaningless episode of life. But as he focused harder on the rifle, eyes locked on the breech, he saw there had been neither round in the chamber, nor a magazine in the stock.

With Sol's first patient in the Sudan on his way to join his tribesmen, the passengers filtered back into the truck, on their way once again, only six, or maybe twenty minutes, behind on a schedule that had them in Umm Balla that night or the next day, or perhaps the one after that, *Insha'Allah*, God willing.

* * *

The bus ground through the desert until 9 P.M. The driver jammed the brakes, jumped from the cab, rewound his *immah*, walked away from the vehicle into the desert, lifted his *jellabiya* to urinate, came back, and without a word of explanation, crawled under the bus, unfolded a blanket, smoked a cigarette directly beneath the fuel tank, and fell off to sleep, the cigarette butt smoldering next to his face. Some of the passengers crawled topside and dug through their luggage for scraps of cloth to transform into bedding before claiming trivial patches of ground next to the bus. They prayed first then settled in to sleep. They were far too close, Sol thought, in the oppressive heat. The UN doctor, spying Sol lying on his back, uncovered between the rows of wooden picnic benches aboard the bus, gave him the extra blanket she had folded to use as a pillow. He demurred, but by ten, when his shivering shook the vehicle, she unfolded the blanket and draped it over him. Despite the half of the thin coverlet he'd placed under his body to soften the high spots of the worn, wooden truck floor, his back ached so from the uneven boards, he could not fall asleep.

At midnight, the cold had deepened to the point that the blanket was pathetically inadequate, and he co-opted the strip from underneath him to double the thickness over him. But that just allowed the frigid air to seep in through the cracks in the rotted floorboards, and twenty minutes later, when the temperature dipped into the mid-thirties, he jumped up in exasperation, wrapped himself in the blanket, and took off at a slow trot across the desert to generate heat.

The passengers were silent when Sol first started off, though they all looked up at the apparition heading into the blackness. The stirring woke the driver, who clucked in indignation, crawled out from under the bus, and rose to holler after Sol, commanding him to come back. He kept shouting the word "*jinn*" something, something "*jinn*," the "*jinn*," and Sol thought for a moment that the man was offering to pour him a stiff drink to help him sleep if he'd only come out of the desert. The thought of a nip, though, culled the image of the UN worker from Holland, the poor bastard sentenced to ten, or was it fifteen, lashes instead of twenty because he was just a stupid foreigner. He had been beaten within an inch of his life, all over two bottles of Ethiopian rotgut. Then Sol thought back to his own wasted weeks in the capital city of Khartoum. He certainly didn't want to wind up in a hospital there, sharing a bed with a man dying of skin cancer, the three-star hotel in that city having been punishment enough.

When Sol started to sweat, and the blanket became damp, he realized it would never dry in the cold, and that he'd have to run for the next four or five hours to survive the night. He considered building a fire and jogged back to the encampment, searching for dried brush and twigs. But the desert was devoid of firewood, cleansed by the nomads who had traveled those plains for the decades since the last plant had been pulled from the earth by a freezing native.

Finding not even a thistle to fuel a fire, Sol climbed back into the bus, slipped under his bench, and contorted himself into the most compact fetal ball his six-foot, two-hundred-fifteen pound, shaking mass could be warped. Covering himself with the now triple-overlapped blanket, he must have fallen off to sleep, for the next thing he remembered was shivering awake in the utter darkness as the passengers climbed aboard for an early morning departure. At first it was too cold for anyone to do other than sit wrapped in their threadbare cotton shells and huddle for warmth, each soul, including Sol, sucking on a twig toothbrush. An hour or so later, however, the sun began to rise behind them, and soon the meager rays warmed the bus to the point that Sol's neighbors gained sufficient control of their trembling hands to pull shreds of pita from their bags; here and there a more opulent pilgrim produced a tiny, brown, hard-boiled egg. A man in front of Sol picked through his belongings until he found an oblong, curved green vegetable, an edible scimitar, from which he cut a slice, turned to Sol, and handed him a hunk. Not a word was spoken. Before Sol could look up, the man had turned forward. As Sol leaned toward the man to thank him, a soul to Sol's left pulled a strip of pita from his round and handed it indifferently to the strange, ill-prepared, pallid man. Sol munched on his breakfast slowly, savoring the dry bread and the gooey produce, smiling broadly at his new friends when they turned furtively to fix in their minds the portrait they would detail to family and friends for the rest of their fleeting lives.

He washed down his breakfast with a half-glass of muddy water, heavily mineralized refreshment, a primitive vitamin pill, he persuaded himself. Though his appetite waned from the taste, he conjured he was back in Whitaker, transforming the liquid muck into a latte, and the sandwich into a veggie sub.

For fifteen minutes, the temperature hovered around a magnificent seventy degrees, the gentle warmth nurturing marvelous scents from the ancient desert. The view, when the bodies bobbed and he could see through the flapping *jellabiyas*, was breathtaking. A distant, towering mountain rose off the savanna, the craggy volcanic peak glowing apricot as the sun crept above the horizon. Minutes later, though, the sun was no longer the mellow complexion of a moist peach, having morphed into a mammoth, fiery tyrant in the eastern sky, all of its radiation focused, Sol reckoned, on the dreary craft crawling across the blowing sands of Darfur Province. Soon, Sol was taking tiny breaths again, though only through his mouth, letting the air cool to body temperature before allowing the broiling gas into his lungs. And so the cycle recommenced.

* * *

Sol became irritated at the UN doctor, who had reassured him the trip would soon be over, and he grumbled "Are we there yet?" And that made him think of his father and mother and sister, Michaela, on their first family vacation, driving out of the city into the Adirondacks for three days. It was the miracle summer, the only time his father's union had been able to garner a wage hike of a few pennies an hour without a strike that always left them poorer in the end.

He smiled to himself, remembering how he and his sister had sat patiently in the back of the '56 Pontiac, she reading, Sol mostly watching the farmland glide by, in love with the greenery and the animals that he knew only from the books that crammed their tiny Manhattan apartment.

Sol tried to remember Michaela's face, the onyx eyes and towering cheekbones, the flowing, raven-black hair. It was hard to summon her image, a protective gift, he imagined, God bestowed on the heartbroken to soften a loss. Then his mind shifted to the memory of Dana's blue eyes, and his reddened. He stopped short, not wanting to remember. At least Michaela and Dana had spent their last moments together, his sister commencing her journey to pay tribute to their father, and Dana, so committed to their marriage that she had gone with Michaela all the way to New York to make sure her sister-in-law got her visa to work as a nun at the church in Korea.

He begged it had been fast, that the blow came from the planes, not the fire and smoke and pandemonium that took so many beings after the crashes. He prayed that they had not been among the bodies leaping from the upper floors of the holocaust. Sol's eyes closed tighter as he fought to control himself, but the tears squeezed through, and at that moment he wished to be done with it all, hoping the Lord would take him that day, that they would all be back together in Little Italy, on Sunday morning, his father making pancakes, the stupid pancakes, and with Dana and her grandfather's stupid vodka company.

The bus stopped again, and several dozen passengers pushed past him wordlessly, climbing over each other to secure a patch of sand for morning prayers. Sol's tears ebbed for a moment, and his anger swelled. He asked himself heatedly, perhaps aloud, "What the hell am I doing here? I give up my life for these people, the ones who murdered my sister and my wife?" Had he been closer to the tailgate, he would have leapt from the bus at that moment and not made his way east, back toward Khartoum, where the religious fanatics were planning the next attacks, but west, across Chad, through Niger and into Senegal, to Dakar, where one of his favorite nurses at the hospital near Whitaker had grown up. He would find her family. They would take him in, and he would regale them with stories of how many lives their daughter had saved and how much she was loved. They would arrange for Sol to jump a freighter out of Africa, and he would work his way home, all of it just grist for a novel he would someday write about the Sudan.

His body must have been trembling, for he heard voices around him, and then from two benches behind. The UN obstetrician called out, "*Doctori*, are you well? You are shaking so. The people are concerned you might have malaria. They are worried about you."

He stood, his head touching the sheet metal roof. "Thank you, Madame, I am fine. I was just..." and he realized his voice was choked with tears, so he didn't finish.

She answered uneasily, "If you need anything, sir, please tell me."

At the next town, he asked the UN doctor again how much longer it would be. Softly, she advised, "Less than a day, or maybe more. *Doctori*, did you not know that Darfur Province is as large as France?"

He laughed, "I do now."

He bought what he could from the shops that were mostly closed on the day after the *suc*, just eight rounds of hard pita left. He laughed aloud, thinking about the day-old bread for which one of his parsimonious colleagues in residency had stood in line for hours at the Pepperidge Farms outlet store in the South Bronx. Sol had gone to the man's tenement to study together for an exam, his friend charging a dime for each slice of rye bread they ate over the eight hours.

Sol also bought six, marble-sized hardboiled eggs, all of which weighed, together, no more than one medium egg back home. A few pieces of the gooey vegetable were on sale at the last stall in town, next to the well, where he filled his canteens.

Here there weren't nomads holed up in the tea shop. In this village, the mud huts were divided from each other by the occasional sand brick structure, two or three of which had roof-mounted satellite dishes convulsing in the howling wind. Modern Japanese pickup trucks were parked in the front of several huts, and at the edge of town sat a gas station where a man reclined in a disintegrating chaise lounge. A rotted tarp blocked a bit of sun. He puffed tranquilly on a homemade cigar—his other hand gripped an AK-47. On a rough-hewn table in front of him were three, one-liter bottles of cloudy, orange gasoline. Under an adjoining tarp, a gaggle of early teens worked with rocks to free flat truck tires from rusted rims. Two of their number sat at the next station patching holes, while three more took turns stroking madly at a bicycle hand pump.

Before Sol was off the bus, a squat Sudanese man in a very old, gray work outfit approached him. The shoulders of his Western shirt were adorned with official patches so faded and tattered they looked more like cut outs of the lint from a clothes drier than the mark of regional authority. Nonetheless, the man puffed his chest and bade Sol with a condescending snap of the fingers. Sol followed to a sand brick building smaller than a men's room in a cheap restaurant.

Inside, a rickety table was obscured under mountains of haphazardly arranged official papers, and in the corner of the room stood a chair with wood so old and dry, when Sol was ordered to sit, a splinter broke off, jabbing him in the butt. He jumped up and protested, but the man motioned disinterestedly for him to retake the seat, so Sol pulled the sliver free with a fair amount of theater and tossed it atop a pillar of documents.

The policeman left without expression, though was back in a few minutes with a tiny cup of bitter, weak tea and a deputy, who dragged in a second chair. The sheriff sat just inches from Sol and wrote in the margins of an old newspaper, scraping letters with such struggle, the stub of his pencil broke halfway through the exercise. The man gave up and pushed the paper in front of Sol, who studied the glyphs but apologized, "*La kelem Arabyah*," his latest phrase, "I don't speak Arabic."

The man clucked his tongue as he thumbed through a beaten Arabic-English dictionary, grumpily spinning pages, finally jamming the book into Sol's face while pointing at a word. Sol pushed the policeman's hand back until he could focus on the entry, "You." The man snapped the book back until he found the entry for "Paper."

"Ah, my papers. No problem." Sol smiled, undid his scrub pants, fished around in his crotch, and pulled free a plastic baggy. Inside was first the translation of his medical degree, his physical examination, and the travel permit, toward which he pointed emphatically at the stamps, indicating that he had already paid, several times, for the privilege of working for free in the mean desert.

The man perused the documents and slid them back toward Sol, who stood, put the baggie back between his legs, retied his scrub pants confidently, and took a step toward the door. The man grabbed his arm and hauled him back, scribbling ٧٥٥ D in the margin of the yellowed newspaper. He asked for the papers again, and Sol went through the process a second time. The officer pointed rather insistently to the duty stamps with the most digits, then at the numbers he'd scrawled in the newspaper margin. Sol could not read them, but he knew he was being swindled, as he had been in Khartoum, in El Fasher, and Nyala.

He snatched the nubbin of pencil off the table and corrected the backwards 7, gathered his documents, folded them slowly, and muttered, "Over my dead body." He jumped up and took a giant step toward the door.

The policeman grasped his arm more tightly this time and called out harshly. The beefy deputy poked his head in, and Sol was ordered back to his seat. The two men left the hut in deep conversation.

In minutes, a handsome young man in a clean, white *jellabiya* stuck his head into the tiny police station. He bowed slightly, losing his *immah*, which he redid before speaking quietly to Sol. "Sir, I am the teacher. It is the law that you pay for travel in our country. That is how we keep the roads. You must pay Policeman Mr. Muhammad."

Sol noticed the two officers peering from the outside through the glassless windows, and he shook his head and smiled plastically. "You see, sir, I have no more money. The government took it all in Khartoum and El Fasher and Nyala, and this is stealing. What am I supposed to do? I have nothing left."

With the translation, the swarthy police officer came to the door, sucked in air through his teeth, and shook his head. The young teacher screwed up his face though spoke softly. "I am very sorry, sir, but you must pay now or return to Nyala, and you will go in handcuffs. They will charge you for the policeman, who has to sit with you on the bus, and then you will travel back to El Fasher with another policeman, and you will pay to travel back to Khartoum. You will have to start all over again. Why do you not pay, sir? It is very small money."

"You tell him it is not small money. I gave up a life in America to come here and help your people, and all you do is steal from me. No more." He strode to the door before the policeman or his helper could stop him and marched toward the bus. He climbed over the tailgate and the benches, dropped down onto his seat, folded his arms in front of his face, and snapped them onto his chest. He smirked to himself that he must have looked like Mussolini, the Italian dictator who had raped the Sudan's cousins in Ethiopia. He knew, though, the overwhelming majority of Darfurians had never heard of Ethiopia, or even dreamed of a land more than a few kilometers, if that, from their home village. Some did not even know they were Sudanese, barely aware that they were of the Clan Fur, for there were no other humans beside the Fur, and such a topic never came up in conversation. While interlopers like Sol passed through their territory, they were nothing more than temporary, human-appearing incarnations of the *jinn*, evil spirits up from hell, Jews that could morph themselves into desert lightning at night and colorless imposters during the day.

Yet with lives paralyzed by interminable boredom, the possibility of a shred of entertainment was so enticing, the crowd shadowed the policeman, who walked single-mindedly toward the bus, rusty AK-47 in hand. Only two crescents formed this time, the nomads miles away.

At the tailgate, the policeman shouted for Sol to get off the bus and pay his levy. But Sol tightened his arms in front of him and stared forward as the

The policeman stepped over the final bench, took Sol's arm, and pulled at his prisoner, but Sol wrenched himself out of the man's grip. "Go to hell. I'm not paying you seven hundred dollars. Period. This is the last straw. I'm goin' home."

The serious tugging began, but an instant later, he heard the UN doctor speaking softly with the constable. She called to Sol. "*Doctori*, do you think it is worth the trouble not to pay the road tax?"

"I'm not paying seven hundred dollars. I'll go home first. No way."

"Why do you say seven hundred dollars?" she asked gently.

Sol, possessed of a glut of adrenaline, stood, hopped angrily over the benches, jumped from the bus, and ran toward the office. He found the newspaper, his anger deepening as he looked again at the numbers, and brought it back to the woman. "Here, he wrote it down. See for yourself." Sol pointed to the "٢٥٥ D" and then to the man. "Seven hundred dollars, and he can't even write his numbers."

"*Doctori*," she spoke gently, "that is not seven hundred. It is Arabic for two hundred fifty-five."

Sol's face reddened. "Okay, two-hundred-and-fifty-five dollars. It's still robbery."

"Doctor," she whispered, "it not dollars. It is how they write dinars in the Sudan. They use a 'D'."

He calculated the value of a couple hundred Sudanese dinars—about three dollars. The rubor deepened. "Is that all he wants? Why didn't his helper over here tell me?"

The woman's head dropped. "He says he told you it was little money, but you ran out before he could figure out how much in your money. I do not think he ever met a Caucasian in his life. It was difficult for him. And I don't think he liked your middle finger pointed at his nose. He wonders what that means."

"It means I wasn't happy. Is it too late to pay the tariff? And please let him know that I was cheated in Khartoum and El Fasher and Nyala, and I thought that was what was happening here. I'm sorry."

She shook her head. "He knows what happens in Khartoum, and in each city, and in the towns and the villages. It has been this way for thousands of years. He has no idea on this Earth that it might be wrong, or that there is any other way. Do you know, Doctor, what corruption means?"

"Of course."

"He has never heard of the word. He does not know the concept."

"What about baksheesh? Bet he knows that."

"To these people, that is not corruption. It is the way the man makes his living. You call it a tip. A person pays what can be squeezed out of him. How is that different than you paying taxes to your government? Does some of that money go to individuals who use it for their own purposes? Do you pay your taxes?"

"Not happily. But people who steal from the government go to jail."

"Have you ever met a person who went to jail for cheating on a government contract?"

"No."

"But you pay your taxes, and you do not think twice, do you?"

"No, ma'am."

"It is no different here. You believe it is wrong to extort money from those who can pay, but it is no different than in your country." Her eyes closed, and her shoulders drooped. She added almost too softly to hear, "I hope you will pay the tariff. Your mission is more important than your feelings."

Sol conceded, "You're right. I made a mistake." He undid his scrub pants and pulled out a plastic bag tied to the string that served as his belt. The smallest bill in the bag was five US dollars. He handed it obsequiously to the sheriff, who took it and ran to his office. Sol held out his hands to the obstetrician. "See."

But the man returned at a trot carrying a fishing tackle box. At the bus, the officer took a key from a string from around his neck and pulled out a 3-inch wad of faded, green dinars and handed them to Sol as change. Sol's face reddened again, and he tendered half the dinars back to the man, adding another half-inch. He whispered to the UN doctor, "Would you thank him for the tea?" She translated, and Sol asked, "Ma'am, if that stamp was only three dollars, why was it five hundred US in Khartoum?

She did not change expression, but the almost indiscernible shaking of her head was not lost on Sol. "*Doctori*, you paid what they told you, not what the stamps said. Had you been able to read Arabic numbers before coming here, that would not have happened." She waited for him to protest, but he nodded and returned to his seat.

Half the scuffle concluded when the officer waved his hand at the driver, shooing him off, and then the other when he dismissed the audience. Some of the locals stayed on, though, standing with expectant smiles, but left when the constable's threats became nearly as loud as the din from the local farm animals.

The driver cranked the engine, spewing a string of grumbled curses, blaspheming his luck for having drawn the foreigner as a passenger out of all coaches that plied the sands of the sub-Sahara. Just as he persuaded the clutch and the transmission to synchronize, just as the first revolution of the bare tires lifted the truck out of the sands, the policeman headed back to the bus. A woman behind him trotted, trying to keep up. She carried a baby swaddled tight in layers of faded cotton cloth, shreds of a long-discarded *tob*. While the mom had a look of dread about her, as if her child had ceased breathing, her expression was tempered with determination.

The driver pretended not to notice, but the woman arrived at the tailgate, and the policeman shouted breathlessly to the UN doctor, who called to Sol. "*Doctori*, he asks you to fix his baby. It has been very sick for three days. Very hot. Will not eat."

Sol asked, "Why don't they want *you* to see the kid?"

"Because, *Doctori*, I am black and you are white. They fear you, maybe even hate you, but they think the white man's medicine is superior to anything a black man can do. And, I am a woman. Double curse, and a Christian. I think you say in America, three strikes and you are out."

Sol smiled while weighing her words. Several of the passengers relayed the message to the driver. There was a growl, but the grinding of gears stopped and the tires locked. The constable raised his voice impatiently, ordering his wife to lift the baby into the air and allow the doctor to make a diagnosis. She did as ordered then made a full circle of the rusted casket of the vehicle until her arms tired. She squatted in the blazing sun, placed the baby under her skirts, and waited without expression. Unable to see past the bodies and billowing *jellabiyas*, Sol crawled over his fellows toward the rear hatch.

Though the driver, like the balance of his countrymen, was the hue of coal, there was a growing ruddiness to his face as he removed the ignition key with an irate twist of the wrist. He muttered a few "*Al hum de le la*s," jumped from the cab, lit a cigarette, threw the match onto the scorching sand, and kicked it in his fury. It caught in his sandal and burned his big toe. After a few fuming puffs, he bristled to the rear of his vehicle just as Sol arrived at the tailgate.

The conversation was quite one-sided, the blasts of heated verbiage from the driver drowning Sol's, "Sir, let me just take a look at the kid. I'll give him some antibiotics, and he'll be fine in the morning."

Forte climbed onto the roof to search his bags for an otoscope, a stethoscope, a bottle of dry amoxicillin, and one of penicillin, just to be sure. He found that chicken-dropping-encrusted duffle bag under the far chicken coop. Sol peered down at the woman, who removed the baby from the safety of her skirts and again lifted it upward toward Sol. He smiled, "I'll be right down."

The driver's scowl grew as blistering as the unrelenting sun when Sol crooked his finger at the woman to follow him to the nearest corner of shade, which happened to be the police station. She stood, rewrapped her *tob* then inched, eyes down, as if being led headed to her own execution. Sol lifted a stack of documents from the table, eying the splinter that still lie on another pile, wondering how many years it would sit there, ignored.

Sol took the newspaper from his back pocket and laid it on the cleared corner of the table. When the mother stepped back to redo her *tob*, he slunk behind her and began to unwrap the infant, though the harder he worked at the interwoven cloth, the more tightly tied it became. The woman leapt forward and whined at the constable who was peering in through a window. Sol appealed with a shrug, and the policeman shouted at his wife to unwrap the boy. She obeyed, eyes downcast, proceeding through a series of steps as complex as folding an origami rose cube. Down to the last rag, she lifted her head and once again petitioned shrilly to her husband, though he clucked his tongue and stepped into the hut to yank at the final strip of rotting cloth. With the tug appeared a small, dusky patch of very brown tummy.

The mother swayed a bit, wailed a dirge, then sprang forward and started rewrapping, slapping Sol's hands away as he parried. The man bellowed vehemently and shoved her when she grabbed the baby off the table. She put the bundle back down and withdrew, head hung nearly as low as if she was genuflecting

With the woman standing in a corner with her eyes cemented to the earthen floor, Sol fully unwrapped the baby and begin the examination, starting, as at home, with the least threatening part of the assessment. He placed the stethoscope on the child's back, catching a single breath before the mother's howling deafened him. The policeman now stepped forward, head cocked in confusion.

The UN physician, who had followed Sol, stood behind the waves of onlookers until the constable raised his voice. She moved forward and muttered to Sol, "He wants to know why you insist upon touching his son. He's saying that Sudanese doctors in Darfur don't lay a hand on patients. To be honest, *Doctori*, he's right. You're acting very strangely. Here, doctors don't look at their patients. They hand out paper packets of pills in one hand and take money in the other."

At that moment, the mother rolled the baby onto its back in preparation to rewrap him. It was Sol's habit at home to take the chill off his stethoscope by running it under warm water, but here, he cooled it by trickling a few drops from what was left of his muddy tea on the diaphragm. The woman stopped and watched Sol, saucer-eyed. He sidled around her and quickly, but softly, placed the stethoscope just a bit above the tummy, at the "orthopedic point." That was where bone doctors insisted they could survey all the organs—the throat, heart, lungs, abdomen, and genitals—all at once, a technique that saved time and delivered the patient to the surgery scheduler just that much sooner.

The mother lunged forward and snatched the baby from the table, clasping him tightly against her breast. This gave Sol the opportunity to listen to the patient's back, but it also meant he wouldn't get a look at the ears. He considered appealing to her husband but rejected that out of hand, for if he uttered a word, he'd be saddled with two patients—a baby with an infection and a mother with a black eye.

He stuck the stethoscope on the child's back quickly. The diaphragm overlapped the edges of the moth-wing-sized shoulder blades. In between howls, he analyzed a rumpus of breath sounds louder than a pot of boiling gruel. He diagnosed pneumonia. That excited and relieved him, for he had found something objective to treat, unlike in the States, where, with pediatric patients, doctors often made up a disease to throw medicine at. Most of the time with children, it was a viral infection, a cold, and the physician found nothing on the exam aside from red eyes, a drooling nose, a scarlet throat, and red eardrums, all likely symptoms of the crying, not the disease. But at home, the real patient was the parent, so when the therapeutic decision was fashioned, the savvy physician nodded comfortably and dispensed all manner of unnecessary poisons to appease expectations. If an antibiotic was not produced, despite it being a medicine of no use in a viral infection, parents often became very quiet and left with plastic smiles, only to scurry, muttering, down the street to the next healer. You did not see them again, nor would you see the co-pay.

Though happy to have a diagnosis, Sol remained a bit bothered that the child had not yet coughed, was not having trouble breathing, and wasn't sucking hard for air, the cornerstones of pneumonia. Even his respiratory rate was normal. It was not that the child was so far gone that he didn't have the strength to cough. His cry was hearty, and Sol let his eyes drift upward in thought. The parents looked up for the object of his attention, and when the mother saw only the thatched roof, she snuck forward to start rewrapping the baby.

Sol ignored her and stepped outside the hut and told two of the dozens of gathered little boys to lift their ragged tee shirts. The first ran away but the second stepped up, and Sol listened. He heard the same raucous amalgam of toxins he'd detected in the baby. It was repeated in the lungs of the twenty other children who ran forward, shook Sol's hand, lifted their shirts, laughed, and begged the doctor listen to them. So, the baby's diagnosis wasn't lung disease, but the synthesis of the blowing sands, second-hand LIFE cigarette smoke, and the thick smolder of the cooking fires that consumed what wood, brush, and lumps of semi-dried camel and goat dung that could be scavenged from the desert.

Sol grabbed his otoscope for a look in the ears. As he placed a plastic speculum on the tip and turned the dials, there was a collective gasp from the audience and a then silence. Not one of the AK-47s, though, was pointed in his direction.

The child's ear canals were entirely blocked with dust, bits of dried grass, and a dead ant on the left. Sol was running out of things to test, and though he knew he ought to examine his patient's throat, the mother's fingers became more flexed. Her nails, though chipped and filthy, were long and sharp. He touched the patient's left cheek with the shaft of the cold otoscope, and the child turned hard the other way. Sol was waiting on that side, and when the baby caught sight of the white apparition, he opened his mouth to scream. Sol stuck his index finger deep into the waif's throat and depressed the tongue for a fleeting glance at a pair of swollen tonsils as scarlet as the setting African sun.

Sol jumped back, out of vomiting and scratching range, and smiled at the mother, who smiled back. He delivered his diagnosis to the UN doctor. "Please tell Mrs. Muhammad that the baby has a sore throat, but he's going to be like new in two days. Have her fill this medicine bottle with clean water, shake it well every time, and give him one, just one, capful *four* times a day until it is gone. And tell her to keep him unwrapped so the fever has somewhere to go. He'll do great. Two days. All better."

The mother listened attentively and grabbed the bottle of antibiotics. Sol waited for a comment, a word of understanding, perhaps of thanks, but she cast her eyes down shyly and squatted on the ground. As Sol left for the bus, he turned to wave at the woman, but she had sprung to her feet and joined a mob of her friends who jabbered as they passed the little plastic bottle around. There was a lot of concerned discussion, but some of the younger women stepped away, giggled, and smiled at Sol.

He thought the chronicle of that oasis might have a happy ending after all, and for the briefest of moments, he felt fulfilled as a physician, but as he neared the bus, he saw the driver glaring at him.

There was a pile of butts at his feet, and his hand gripped the rifle so tightly, his fingers were nearly white.

Sol broke into a trot toward the tailgate, but half a stride from the bus, a commotion built behind him, and he turned to see the policeman sprinting forward, his fist clutching a lump of dinars.

The policeman tried to hand Sol the pile of cash, but Sol pushed the man's hand away. There were head nods and murmurs from the crowd on the bus and from the locals in their crescents, but only an angry growl from the driver, who had restarted the vehicle. The officer jammed the bills at Sol so hard, he had no choice but to put his hand up. The man let go of the bills, and Sol had to take them or let them flutter into the wind. The driver popped the clutch and Sol pulled himself over the tailgate.

Passing the police station, Sol peered through the blowing robes of his fellows to see the mother rewrapping the baby tightly in the cloth, adding an extra layer of swaddling.

On board, Sol went through his inventory of purchases and returned a whole round of pita and a shaft of the viscous vegetable to his benefactors. They accepted the principle and interest without thank yous, but this time he saw in their eyes and subtle nods the connection he had missed with the angry nomad several towns ago.

Through the spider-webbed front window of the driver's compartment, Sol counted several new pairs of dangling, calloused toes and heels. He could occasionally see the feet when the bus jolted and the bodies of his fellows were tossed about, opening a tiny, visual wormhole to the outside world. Sol also caught a glimpse of the miles of mesmerizing yellow desert broken by an occasional farmer's field. Where, he wondered, did the water come from? But soon the monotony overtook him, and he fell into a rocking sleep. In his next lucid moment, several people shook him gently to get past for prayers. They had arrived at another town, a bit larger than the last, and he stood to stretch his legs but thought better of it and settled for a few push-ups on his bench.

When the passengers reboarded, Sol smiled that he had gone through a Sudanese village without incident. He watched the driver pull himself into the cab and start the reluctant engine, and with the first lurch, his fellow commuters calmed, aware that in just a day, or perhaps two, they would rejoin their lives in the fields and crumbling mud huts of central Africa.

Sol closed his eyes and let his mind drift to past girlfriends, but there was sudden yelling, and the driver jammed the brakes, shut the motor down, jumped from the cab, and pounded, rifle tightly gripped, to the rear of his coach. Sol was able to twist himself enough to see a figure in gray pants and shirt engaged with the driver in a high-pitched shouting match. Sol stood and stooped forward at his seat to pull out his plastic baggy.

The UN doctor called to him. "*Doctori,* sit down. This is a problem with another passenger. It is better if they don't see you."

Sol laughed at the squirming man being carted off the bus by a deputy for having failed to pay his fare. He could picture the stuffy, mud-walled room in which the prisoner would sit until a settlement was reached. Sol wondered if the thief would be offered a cup of tea.

The constable, however, walked to the side of the vehicle and looked over the tinfoil sides, nodding as if confirming what he thought he'd spied during the arrest. He passed word that the visitor would pay the road tax or be taken off the bus and manhandled as had the last miscreant. Sol handed his neighbor a swell of sweaty dinar bills. That man passed them on, until they reached the keeper of the water bladder, who handed the money to the policeman, but not before skimming a five-dinar note.

The truckload of civilians sat frozen, eyes wide. Not a word of controversy arose over the road tax, the stolen pennies, or the ticketless man. The cop waved his hand for the driver to set out, but Sol yelled to the UN doctor that he would pay the nickel for the man who had tried to stow away, and the bus idled until the soul climbed up to take his place, hanging on to the outside of the coach. The passengers relaxed; one smiled. An old man rolled beads in his fingers and hummed prayers. Another man called out in English, "Soon, Umm Balla!"

There were rounds of "*Bookerah, Insha'Allah,*" tomorrow, if God wills it, followed by a wave of "*Al hum de le la*s," Praise be to Allah, as the bus ground on for a quarter of a mile. It stopped at a lone hut in the desert scrub. Sol tsooked impatiently, wondering aloud, "What now, and how much is it going to cost me?"

After a minute, a skeleton of a teenaged boy shuffled from within the hovel, stopping in his tracks, as he was hobbled by spasms of a hacking, wet cough. As he regained himself, a thick, yellow muddle dribbled from his mouth. Before it hit the earth, the cough again overtook him, nearly dropping him to his knees. As that fit passed, the boy shuffled to the tailgate and was pulled aboard by the back row of passengers then nudged forward until he stood next to Sol. A man touched Sol on the shoulder gently from behind and made hand signals to let the boy sit next to him.

The driver turned the key, but the boy began to cough so deafeningly, the driver half-stood, turned to the mass behind him, and dropped from the cab. There were grumbled words from the driver to the passengers around Sol, grumbled replies, and a final gripe from the driver as he crumpled back into his seat.

As the engine burbled to life, the boy pointed to Sol's half-full water glass, then to himself. Sol hesitated for a moment, having already diagnosed the child as suffering from advanced TB, but chastised himself and handed the glass over. Between the tremulousness of the boy's hands, his hacking, and the lurching of the bus, the water shot forward, sloshing against the head to their front. Sol braced for a menacing interchange, and he tried to recall just how many dinars he had left in his pocket, but there was only a gentle "*Al hum de le la*," and then a refrain of "*Al hum de le la*s," wafting from the corners of the truck bed.

They followed sand tracks that ran along a succession of ancient, scorched telegraph poles, the wires lines long since stolen for the copper. Perched on top of each was a single vulture facing into the unceasing wind. The birds turned their heads, soon dipping and bobbing as they appraised the potential of the ship rolling across their domain. The vultures which had followed the bus for days began to scream so madly, they could be heard over the din of the engine and the wind. The local flock leapt into flight, closed into battle formation, then began a climb to engage the interlopers. The intruders, though, maintained their altitude and soon gained the advantage by feinting and diving, forcing the locals further into the desert, until the bus passed.

By sunset, Sol had drifted into a stupor and was nearly asleep, though the report of distant rifle fire drew him back to consciousness. Through the open sides of the bus he could see green tracers and muzzle flashes dart across the desert. The activity went largely unnoticed, or perhaps ignored, by the comatose passengers, and soon he turned back and let his head fall, praying to return to the escape of sleep.

CHAPTER TWO

At 10 PM, the coach squealed to a stop in front of a rectangular, mud-walled, twelve-foot-square African hut. One of Sol's neighbors shook hands with his bench mates and worked his way gently over dormant figures, finally making the tailgate and freedom. Several of the people on the roof got off as well. From the man next to Sol, who had returned to life with the gentle hubbub of the disembarkation, came a weak, "Umm Balla, *al hum de le la*," and then the chorus. With the driver mystically assured, for he hadn't bothered to look out of his cab, that the bodies of those who had climbed off were well away from the vehicle, he started off with a lurch, the barely functional headlights brightening a candlepower or two with the increase in engine RPM. At another set of huts, several more of the weary disembarked, amongst them the frail teenager with TB. The young man started to extend his hand to shake Sol's, but was wracked by a cough and left a puddle of yellow-green-brown sputum on the floor as he teetered off the truck.

At the next set of huts, the UN doctor gathered her things and left, calling quietly to Sol, "*Doctori*, I hope I will see you in Umm Balla town. Be well."

Sol answered, "*Insha'Allah*," throwing in an "*Al hum de le la*," to be sure the sentiment was precise.

The bus rolled a half-mile to the front of a compound. A dozen or so thatched sheds were enclosed by an eight-foot-high wall of desert brick. The arrival triggered another reprise of "*Al hum de le las*" as the passengers pointed energetically at Sol and then to one of the huts. Several of the boys helped lower Sol's bags, and he reached up to the roof to hand them a few wrinkled bills. That brought gentle smiles from the kids, more "*Al hum de le la*s," a grind of the gears, and a shout from Sol to stop the coach. The driver growled angrily but hit the brakes, and Sol trundled forward with five US dollars. The driver was barely able to grasp the unexpected largesse in his tremulous, nicotine-stained fingers. In one fluid motion, he lifted his *jellabiya*, slipped the bills into his shorts, jammed the bus into gear, slammed the gas pedal to the corroded floor, ignored the puffs of black exhaust belching from several rusted holes in the engine compartment, and drove the rattling coach into the dim moonlight.

Though the lunar outline was as colossal in the evening sky as Sol had seen in photos or imagined from the words of the poets, the haze was so thick with the settling of the day's sand, he could barely make out the entrance to the compound just feet away. He wiped the layers of gritty sweat from his face, combed through his soaking black hair with his fingers, and called out toward the inside of the complex. With no answer, he tried the metal gate, which rasped open far enough to allow him to squeeze through and walk toward the largest hut, drawn by the flickering of a candle. The woven-grass door was slightly ajar, and he knocked with the slightest tap, pushing on the straw portal very slowly. He sensed there were beings in the room and announced his presence with a whispered, "Hello? I'm sorry to bother you, but I'm the new doctor."

In the dim light, Sol barely made out the form of a petite woman reading by the sparse light of a gloomy electric bulb, one producing less radiance than the candle across the room. The bulb blinked in concert with the rhythmic droning of a distant generator, and as she sat up, her face sputtered as though part of an old-time movie. She said nothing.

When Sol's eyes accustomed to the bare wisps of light, he discerned the form of a man sitting across from her, head buried in a book as well. He looked up only after he had finished his paragraph.

Sol dared venture one step into the room, stopping with his back to the door, at attention, as if to await further instructions. The woman joggled her head, shaking away the apparition, just another of her ludicrous fantasies—a white man claiming to be a medical doctor materializing in the furthest reaches of humankind. He had come to transport her away from a ghastly dream. She shook her head a second time, asking reluctantly in an upper crust British accent, "Who are you again?"

"I'm Sol Forte. I'm the doctor from America."

The man at the table looked at the woman questioningly then stood stiffly and walked toward Sol. He extended his hand, perhaps a bit cautiously, clicked the heels of his flip-flops, and mumbled in a thick French accent, "I am André Pierre Anseau. I am ze medical student on leave from ze France. Lila, 'ere, is ze nurse from London. We were assured you were not coming, zat a cable was to reach you in Khartoum, one to stop you."

"Stop me? There was nothing in Khartoum. But that was quite a few days ago."

"Only days?" Lila asked in surprise.

"Yeah, I hopped a Belgian Air Force mercy flight to El Fasher. Then I took that so-called bus down here. I've been on the desert for days."

"Bloody hell," Lila groaned. "Well, let me brew a pot of tea."

"Maybe you want ze coffee." André asked. "Any 'ow, please you take ze seat."

Sol's eyes surveyed the room, perhaps twenty by twenty, whitewashed walls outside, the interior bare, dried mud. The ragged under-surface of the thatched roof was barely lit by a fifteen-watt bulb, one suspended far from the tinder of the roof. The wire was so long, the light swung in the wind at nose level. He nodded, remembering the warning from the administrators in London. Sudanese light bulbs exploded for no reason, sometimes even when they were not lit. Propped in a metal pie plate was a skinny candle surrounded by an inch of water. Its light flickered off a full-sized fridge, the once-white door crusted in sundry tones of off-green mold. The machine was older than the one he'd grown up with in Little Italy.

Sol studied the walls—jagged sand-brick supported by an internal skeleton of tree-branch rebar. The corners, reinforced with root wood, formed bookshelves, all sagging with the weight of worn paperbacks. With the meager ambient light now curiously sufficient, Sol could read the titles—a hundred recent British, French, and

German mystery novels intermixed on a shelf lining one side of the hut. A dozen American paperbacks across the way sat in a sloppy pile on the earthen floor. Stacks of well-read newspapers and pop-culture magazines served as bookends for a set of European medical texts sitting in the dirt of the final corner.

Sol turned to Lila and smiled, "You know, I think I'll take some ice water."

She paused, her face twisted skeptically, until Sol nodded at the refrigerator. "Oh, that," she scoffed. "Not working, never has, the freezer, that is. The fridge works, sort of, when we have the generator on full tilt, but it's been on the blink for a week. Only a few revolutions per minute, or such. Lights the light. That's about all. Our houseboy hasn't quite yet got the hang of tearing it down." She turned to André. "He's not that keen on devices that have moving parts, is he?"

André rolled his eyes. "He is not zat keen on ze devise wis out ze moving part, like ironing." He pointed to his hospital scrub pants and the burned out, half-football-sized gap in the material of the left thigh. It was the perfect shape of an iron. "You are ze mechanic, Doctor?"

Sol smiled. "I'll take a look at the generator in the morning. No problem. Is it gasoline or diesel? Diesel's hard."

André turned his head, contemplating the question, but before he could answer, Lila snapped, "I think before the generator we need to explain that we have no need for a doctor here. London was to contact you in Khartoum and send you back to the States. A telegram should have been waiting for you in at the Acropole Hotel."

"There wasn't. Not a reservation either. Your people in London promised they'd take care of that. Hotel probably received the telegram, got confused, and cancelled the room, not me. Spent the first night on a chair in the lobby. And it's been downhill ever since."

André growled. "Ze Acropole 'otel? Ah you mean ze Crap 'ole 'otel? I will tell you about zis one."

Lila sighed. "André, please. You've been here far too long. I'd give my right hand to be in Khartoum at this instant at the Acropole. The food was fine."

"And you are ze English to talk of ze food. Doctor, you know ze old story of ze definition of 'ell?"

"Umm Balla?"

André sniggered. "*Mais non, mon frere.* Well, it is partly true. No, it is where ze British are ze cooks, ze Americans are ze lovers, and ze French, we are ze mechanics. Ze food at the Crap 'ole is ze poison. You can be sure. And ze next sing to tell you…" He stopped in mid-sentence, for Sol took several staggering steps toward a broken wicker chair. As Sol's eyes glazed over, André jumped forward, took Sol's arm, and walked him to a battered couch next to the medical books. Lila rose as well and stared then struck a match to a kerosene hotplate that sat in the middle of the floor, also far from the dry-straw roof. She filled a tiny pot with water and set it on top to boil. "Tea in a jiff." She forced a smile as Sol eyed the liquid in the open kettle, instantly dispirited that it was murkier than that purveyed in the long-gone bus.

Sol began to drift off, reliving through a gauzy dream the Africa in which he had been entrapped for so many days. He felt the life and heat, the incessant blowing sands blasting the lives of the innocent, and the tattered prayer rugs. He heard grouchy constables harassing the public, no different than in the Bronx, or Whitaker. He saw defeated children and frail, blameless old ladies brandishing skeletal fists over three broken, marble-sized eggs. All that had been so critical for the interminable days was now just so many scattered, vanishing mirages.

He flashed to the nasty shouting match in which he'd found himself embroiled in the Nordstrom parking lot the Christmas before. "Over a parking space. Over a parking space! Never again," he whispered to himself, "never again."

Lila placed a cup of weak tea before Sol. He looked up and caught her peeking at his left hand, but she quickly averted her eyes and spoke curtly. "Sorry, we'll put you to bed straightaway, but back to business for a moment. Solomon, is it?"

He nodded. "Or just Sol—either is fine."

"London's cable was supposed to inform you that the camp is closing, or at least our role here is ending. Quite tragic, this."

"Closing? Disease?" Sol queried.

"No, though everyone is sick to some degree. It's the food, actually. We don't have any. There's not been a single delivery for the past three or four weeks. We're almost down to feeding the kids sweet tea and..."

André interrupted, "Green pee water, and when I say pee, I do not mean ze legume. It is what is left of ze water in ze great river of ze Wadi Azum. *Une flaque d'eau.* I sink you say ze poodle."

Lila shook her head, "That's puddle, I believe." A wisp of a smile brightened her delicate lips. "André, André, what are we going to do with you? Trouble is, he's quite correct. The water left in the *wadi* seems to bubble up green and thick."

Sol screwed up his face. "There's tons of food in Port Sudan. It's on the docks. I saw it just a month ago. You could feed all of Africa with what's sitting on a single pier. I never dreamed there could be so much of anything piled in one place. And there's tons at the UN warehouse in El Fasher. I just saw *that* a couple of days ago."

"It's there, no doubt," Lila agreed, her jaw set, "but getting it here, a few thousand kilometers from Port Sudan, and a few hundred from El Fasher, that's the rub. There's no war in the East, out there by Port Sudan and in Khartoum, but out here there is, and in the South, it's even worse. New here, though." She raised the teapot toward André.

He shook his head no. "I prefer my cocktail, sank you very much." He sipped from a glass of orange liquid, looked at Sol, and laughed, "Screwdriver."

"Is not," Lila laughed sardonically. "It's almost the last of the powdered orangeade. Don't listen to him, Sol. There's no alcohol here. A crime punishable by death, drinking is, you know."

"I've heard."

"So, welcome and farewell to the Umm Balla Please Help the Children Feeding Team. A Garden of Eden. A feeding team without food. And that's the easy part of the problem." Lila's eyes hardened. "There's simply no work for you, and soon for us. It is not personal."

Sol's hands began to tremble, and one balled into a fist. He smacked it against the table. "I can't believe this! I'm sitting in that so-called bus for like a month, eating dust, and all I can think about is not getting murdered by the locals and maybe helping a few kids. Not save the world, just a few kids. And now, I gotta get back on that tub before it turns around for El Fasher and then find a way back to

Khartoum? This is nuts. I'm not going. I'll find something to eat on my own."

Lila and André stole wary glances at each other, startled by the outburst that was so decidedly American. But Lila waited for Sol's face to relax before warning softly, "Yankee ingenuity, eh what? Good luck. Look, the province is barren. It hasn't rained in nearly five years. Nothing grows here besides a bit of brown grass. Even the sheep and camels have trouble eating it. What pushes through the sand's got barbs, and they hate it. Makes their mouths bleed. Most of the livestock the refugees brought with them from Chad have died, starved, just like their kids. With our supplies drying up, the only food is handouts from the locals, and they've mostly stopped since their own food supply is nearly gone. And now their cattle are dying. Then there's the government in Khartoum and the raiding parties they commission. This is not a pretty place, sir. It's a blessing we have to abandon it. Let's hope we escape before one of us, or likely both of us, are murdered."

The air puffed out of Sol's chest, and he spoke calmly. "Murdered? Didn't realize things are that bad."

"Oh, they're worse. We have to sit by and simply wait our turn. The Janjaweed patrols kidnap whole villages, take them out into the desert, and slaughter them. We've been lucky so far, probably because they know that if they gun down foreigners the government is going to have to answer for it. Plus, we're keeping these people concentrated, and that means under control. Easier to round them up when the government gives the word to their clients, the Janjaweed, to take this group or that. And those militias are getting bolder. They've begun coming to villages a dozen miles from here, raping the women in broad daylight then slaughtering them. Sometimes they only kill some and haul off the rest to sell to slave markets in the Middle East."

Sol asked, "Don't the men fight back?"

"There are no men. They've gone off to those same countries in the Middle East to work. There's no money here, barely any food, and a lot of blowing sand and disease. I told you, this is an ugly little patch. I'm surprised you didn't know what was happening. I've sent a dozen letters to our London office."

Sol thought back to his meetings with the directors of Please Help the Children, first in Los Angeles, then New York, and finally in England on his way out to the Sudan. In London, world headquarters, they had placed him in a large meeting room and poured cheap sherry, "club house pee," they remarked. Steak and kidney pie was served with fanfare, but it was just flour-and-tiny-bits-of-unidentified-meat pie so thickened with raw starch, it was hours before Sol was able to rub the patina of swill from his teeth. Dessert was a sodden custard, after which the director leaned back, belched, and warned Sol that might be the last good meal he'd enjoy for half-a-year.

When a sufficient number of sherry bottles had been exhausted, the directors finally got to Sol's assignment with the feeding team in Umm Balla. "Lila," they remarked, "is a good nurse, solid family, firm medical education, but given to flights of gloomy imagination and unfounded anxiety. Tends to catastrophize, so take it all with a grain of sand."

"After all," one of the grey-haired, paunchy men leaned toward Sol and whispered behind his hand, "what kind of woman leaves a good position at Addenbrook's Emergency Ward in Cambridge to live out in Africa with a crowd of other *female* nurses? Nearly thirty-three, question if she's ever been married, well, to a white that is, if you get my drift."

Sol nodded at Lila. "Yes, they told me it was a challenging assignment, but they never hinted it was unsafe."

Lila snapped, "How would they know?" They've never bothered to come out here. They claim it would drain the coffers to make the trip. They're rather soft is what I think."

Sol nodded then asked, "Have you witnessed the Khartoum militias doing these things? The government denies they have anything to do with the raiders. They say they're just highwaymen, and they have no control over them because they fade over the border into Chad or the Central African Republic. Khartoum swears there's no rule of law in the tribal areas in Chad or the CAR, and that those governments have forced the refugees across the border into the Sudan, just to get rid of them and weaken the Sudanese regime. The government in Khartoum turns around and swears they're the good guys for taking in the refugees."

"That's a bunch of rot," Lila hissed. "These refugees tell me every day what's going on. Indeed, they were forced out of their own countries by the militias. Those who didn't go were shot right there in their huts, babies first, or the babies were thrown into pots of boiling water."

Sol winced and held up his hand for her to stop, but she countered, "Don't like hearing it, eh what? Makes you want to run away, yes? But you need to hear it. The world needs to hear it. This isn't your Saks Fifth Avenue."

Sol managed to tighten his shoulders and ask, "Why? They're all Africans, all Muslim, all in the same boat."

"Well, in Chad at least, it was because the land they farmed was valuable. There was *some* water on it. So, the government came in trucks with soldiers and just took it. Gave it to the people from their own tribes, for a big cut. Everything is tribal here.

"Then the Khartoum government had to deal with the refugees, but they were smart. They allowed the good-intentioned foreigners to concentrate the refugees into camps, receive money and food donations from the Christian countries, pocket most of it, and skim the rations to feed their army and the Janjaweed. They let just enough food through to keep the locals and the refugees alive, barely, then sent their mercenaries out here, the Janjaweed, to pick the strong ones and send them off on lories, I think you Yanks call them trucks, to be sold. The weak, they murder where they find them so they don't have to waste food keeping them alive on the lor…trucks."

"Trucks?"

"Yes, the trucks that cross Africa carrying the slaves to ships hidden on the coast—both coasts—the ones they commandeer, boats that were bringing us food."

Lila took a breath to continue, but André, who had begun to nod off, looked up. "Lila, my dear, you don't believe everysing zese people say, do you? Ze worse ze story, ze more food we give zem. Is true, *oui*? Zey are smarter zan us."

Lila set her jaw tightly and glared at André. "They may be, but where's the food if the militias aren't taking it?"

"Lila, Lila, you needn't be so cross wis me."

"Well, you just don't seem to understand what's happening here. You never have. It's all just one big joke to you, isn't it? No one understands. Not New York, not London." Her voice began to waver, and she rubbed her hands together harshly.

"Now, now, Lila, we must not be so upset. We 'ave ze new guest 'ere. He can 'elp us finish ze feeding. We will stay for a few days more and zen go home. All will be well. Soon it will be done. Soon a proper English breakfast for you. Bangers and ze fried bread, and what is it? Ah, *oui*, ze toasted tomato and maybe even ze kipper or two." André rolled his eyes to the shaggy roof and added, "It is ze stress zat is eating you up."

"No, it's you and your jokes about these people. How they're dying by the tens and twenties every day under our noses. And all you do is..." She jumped from her bench, weaved around Sol, and bristled, sobbing, out the door. Sol and André stood and watched her run across the sandy yard into an eight-foot-diameter mud-walled hut. A set of rickety wooden planks tied together with strands of nylon thread served as the door to her whitewashed *tuchel*. She slammed it closed so hard, a length of balsa wood ripped loose and blew along the ground, floating with the dust, coming to rest at Sol's feet.

André shook his head. "Ze English, and zey say we are ze ones with ze emotion. *Mais*, you cannot blame 'er. Zis place is like ze 'ell, Doctor. Ze food is not food."

Sol almost laughed. "It seems everything is the food.'"

"Solomon, maybe you talk wis me again in a week...if you are 'ere zat long."

"I'll be here. I didn't come all the way across the planet to quit that fast. Tell me though, really, when do you plan to leave?"

"We've to stay to ze end. We can 'old out for a few days, maybe a week, maybe two, maybe one mons if zer is ze miracle. It is our commitment. But for you, zer are much better ways to do ze work. Umm Balla does not need a trained doctor. We need ze supply."

"It is André, yes?"

"*Oui, je suis* André." He raised his chin and again cracked together the heels of his sandals.

Sol touched the man's shoulder gently, sighing "Well, for all it's cost me to get here, it's my commitment, too. Maybe I'll just rent space from you and do my own thing. Do a little family practice in the field. And André, tell me, what would happen if I went back up to El Fasher and bought food?"

"*Mais*, 'ow are you going to get zer? I sout you 'ate ze bus."

"I do. But I'll figure it out. I know how to do it now. Ain't rocket science. Bring your own water and food. Keep a roll of five dollar bills in your pocket. Stay away from nomads at the pit stops. Keep to yourself. I can do it."

"'Ow are you going to pay for ze food if you find any? Take a job on ze side washing ze dishes at ze local guest 'ouse? Sorry to tell you zis, but zey do not wash ze dishes 'ere. They rub zem wis ze sand once in ze week, and zat is if zey get too dirty. Ozerwise, if you wash zem, you are losing ze good calorie."

"Money isn't the issue. I've got plenty of US dollars in the safe at the UN office in El Fasher. I can buy food there and rent a few of the busses to bring it down here. That's not a problem. It may be security, if what Lila said was true. I have no idea what's going on…"

André interrupted. "How did you get ze money past ze customs in Khartoum? Zey are awful. When I arrived, I had over a souzand bottle of ze powdered amoxicillin. They broke ze seal and stuck zer dirty finger in every single one of zem to make sure it was really ze medicine. Ruined ze 'ole lot."

"No, it's still good. You didn't throw it away, did you?"

"No, no, no, but ze money, tell me."

"I snuck it into Khartoum inside my two cans of shaving cream."

"How you do zat?"

"Did you see the movie *Jurassic Park*?"

"*Mais*, of course."

"The kid who did the job for me was an MIT grad. One of my patients. You know MIT?"

"*Mais*, of course."

"Well, he took my shaving cream cans, cut out the bottoms and stuffed them with hundred dollar bills. He even brazed a false bottom halfway up the can and left a little pocket of pressurized cream at the top, good for maybe ten squirts. So, when the dung ball customs officer in Khartoum checked it, I let out a little puff of foam to show him. Funniest thing he ever saw. He grabbed the can away from me and squirted it at his buddy. Then his pal grabs the second can, and they start a war. And all the time I'm counting down, nine, eight. That's when I let my New York temper get the best of me. I hopped over the counter and grabbed the can away from the first guy and chewed his ass. Demanded to see his superior. So, they let me go through without any more fuss.

"Nobody bothered to check me when I got on the Belgian Air Force C-123 in Khartoum to fly out here. In El Fasher, I went right to the UN and put my passport and most of the money in a shoebox, wrapped a rubber band around it to make it look innocent, and the UN people let me leave it in their safe.

"Now you know, so if anything happens to me, you can go up there and get it. I'll give you a note on my letterhead saying that I grant you permission to collect my things. There's a letter with my signature on it in the shoebox—instructs them to compare the signature to the one on the note I'll give you."

André asked, "May I be zo rude as to ask 'ow much zer is?"

"Of course. You need to know. We squeezed forty-six thousand in U.S. hundreds into two cans. But in Khartoum, you can't imagine the hassle of changing the hundreds into small bills."

"Your embassy will not 'elp?"

"First day, couldn't even get past the Marine guard outside. Guy wouldn't let me near the compound. I came back the next day and waited until a change of the guard and told the new guy about my father."

"Your fazer is ze diplomat?"

"No, he was a Marine, at the Choson Reservoir during the Korean War. Got shot. Almost died. As soon as I said 'Choson Reservoir,' everything changed. He grabbed my arm and introduced me around. Then the ambassador's aide de camp sent me to the Quatar Animal Bank. He told me to tell them I was there to buy livestock for a government program. If I had told them it was Darfur refugees, they would've kicked me out. Apparently, the refugees aren't religious enough, but animals are okay. The guy at the Quatar Bank told me I would hate it here in western Darfur because the people are *kafirs*. They say they are Muslim, but they're really infidels.

"No, no, ze are ze Muslim. You can be sure."

"Well, anyway, the bank took a three percent commission on top of a crappy exchange rate. Made me buy a carton of Sudanese money. Then I had to run through the streets with the box to the Bank of Khartoum to change it back to small US bills. Four percent this time, and a worse exchange rate. So, that left a few thousand less. Then there were the fees in Khartoum…"

"You do not need to tell me. Zey are ze pig."

"So now I'm down to about forty-one thousand before I even get started. I have a few thousand in my bags here, the rest's in El Fasher."

André sighed, "My Got! It is too much. It is dangerous to 'ave money like zat 'ere in zis awful place." He was silent for a moment then shook his head. "Zen zer is anozer problem. When you buy ze food, if zey will sell it to you, you must transport it 'ere, and ze 'ighway man will get you for sure. Zey know everysing."

"I can hire a security force. Or maybe I can get the government to ride shotgun."

André clucked his tongue and shook his head no. "Zat is ze point. Ze government want zese people to die, or at least go back into ze Chad and never come again. Zey will starve or murder if zey 'ave to. Sell ze rest like Lila say. Ze government is ze reason zere is ze famine 'ere. It is *not* ze lack of ze food. Zer is plenty of it. You saw. *Mais*, zey will not let it to come 'ere. Zey want to cleanse ze 'ole province of ze peasant. Soon even ze Sudan people will be murder, not only ze foreign refugee. Zer is oil and water 'ere."

"I thought you said Lila was overreacting."

"I cannot 'elp it, to tease 'er. *Mais*, she is so serious. I am trying to make 'er life better. To make 'er ze calm one wis my 'umor. You may not see it, but she is ze special woman. Maybe ze most special in ze world."

Sol was silent for a moment trying to picture Lila and what André found so singular about her. It came to him that she was so striking, he hadn't dared take a second look. He remembered that when she got upset, he had averted his eyes to the far wall.

André went on, "You will see."

Sol shook his head, feigning disinterest, and spoke quickly. "Okay, but are you are saying, if I buy food in El Fasher, I could get murdered on the trip back?"

"*Mon frere*, it is not ze 'could get.' You will be murder by one side or ze ozer." He paused, and the color drained from his face. Finally, he grunted, "It is too much for now. Come, let me give you ze room for zis night. Maybe tomorrow you want to leave."

Sol asked if he could just sit in there quietly for a few minutes, and André nodded.

"I am sorry we do zis to ze new doctor. I come in five minute for you."

Sol leaned back on the moldy couch and closed his eyes, content not to be moving. He stayed like that for ten minutes, until André stuck his head through the door. Sol nodded and rose. André grabbed a few of the duffle bags and lugged them to a *tuchel* next to one into which Lila had escaped.

When he came back for another load, Sol blurted, "Hey, wait just a minute, my medical colleague, I want you to see something. There is *some* good news." He peeled away a scale of bird droppings garnished with feather filaments from one of the bags and pulled out a cloth-wrapped softball. He unwound the fabric, carefully lifting three bottles of clear liquid, tilting them for André to peruse in the feeble light. Sol declared, "Five hundred, U.S.! It'll take a big bite out of the malaria in the camp. A gift from the CDC, though they had no idea they were contributing."

André focused fleetingly on the labels and mumbled, "Not bad," then glanced at his watch uncomfortably. 'It is late, even for ze young man like me." He grabbed the rest of Sol's bags but thought for a second and put them down, walked to a corner of the common hut, and tugged a bolt of dusty white cloth from behind a stack of old newspapers. He used his teeth to start a tear then sheared off a four-by-eight-foot length and rolled it into a loose ball. Tossing it to Sol he laughed, "Ze finest of ze silk sheets for our guest. Usually zis is ze death shroud, but who will know? We don't 'ave enough anyway to bury our dead. Zer is not enough in ze 'ole world to bury our dead." André lifted the luggage and kowtowed to exit the low common room door.

Sol held the medicine in his right hand and followed André to the primitive hut. André went in first and pulled a string hanging by the door. A single, bare light bulb came to life, though it was watts fainter than the one barely lighting the hut. It sputtered, resonating to the beat of the camp generator, revving from the luster of a birthday candle down to that of a dying charcoal ember and back up.

André laughed, "We give you ze best room in ze 'otel, *oui*? Even you get ze mirror from ze last *mademoiselle* to live 'ere. *Mais*, Doctor, you must look quickly. Ze generator it is failing, like everysing 'ere. Look fast."

There was an abrupt, high pitched whine from the generator, and André smiled, "Finally, ze sing goes fast." The light bulb glowed with relative brilliance for a couple of beats, but the machine quickly gurgled to a halt. The two were left in perfect silence and utter darkness. For a reason he would never understand, Sol felt the need to take a step forward into the hut, and André felt the need to take one out of it. They collided and landed on the earthen floor. There was a thud and then the tinkle of breaking glass.

The final sound was André hissing wrathfully, "*Merde! La Afrique*! You are okay, Doctor?"

Sol answered sharply, "Shit. That was good stuff. What next?" He reached down as if to salvage what remained of the liquid, but it had soaked into the dirt floor. "It's mud now. Roaches won't be getting' malaria." He sighed, "Well, two of the bottles made it. Maybe we can get some more. I got friends in high places. You know what, I think I'm just going to go to bed, and maybe in the morning we can all start over."

André pulled a flashlight from his pocket and played it on a simple bed. He warned, "Ze mosquito net. Important. Ze last British doctor, 'ee forgot, or maybe 'ee was so tough. Big machismo, zat one. He leave 'ere very sick wis ze malaria. Zen, it takes so long to go back to Khartoum, ze malaria spread to 'is brain. He die on ze trip home to London. 'Ee was ze lucky one. So please, you will use ze net, *oui*?"

"I will use the net. I promise. Is that story true?"

André laughed. "*Mais non*, it is my 'umor. But in ze morning, you shake ze shoe for ze scorpion and tarantula. Sometime ze Green

Mamba, 'ee get in zer first, so to be very careful. Is ze two-step snake."

"Two-step snake?"

"*Oui*, if 'ee gets you, you 'ave two steps before you are dead."

Sol laughed, "Better make 'em big ones, huh? I'll be careful."

"One more last word. If you see ze bastard bug, you get 'im off you so fast. If not, ze skin die where 'ee walk on you. Just ze walk on you is suffice. 'Ee does not even bite, zis one. But, welcome to Umm Balla, Doctor, ze Garden of Eden, the spot on ze Earth where life come from, and we do ze work of God—ze cradle of man."

André shook his head and took a step to leave, but Sol laughed and exclaimed, "André, you know what, I'm still glad to be here. Crazy, huh?"

"Maybe crazy, maybe not. And make sure you close ze door before ze rise of ze sun. And be sure to lift up ze mosquito net before ze sun and put 'im away. *Bon nuit, mon frere*, good night, my friend."

Sol took a seat on the edge of the frail bed and picked through another of his bags. He fetched a flashlight and pulled free a small framed photograph. "Crazy, Dana, huh?"

The bed was hard, just a few planks of coarse baobab atop a rusted metal frame; the mattress, barely an inch thick, was a lumpy sack of shredded rags stuffed into a mildewed, bristly bag of the same material André had given Sol as a sheet. Sol brushed his teeth outside the *tuchel* but ignored André's admonition and left the door cracked to quell the heat. He pulled the mosquito net over himself and shut his eyes. At first it was magic, to relax after the nights of wooden floors, but he woke every few minutes during the first hours to wipe sweat from his face, and, after midnight, every few minutes to double over André's sheet. At two or three, a thin but intense streak of light from the full moon burned through the glassless window into his face, and when that passed, he was roused by spasms of animal bleating and snorting that ebbed and peaked every fifteen minutes.

At the first inkling of dawn, the door he'd left an inch ajar had blown completely open. Sand and trash blustered in. At first, it was just a dusting, but by full sunrise, the laws of thermodynamics applied themselves more brutally to that patch of star-crossed land than anywhere else on Earth. With the uneven heating of the Sahel, Sol's hut was soon churning with a freezing gush of wind, and in seconds a burning surge of air. When the two merged, a tornado roiled inside the hut admixing his papers, clothes, and bedding.

By the time the sun climbed to fifteen degrees above the hazy, indefinite horizon, the passion of the African heat had grown exponentially. Sol's sweating did as well. In minutes, the finer blowing sand sieved through the mosquito net, crusting Sol's exposed skin with a patina of what looked like toasted bread crumbs. With a few more degrees of the sun's elevation in the dust-choked sky, the air swirled so violently, gravel whooshed in, pelting the mosquito net. A few jagged holes appeared in the fabric, through which the mosquitos were drawn magnetically.

That finally woke him from the exhaustion of the weeks he had not slept, and he jumped from the cot, becoming entangled in the netting. A piece ripped from the bedpost. He took two steps into the center of the hut and jerked the mesh from his torso.

He surveyed the contents of his life: a two-by-three metal table, a rusted metal chair, and five duffle bags crammed with outdated medical books, expired medications, and antiquated healing tools. Every scrap of which had cost him an episode of prostration before hospital administrators across several states.

Even the three pairs of operating room scrub suits had been a misadventure. The medical director of his very own beloved hospital, the one to which he had brought millions and millions of dollars of business over the years, snapped at him that doctors who borrowed scrubs for voluntary overseas missions never returned them, the financial loss to the corporation unconscionable. When Sol mentioned he had never heard of a single physician or nurse who had ever gone on a foreign mission, the medical director barked, "I don't care. I *will* maintain discipline in my hospital. The answer is still no."

The volume of fine grit filtering into his new house rose, much of it clinging to subsequent layers of sweat. He pondered his next task—a shower. Wrapping himself from head to toe in the bed sheet, he took a step toward the door and caught his reflection in the shard of mirror, a Grand Wizard of the Klu Klux Klan.

The sand, though, would not be denied. It sifted through the cheap muslin, pasting to his face and grinding into his tightly closed eyes. He threw off the sheet and sat on the side of the bed, his eyes encircled by thin brown crusts. He spit out sand and wrapped himself in a towel then staggered in the whipping air toward the latrine shed. Already open a crack, he didn't knock as he yawned and gave the rope handle a pull.

He saw a dark form squatted over the little hole in the cement -capped floor and turned away quickly. As he pushed the door closed behind him, a woman's voice murmured without emotion, "I'll be done straightaway."

A moment later, Lila pushed out of the latrine, a towel wrapped only around her waist. Sol scolded himself not to look but could not pull his eyes away. The blunted sun reflected off her face— she was exquisite, a mirage. She had the most beautiful nose he had ever seen. Her towering cheekbones and lips were flawless. He told himself to stop, but his eyes lowered and brushed her perfect breasts. It was for but a trice, and he lifted his gaze back to her face just as she slowed and turned to look at him.

He perceived great sadness in her onyx eyes. They radiated such cheerlessness, and Sol sensed a disquiet wash over him, one deeper than the pall brought by the already-squandered weeks he had passed in the Sudan. The spirit leaked from his heart, and he sensed a darkening of his peripheral vision. The world narrowed to a black-walled tunnel even longer than the one in which he had felt himself as he stared at the nomad's rifle. He understood that over the past weeks, he had begun to sink into a state of depressive illness, but his lips tightened as he realized there was nothing to be done.

André exited his hut clad in boxers bulging at the crotch. He walked to the latrine without a word, and when he drifted out, the bulge was gone. He nodded to Sol. "*Bon jour*, Sol. You pass ze night well?"

"Very, thank you," Sol smiled.

"You are okay? You sound tired, like Lila."

"No, I'm fine. I just need to wash up. Where's the shower?"

André pointed a few feet away to another telephone booth-sized hut and laughed, "If you wish to baze."

"I think I'd feel better." Sol nodded a thank you and looked at the stall. A half, fifty-five-gallon oil drum teetered on the roof, an edge of the rusted barrel pushing through the rotting wood.

"Yes, *mais*, ze water is very cold in ze morning. Zos who wish to wash zemselves do so at night while ze tank is still warm from ze day. But you must take ze caution, Sol. If you wash before ten-sirty at night, you will burn your body. If you wash after ten-forty at night, you will freeze your body. But everysing is good 'ere."

Sol opened the door of the sheet metal shower stall. He gasped as an army of insects buzzed into his face, and though he slammed the door shut, several more legions crawled under the door and took flight to whirl about him. Though he slapped madly, and a pile of bodies collected at his feet, more and more of the vermin, drawn by the scent of fresh meat, escaped through cracks. A species of beetle crawled toward his feet, a dozen or so trooping past the flip-flop he used to dispatch the majority. A few made it to the top of his foot. They succumbed to his battering, but not before leaving a crisscross of cloudy yellow effluent that squirted from their rear ends.

He kicked the dead and dying into the drain, a gully cut in the dirt that coursed under the back of the stall. It was soon clogged with carcasses, and he went outside to clear the channel. He followed the thin trench with his eyes as it ran along a shallow hill, through the middle of another hut, out again and further down the hill, under the compound's mud wall, and into the neighbor's yard, where it ended in a runty vegetable garden. Lashed by vine collars to the wall were a half-dozen monkeys. They screeched at Sol as he pulled the shower door open.

Inside the tin closet, a half-inch lead pipe poked through a piece of the curled plywood ceiling. Sol pulled the rag from the tube slowly and a bare trickle of freezing water dripped onto his head. He poked it with a stick, and a lump of red mud broke free abruptly to thump him in the eye. A gush of frigid red water and sludge followed, and by the time he jammed the rag back into the pipe, most of the team's daily wash water had been squandered.

He tried to dry off with his new towel, a five-foot square of threadbare nylon he'd bought in a bazaar in Omdurman, a suburb of Khartoum. That was where, on the Friday Sabbath, hordes of the curious crossed the Nile to watch the whirling Dervish, religious disciples who spun in the immense heat while pacing in a circle, twirling towards the Truth, the Perfect, their egos deserted. After twenty minutes, the devotees, six men in soaking *jellabiya*s, frothed at the mouth and, ten minutes later, fell to the ground, having returned from their spiritual journey. The locals approached with cups of water.

Sol stumbled upon the bazaar after the ceremony. As he went to pay for the nylon towel, he discovered that his pocket had been picked of all but a dollar. He spent fifteen cents on the towel, and fifty cents on a taxi back to the Acropole Hotel.

This morning, he cursed himself for having wasted the money on the towel, for it was impermeable, useful only to squeegee sheets of ice water from one patch of skin to the next. As he ran back to his hut, he noticed the monkeys were on the ground drinking the water in the drainage ditch. He was shivering so violently, he thought he would chip another tooth. Inside, he was met by a cyclone of microscopic dust filtering down from the weed roof; a barrage of larger particles hurtled through the windows. He was instantly recoated. He dropped onto his bed shaking and cursing, his eyes burning from the sand. Covering them with the towel did nothing, the blowing sand easily grating through the porous nylon.

As the sun rose another fifteen degrees, the temperature hiked the same number of degrees Celsius. The warmth rekindled his hope, and he wrapped himself in the towel to dash back across the yard to the shower. The monkeys squealed rancorously as he entered the metal box. He could hear them as he pulled the rag slowly, only partially free. He soaped up and washed away the latest iteration of grime, and there was sudden quiet from the neighbor's property.

In between loosening the cloth and the seconds he allowed himself of the water supply, the sun rose precipitously. The temperature soared to the point that he was dried by a howl of blistering air the instant he opened the door. But as he trotted the thirty feet back to his hut, he began to sweat, and the flapping of sandals kicked up sufficient filth to coat his legs. When he dove inside his *tuchel* and pulled off the towel, the spinning cloud of finer particles fused to his sweaty body. His veneer was now thicker than before the second shower, and he spent many minutes brushing away what he could of his gritty patina before dressing in clean clothes. He chose from one of four tee shirts contributed by the D.A.R.E. officers at his sendoff.

Before he left the *tuchel*, he began itching from the sand he'd been unable to scrape off. He worried he would spend his first day saving the people of the saddest corner of the Earth scratching like one of the leashed monkeys glaring at him from the neighbor's mud wall. André watched with a droll expression, though his fingers began to drum the roughhewn breakfast table as Sol dashed from his hut back to the shower, a new set of clean clothes wrapped in a compact ball jammed under his arm. When Sol disappeared back into the stall, André walked over and yelled in, "Doctor, we must be going to ze camp before ze end of ze new century."

Sol stripped quickly, jumped under the lead pipe, and pulled the rag loose. The still-frigid water petered out before it reached his waist. Drops of muddy liquid mixed with the fine dust that had filtered through his clothing to form a plaster of Paris mold around his chest. It dried instantly as waves of burning air were drawn into the shower stall.

Sol redressed in the first outfit and joined André, who had retaken his seat on a wooden bench at the table. Lila came from inside the common hut carrying rounds of pita wrapped in newspaper, a bottle of orange marmalade, and hot water for tea. Sol squeezed in, reaching expectantly for the bread, but stopped in mid-grab, remarking, "Whoops, there's sand in the bread. Did you see that?"

Lila smiled caustically. "Doctor, those are toasted sesame seeds."

André groaned, "Oh, Lila, you must not tease ze new 'ealer." He turned toward Sol. "Zey are your ration of ze insect. It is ze Umm Balla protein allowance for ze day. No B-12 deficiency on zis trip for you."

Sol eyed the jelly bottle, impressed with the English crest on the label, and noted that the box of Earl Grey tea was also from Great Britain. He smiled. "Marmalade. Excellent."

His breakfast companions did not comment, but André opened the bottle and pointed to a web of moldy filaments. "You are still 'appy?"

With a glimpse back at the bread, Sol stood and grumbled, "I think I'll wait for lunch. Not that hungry anyway."

But Lila warned, "This is all there is of fresh food until supper. Only tinned goodies for dinner. I believe you call that lunch. And you refer to our supper as dinner. All very confusing. Two very different languages. And we never bring pita or sweets like the jam to the refugee camp, ever. We used to take a dozen rounds with us in the morning, cheese, yogurt, but when we got out of the Land Cruiser at camp, the kids found the food. They put out the word, and there were stampedes, especially when it was something new, like the day one of the Americans tried to sneak in a bottle of ketchup. You'll wind up trying to throw it as far as you can to get the crowds off you, and then the kids'll fight over what you throw away, and some will get trampled, and one or two will die, and their mothers will blame you, and there'll be yet another riot in camp, and they won't bring the kids to be fed, and that means more of them will die, and your embassy will get word straight-away, don't ask me how, and it will be classified an international incident. The UN will say we Western bastards are killing the third-world's children while throwing balls during our cricket matches. And you, Doctor, will have caused it all. You may even be charged with crimes against humanity. You'll be put on trial in The Hague. Better eat something now."

Sol nodded unhappily, asking if he could try one of the tinned items. Lila smiled, and Sol reached for a can marked in an Eastern European letters and a smudgy photo of peas and carrots.

André shook his head. "You do not want zis one. It is like ze roulette. Zis is better." He handed Sol a box full of paper pouches, these labeled in Cyrillic characters. "Ze packet of ze oatmeal Russian. Maybe you take zis now wis ze bread. Try it, it is delicious. Cereal and toast. Not ze American steak every morning, but maybe you keep alive."

Bits of baked insect pulled easily from the still-warm pita round, fragment by fragment, until Sol amassed a pile of abdomens, feelers, and legs, which he heaped on the square of newspaper that served as a napkin, a tiny piece of paper that was peculiarly similar to the shredded Arabic language tabloid that had performed a relatively analogous function in the latrine. He boiled a cup of water in the common hut, made oatmeal, then, avoiding the iridescent, spidery fluff around the periphery of the marmalade bottleneck, scooped a teaspoon onto the pock-marked pita. He pinched his nose and ate quickly, tasting nothing. *"Al hum de le la."*

He washed the meal down with the sweet tea Lila brought to the table. She'd pushed the floating sesame seeds to the side of the tea and drew them out with a finger before placing the cup in front of Sol. Lila smiled blandly, "In the sugar as well, I'm afraid."

"And so passes ze premier *petit déjeuner*, zat is ze breakfast, of Dr. Sol in Umm Balla. Is very good, *oui?*"

They boarded a Toyota Land Cruiser. Next to it, partially covered with death shroud, was a British Land Rover on blocks. "When the team had twelve souls," Lila mumbled, "we needed both, but now we only use the Rover once a week. André says it isn't smart to let it sit. I say who cares?"

They bumped along a road worse than the desert track that had carried Sol to Umm Balla less than twelve hours before. Here, however, there were acacia trees and bushes, a painted world unlike the monochrome of the past days of wasteland. Sol rubbed his eyes in surprise at the hues of life, the varied shades of jade on the road to the Umm Balla Refugee Camp, colors brighter than any he'd ever seen. But in a few moments, the shock of a colored world wore off, and he realized the tinctures were really quite drab.

André drove. He slashed violently at the steering wheel, left and right, white knuckled, avoiding potholes, though the entire road was one grand catacomb, just a bit deeper or shallower in places. Some of the gaps were so large, André had given them names, barking with disgust, "Zat one is Eduard, and zat bitch is Jean Paul." Lila sat silently in the back, eyes closed.

The Land Cruiser rocked for a mile before coming to a village with topless, ragged African women, mothers kneeling in front of mud-and-thatch huts, their hands busily grinding grain with fist-sized rocks in two-foot-diameter, slightly hollowed out stones. Nude, three and four-year-old kids circulated along the road in bands, some yanking along luminescent green beetles tied to thread leashes. Others dragged diminutive cardboard models of the very Land Cruiser in which André and his two passengers jerked through the settlement at seven or eight miles an hour. The vehicle raised dust bowls that blocked most of Sol's view. With the road a bit smoother, they approached another small settlement of sand-brick huts, the actual village of Umm Balla, after which the camp had been named. Sol asked, "Does anybody know what Umm Balla means in Arabic? I know *umm* is mother."

André had kicked the Land Cruiser into third and was accelerating. He took his eyes off the road and turned to Sol. He laughed, "*Oui*, ze meaning is somesing you greatly do not want."

"No, I would like to know."

"*Mais non*, zat is it: ze meaning *is* somesing very bad, like, I hope zis does not 'appen."

Sol chuckled, "So it means Mother of Your Worst Fears."

André slammed the Cruiser into fourth, speeding to nearly thirty before turning back to Sol and nodding, "*Oui*, yes, zat is it."

Lila opened her stunning eyes and snapped at André, "You simply won't be satisfied until you hit a child or two, will you?"

"I am ze Grand Prix driver in ze France."

"And also a mountaineer, you told me," Lila snarled sarcastically.

"*Oui*, I am knowing what to do wis zis car and to climb ze mountain," but he slowed to twenty when they came to a bull mounted on a bony cow in the middle of Highway 46, a quasi-road as primeval as the footpaths trod by the first humans who sought to flee the horror of Africa seventy thousand years before. At first, André raised his eyelids several times to Sol, grinning lasciviously, but he became impatient and honked, though the animals did not look up, and he turned off the road to bounce through the front yard of a grass hut. They passed feet from a sloppy, mud and straw heap of earth encircling a crude shelter, a wall of sorts, the six-foot crest patrolled by a monkey leashed about the neck with a short tether of woven vines.

Sol bade André stop. He exited the Cruiser and beckoned in a falsetto, "Here monkey, monkey." When Sol offered a shred of the pita he had slipped into his pocket for lunch, the creature screeched, ground its teeth, and the fringe of white around his face stood erect like a porcupine preparing to strike. As Sol inched closer, the monkey's shriek decayed to a rhythmic growl. André jumped from the jeep and yelled, "Doctor, you must leave 'im alone. Ze minkey 'ere is like ze cobra. You will be killed. You must take my words."

Sol stopped in his tracks and laughed. "Excuse me, Inspector Clouseau, it's *monkey*, not *minkey*. And don't worry, I can handle myself. It's a vervet. Very social. Smart. We used them in medical school. Treat them gently, and they're gentle back."

But before he could take another step, a coal-black woman emerged from the hut wagging her finger at Sol, then at the monkey, finally shaking her head and protesting, "*La, la, la, la.*" Sol handed her the strip of pita and pointed toward the monkey. She was stunned for an instant but locked her eyes on the scrap of bread and jammed into her mouth.

Sol shook his head. "That was for Mighty Joe Young, not you." He pointed at the maddened primate who was pulling so franticly on his leash, the grey body whirled and his mouth foamed like the Dervish of Omdurman.

The lady stuck her hand out for the rest of the bread, but Sol grumbled and returned to the jeep. He nodded for André to move on and glanced back at Lila, her eyes now sealed more tightly, her breathing so slow, she seemed to have placed herself in a state of suspended animation.

A bit farther on there was a patch with several dozen more mud and straw huts, the entire clutch surrounded by a much thicker, tidier mud and straw wall. Sol assumed they had arrived at the refugee camp, but André sped up and announced, "Ze City Hall of Umm Balla. Zer are many little family settlement along ze road. Zese are ze Sudan people, not ze refugee. But zey are next to go. You will see. When ze Khartoum government come for zem, zey will run to ze Chad, and zen we will 'ave ze Chad refugee 'ere, and ze Chad Please Save ze Children will 'ave ze Sudan refugee zere."

Sol turned to Lila for the other side of the argument, but her eyes remained cemented shut.

They drove through the browning tropical countryside for another mile until the water-starved trees and brown grass faded, leaving an open panorama of rolling hills as far as Sol could see. When the jeep crested the next hillock, there opened before them a shallow valley studded with countless blue dots huddled into two square miles, an immense, though tatty, cross-stitch blanket. It was not until they were closer that Sol realized the blue was a montage of thousands upon thousands of sheets of eight-foot-by-eight-foot azure plastic tarpaulins, roofs, each defining one family home which sat two feet from the next.

Just yards from the camp, Sol could make out the hut walls were rotting, grass pads, beach mats, the kind he had enjoyed for an afternoon at the Jersey Shore then stuffed into the parking lot trash barrel. At twenty-five yards, the framework of the hovels came into view, four-foot long tree branches, a commodity so precious in the sub-Sahara, each had been quartered lengthwise, now skinny sticks to support the mat walls and truss the plastic roof. That left the structures as well supported as a paper kite, and so close to the desert floor, the tenants, all but the toddlers, dropped to their knees to crawl in.

After thirty minutes on the road and less than three miles covered, André sped up for the last fifty yards so he could bring the vehicle to a skidding halt. The maneuver lifted a cloud of dust so thick, Sol couldn't see beyond the windows.

"It must be zis way, Doctor," André said softly. "Ozerwise, ze kids, zey surround ze cah, and you cannot get out."

Lila groaned, "This, Doctor, is why you came halfway around the world?" Her eyes rolled as she went on, "Welcome to the heart of the Umm Balla Refugee Camp. Give it a minute."

As the grime settled around the Rover, Sol peered out at four massive, primordial structures, each five thousand square feet and fifteen feet high, all crafted from the very same materials and techniques by which the individual huts had been hewn—just sticks and woven grass.

Lila let him peruse his new world, but when Sol started to open the door, she warned that they had to wait until the kids became bored and went off and allowed the team to exit in peace. She went on drolly, "This is the nucleus of the camp, our feeding centers. This is where the kids and their mums come three times a day when the cowbell rings."

"So, you *are* still feeding them."

"For a bit longer. The kids get a bowl of lukewarm swill: powdered whole milk, raw sugar, and cooking oil, all boiled, or at least warmed, in the green water from the wadi. They drink it, some of them do. But we're nearly out of sugar, and there isn't much oil left."

Off to the side were two only slightly smaller grass mat structures. Sol asked, "And those?"

"Quasi-hospitals. That's where the same kids go to die when their guts give out, and they don't tolerate our slimy fare any longer."

On the periphery, fifty yards from the hospitals, were two more woven grass buildings where Sol watched men in *jellabiyas* moving great, white bags of food from one ten-foot-high pile to another. He pointed. "And?"

Lila mumbled, "Food storage and distribution." She pointed up a hill to a three-hundred-square-foot grass-mat structure in two sections. "And that is what is left of our clinic and pharmacy. When we were at full staff, we had a medical center. There were four doctors and two dentists. We worked around the clock."

"What happened to them, the doctors?"

Lila's face tightened, and she turned away. André sputtered, "What do you sink? It was time to go 'ome when everysing you do is only to preserve ze pain of ze dying. Zey could not take it. Zey said it is better to let ze weak die and only feed to ze strong. Zey know zat when we leave, ze weak baby die in few days. And zen ze mama must go srough ze terror two time of zer child to perish. For ze foreign man, six weeks, maybe two monses in Umm Balla, *il suffit*, it is enough."

"You're still here. Miss Lila's still here."

"You will see. Okay, Doctor, we are ready. Please, use ze caution."

Sol opened his door and slipped from the vehicle. As André had warned, the moment he reached the outer limits of the still-settling, filthy cloud, hundreds of dust-encrusted, potbellied children with twig arms and stick legs descended on him. As they recognized a stranger, instead of running, they jammed closer. A few tugged the dark hair of his arms; others pointed at his deep blue eyes and laughed. Several ten and eleven-year old boys, though, appeared to push the unruly back into the crowd, chastening them to behave politely.

At first, Sol withdrew a few feet, considering a dive back into the Land Cruiser, but there was a gentleness and warmth about the children that swept over him, and he could not help putting his arms around one of the boys, wrestling gently, and then with another.

André came up behind him and spoke in a near whisper. "Welcome, Doctor, to ze sickest, most deprived children on ze Earth. And still zey smile at ze foreign man, and one by one, zey will be shaking your 'and."

Even the few male teenagers at the back of the crowd smiled, though guardedly, and Sol knew, instantly, they were there only to size up what they might purloin from him.

The three Westerners made their way slowly toward a structure, the swarm of children moving with them. A pack of pre-teen boys patrolled the shifting mass, insuring an inner perimeter of clear passage. The mid-sized, grass-mat, administrative hut was filled with well-fed Sudanese men, all in their twenties, most dressed in worn Western slacks and long sleeve shirts. A few wore *jellabiya*s and *immah*s. Each chewed on a toothbrush twig.

Lila announced, "*Doctori* Solomon, these men are our very, very good checkers. Everyone, this is Doctor Solomon Forte. He is from America. He will be here for today."

The room became relatively quiet, though two or three of the checkers continued to speak and laugh loudly, their backs turned to Lila. She took a clipboard from the oldest of the men and read from it distinctly, the men nodding and dispersing to their assignments. As they walked out, Lila explained that these were the literate, the cream of Sudanese society, men who had had to prove to André they were high school graduates from the larger cities, and that they could read, write, and speak English.

When Sol asked if the women checkers had their own office, André smirked, "Zer are no woman checker. Ze female are forbid to travel more zan one 'undred meter from zer 'ome. Zey not allow to live amongst ze unmarried man, and where would we find even one who has been to school, even ze first year?"

Lila interrupted. "André, please. Many of the girls in the cities get some basic schooling. They're just not allowed out of the house alone, ever."

Sol turned to André. "The way you described it, I thought these people would be lying on the ground dying. Looks like there's enough food for right now. Gives us some time to get more, yes?"

André laughed. "*Mon frere*, I told you. Zer is food, but no way to get it 'ere. It looks like ze banquet, but every day 'undreds of zem more walk over zat 'ill down to ze camp." He pointed to a hillock a mile from the camp. "What is on the ozer side; I do not want to see it.

"But we 'ave not received ze shipment in sree weeks. Zat means in ten days it is over. Zen ze people 'ere will turn on us. We must leave before zat 'appens. Very soon."

"André, I have only known you for a few hours, but you seem like a good man. You must have believed you were going to help these people when you first got here. You had to know it was going to be hard, but you came and you stayed. What changed your mind?"

"Ze reality."

"Well, wait a minute." Sol went to the doorway and pointed at the stacks and stacks of food being moved by coolies from one pile to another. "Did that come from the stockpile I saw in El Fasher?"

"I am sure. But ze road is so bad, ze trucks zey cannot get to Umm Balla."

"I got through last night…in a truck."

"*Mais oui*, but ze drivers of supplies tell us ze road is closed. Mud and ze 'ighwayman."

"Mud? There isn't a drop of water out there. It's dry as a bone."

"Where you are, maybe dry. But ten kilometer away, and zere is ze flood. I tell you, zis is Africa. God is mad wis zis place."

"What about the 'highwayman'?" Sol made quote marks with his fingers. "Do you mean the supplies are being stolen?"

"Somesing like zat. But we go over zis last night."

"Have you contacted the authorities—the police?"

André shook his head sadly. "Doctor," he said barely above a whisper, "you are ze American. You do not understand zees sings. To you, all ze life is ze good one, wis ze big cah and ze shopping center.

'Ere is not ze States. Ze camp is over. We go soon, before ze Janjaweed." His face hardened. "And you must go *now*. I do not wish your blood on my 'and."

Lila had been watching quietly, but as André's tone became progressively forced and louder, she placed herself between the two men. She spoke first to the Frenchman. "André, don't take it out on Doctor Solomon. He's never seen the Janjaweed. He knows nothing of them. Leave him be."

"No," Sol barked, "I want to know. Tell me why we can't get food here. I know about the Janjaweed. They torture and rape the locals and the refugees. I know there's no way to fight back. I did my reading, and you filled in the blanks last night. But if they wanted to close *this* camp, it would have been burned to the ground months ago. Our job is to feed these people as long as we can. Isn't that why you're here? When it's over, it's over, but not until then, right?"

"You fool," André responded louder. "You do not understand. Zey keep ze camp alive to get ze supply from ze truck. And to take ze women. You fool zem to get ze food into camp so zey cannot get zer hand on it, zey will take you and cut you from ze top of your 'ead to your ass. Zey are ze devil on ze horse."

Lila faced Sol, her expression vague. "He's right you know. Forgive him. We've lost several of the checkers who tried to ride, as you Yanks are fond of saying, 'shotgun' on the supply trucks; good men who spit in the face of the Janjaweed by trying to outrun them. They disappeared along with the trucks, the drivers, and the supplies. Not a trace, though no one went looking."

"Have you tried having the government provide security? Force their hand. See which side Khartoum falls on."

"The Janjaweed *are* the government," Lila now snarled impatiently. "We told you that. The ministers in Khartoum don't deny the existence of the Janjaweed. They just don't admit to having anything to do with them, and then they snivel they don't have sufficient manpower to stop a nomad army, that they're putting all their money into caring for the refugees. But everyone knows Khartoum isn't spending a farthing on anything but their own fortunes. They want these people out of here, the locals *and* the refugees. They will do anything they need to get rid of them. No one cares about them. End of story."

Sol demanded, "Why doesn't the Red Crescent act? These refugees are Muslim, yes?"

"Yes and no. Depends upon who you ask." She shook her head. "They're part Muslim, but also animist." Sol's eyes tightened in confusion. "I mean they mostly worship animals and spirits and only occasionally Allah, but just enough to stay out of trouble, or so they were able to in the past. There are the ridiculously religious, but most are not. That's how the Janjaweed can murder hundreds of these people at one sitting, and no one cares. It isn't really any different than slaughtering cattle. To them, and to President Bashir in Khartoum, they're not killing people. They're disposing of subhuman monkeys, non-Arabs…"

Sol interrupted, "Everyone tells me these pastoral people aren't Arabs, but the Janjaweed, the nomads, are. To me they're all just as black, and they speak the same Sudanese Arabic as the villagers they destroy. Educate me, please."

Lila shrugged. "I'm not sure there *is* an answer, or one that any objective foreigner can come up with. Mostly, the Arabs out here are camel herders, but they intermarry with the farmers and have for centuries, so it's what each tribe decides to call itself. I've heard of some men who take multiple wives, one who's Arab, the other not. Also, if you rise to a certain level of wealth, which means you that own a lot of camels, you can call yourself an Arab, call yourself anything you want. Who knows?

"And then some people claim this is all about Bashir's fight with his political enemy, Turabi, who supports the rebels in Darfur, and all of this genocide has nothing to do with religion or ethnicity. But he, Turabi, is always in trouble apparently, locked up in his villa in Khartoum, so why does Bashir even bother with him?"

When Sol did not answer, because he'd never heard of Turabi, Lila went on. "The indigenous Sudanese, like the people who live in Umm Balla, where we just drove through, the Furs, now they're complaining that the refugees are taking their food and water, and that Khartoum has to do something. They sent elders back to Khartoum to plead their case, but they haven't been seen since. Then, all of a sudden, Khartoum sends troops out here to 'manage' the land, but all they do is run the locals off their so-called farms in the name of finding places to feed the refugees from Chad. When the locals run, they go to Chad, the ones that survive the raids. Then Bashir's troops run the refugees from Chad off as well, declare the land abandoned, invoke eminent domain, confiscate the water, and now the oil resources. This is not a stupid government. And, I will give the Janjaweed some credit for their enlightened attitudes."

Sol screwed up his face. "Enlightened?"

"Indeed. When they arrive to move people off the land, either group, they rape the women before they cut their throats. They must see *something* human in them. I mean, they wouldn't screw a sheep in public, would they? A bloody lot of lashes for that, I imagine."

"A hundred for adultery, I heard." Sol quipped.

Lila relaxed her face a bit; the edges of her lips, while not curling upward, drifted back toward neutral. "You might want to keep that in mind, sir."

Sol tried, though he could not help but answer her jibe with a tiny smile. His face, though, suddenly tightened, and he faltered to the rear of the grass-walled office to crumple into what was left of a folding chair. He let his head drop between his knees and sat hunched, motionless. The two stared at him, expecting the strange man to draw a deep breath and shout back at them that they were weak, that he was an American and would show them how to get a job done. Instead, he sat winded, the bravado having leaked from him over the past year and months and weeks, with the last of his spirit finally snared in just a few days.

He wanted so badly to call Dana, to ask her what to do, praying she would summon him home, granting him the excuse to abandon his folly, his delusion that he was to be part of a great and noble rescue. Would she tell him he was still a great man and still love him even if he ran from the futility of Africa? But there was no Dana anymore, and his head sank even farther as he rebuked himself for holding the sliver of hope that life promised more than a venal crushing of the heart.

He thought back to the admonishment his partners had dispensed when he took the rest of last September off—their sage advice that he was not the first man in history to have had his life crushed in a single breath. The department head counseled that Sol return to work and embrace his professional responsibilities, calling in the other members of the orthopedic department, all prophesying he'd feel much better if he stayed busy. But his colleagues never mentioned, aloud at least, that they needed him to get back to seeing the state industrial patients they refused to treat. So he did go back the next Tuesday, September 18th, though, after a couple of months, when their advice did not bear fruit, he ran away, convinced by his reading of the epic parables of human sadness that when he arrived in Africa, he'd walk off the 747 and finally be met by a new life. He had assured himself that if a soul sacrificed avarice to do God's work, spiritual rewards were inevitable.

But it turned out he could not run away to the furthest reaches of the Earth and escape his heart. The lone soul to greet him at Khartoum Airport was Solomon Forte, lugging the same emotional baggage with which he had fled the city of Whitaker. There was no escape, just like as there wasn't for the boys in the *madrassa* a hundred miles back in the desert.

Dana was gone, and with her Michaela. Lila and André apparently did not know, and he vowed not to tell them, for even if they were aware of what had happened, they would gasp fittingly, and a moment later get back down to business, explaining why he was not welcome. They cared not a fig for his troubles, for his cares were personal and meaningless in the African scheme of things. There was no one, African or Western, in the thousands of square miles surrounding Umm Balla, capable of investing the energy to do more than bat an eye at a loss as trivial as his.

He calmed for a moment and looked up at Lila and André. They stared back, wondering what to make of what appeared now to be a little old man, the one who had demanded, just seconds before, to be told why the mission could not be salvaged.

Sol suddenly imagined his pop perishing in the primitive field hospital in Korea, and how he had fought to survive and come home to build such a simple but happy life for his wife and two children. If it were Jimmy faced with Umm Balla, he'd just downshift the cement truck and grind on slowly up the hill, never looking back, never tripping on the past. Then he actually heard his father in the primitive room, prodding, maybe even badgering, and Sol jumped to his feet as if he had been tasered, his fists locked tightly, fingers blanched as colorlessly as the dust-choked sky.

Lila and André stared as Sol braced. They stiffened for another outburst, expecting the shrieks of maddened cops and drug dealers, the fare of American TV. The two paced a protective step backward, André moving his shoulders almost imperceptivity in front of Lila.

Though they had lived with a dozen Americans in camp for several months, the Europeans and the Yanks had remained exclusive factions, with separate campfires at night, and food prepared by different cooks in different huts. They even had distinct libraries of mildewing paperbacks. With such sparse contact, Lila and André remained unfamiliar with Americans and their moods. In fact, neither of them had spoken more than a "good morning" to their American colleagues, the British nurses working with the British doctors, Americans with Americans.

But Sol sat back down on a pile of woven nylon, hundred-pound sacks of *durra* wheat. He leaned against a thick tree branch that supported the sheets of blue roofing plastic and mumbled gently, "So why don't we just sneak out of here during the night and go back to Khartoum and fly off in the morning to the border with Tigré Province in the east? One of the American agencies is doing a vaccination program back there in Ethiopia. I understand they're well-funded. And I've got all that money in El Fasher that I told André about. We'd have to stop there first anyway. Don't worry, I'll pay for you." When André and Lila raised their eyebrows in unison, Sol added, "I mean the money I was given was for 'our' project. It'll be okay, legal."

"Don't you need authorization?" Lila asked.

"I guess, but it's easier to beg for forgiveness than ask for permission. My wife's father taught her that. Crazy Russian." And Sol smiled, shaking his head.

Lila's eyes widened ever so slightly, flashing down to Sol's left ring finger. It was still bare. She did not ask, but spoke softly, "Perhaps we should talk about it tonight. There is *some* time left. Meanwhile, Doctor Forte, as long as we've got you here, let's have you take a look at a few of our problem children."

As they walked to the hospital, Sol noticed the morning warming fires had been extinguished, each twig of unburned wood collected and wrapped in burlap for the next morning. The throngs who had hugged the edge of the flames were dispersed, most back to their four-foot high, eight-foot diameter huts, to evaporate the rest of their day in the insufferable heat.

Inside the hospital, Sol got a better look at the construction techniques common to central Africa. The walls of the structure were fashioned of the same grass mats out of which the rest of the camp was built. The reed pads were sufficiently thick to block nearly all the sunlight and most of the swirling sand. The dirt floor had been leveled, of sorts, and pounded, but no water had been used to harden the earth, and each step raised a cloud of silt. Lila watched Sol's gaze as the powder settled, revealing dozens of minute patients spread along the ground.

"Water is for cooking and drinking here, you know. Far too precious to waste on controlling dust, especially in a hospital where no one ever lives long enough to be discharged."

As a young man in Western clothing, the checker assigned to the children's hospital, closed the hanging plastic curtains behind them, Sol was blinded by the sudden darkness, and the best he could do was follow the back of Lila's white blouse. He soon tripped on the nubbin of a felled tree that had not been pulled from the ground. Desperate to regain his footing, he wrenched around semi-upright for several steps, though lost his balance. Sol's landed abeam a dozen pediatric patients lying on grass mats in the dirt. The crash aroused a new mushroom cloud, one that set off fits of hacking amongst the few patients sufficiently alive to mount a cough. He moaned, "This is the hottest place on Earth. It's hotter than in the bus. Can't be."

Lila laughed sourly, "The imam made us seal off this part of the hospital—mats all the way up to the ceiling. Supposed to limit access to the death spirits. But they manage to get in quite easily, eh what? Bloke comes 'round, he's got this stick, points at the holes where the mats have rotted and shouts, 'See, see?'"

What silt Sol had kicked up that didn't stick to his sweat-drenched body hung as a layer of fog in the unstirring air. He noticed, though, that the tiny patients were dusty dry, and he turned to query

Lila. "They're not sweating. Are we letting them get that dehydrated?" She ignored the barbed question and waved him deeper into the sanatorium. They entered a section in which twenty even sicker children lay atop even filthier grass.

Lila grunted, "This is the ICU."

Sol stopped to kneel beside one of the patients, a waif whose mother lay motionlessly on her side next to the child, her hand resting on the boy's bony shoulder. As Sol's fingers moved along the mat slowly to touch the boy, his nails caught on a light-brownish patch of metallic crust. It startled him.

He examined his skin to see perhaps if he had cut himself, and Lila smiled faintly. "Not to worry, Doctor. It's just the dried feces and vomit of the kid who died on that mat yesterday."

Sol's head dropped further. He took a breath and turned to the woman lying by the child's side. "Madame, how old are you?" He assumed this was the child's grandmother, and expected her to say thirty-five or forty, but the woman did not respond. Sol turned to the African man in Western clothing and spoke softly in English, "I guess my Arabic isn't very good."

He did not answer Sol but turned to the woman and shouted in Arabic. "How old are you, stupid cow?"

Sol understood the answer that was barely audible. "I don't know."

Lila added, "She's nineteen or twenty at best. Her child's maybe thirty pounds. That's about five or six years old."

A dozen other gaunt, teen girls stared straight ahead, hunkering on the dirt next to their wasted offspring. Sol stopped at one of the skeletal pediatric patients, a little boy with a large bore hypodermic needle sticking through the skin of his protruding abdomen. His eyes followed the dirty tubing up to a plastic IV bag suspended from a tripod of tree branches. "There's no flow."

Lila shook her head and kneeled to the dirt floor, yanking at the mid-portion of the tubing which was bent over on itself, the fold jammed into the marrow cavity of a silver-dollar-sized wedge of sheep bone. "Some busybody," she snipped, glancing at the young woman now squatting by the child's mat, "has wound our IV tubing around and into, what is this, a talisman?" She grabbed the tubing, pulled it free in front of the mom's eyes, and turned to Sol, smiling sarcastically. "How did this woman discover, when she can't read a single letter of our medical books, that the sacred power of this sheep bone swirls in the hole? Doctor, did your medical school teach you that pinching off IV tubes in the middle and stuffing them into pieces of animal bone endows the magic liquid we give these children with even greater spiritual nourishment?" Lila did not wait for an answer. "I didn't think so." She finished untangling the tubing roughly, allowing the saline to flow again from the IV bag, but drew a deep breath, calming herself before curling the tubing loosely around the outside of the fragment of bone, ensuring the flow was not disturbed. She took a roll of dirty adhesive tape from her pocket, pulled a small piece free, and wound it around both the tubing and bone. She presented the contrivance to the woman, whose eyes were following just inches from Lila's fingers. "Hope that meets your learned approval, Madame."

Though the fluid began flowing, it was but a trickle, and she dropped her hand onto the needle poking into the child's belly to shift it left and right, shallower and deeper under the paper-thin skin, until the saline flowed in a steady current. The child barely moved his lips.

The mother watched for a moment then turned her head away from Lila, squeezing her eyes shut. Lila stood and started back toward Sol, though the instant she turned her back, the woman rose, redid her *tob*, dropped back into her hunker, picked at the tape with her beautiful white teeth, unwound the tube, and pinched off the same section, which she threaded back into the hole. The tube cracked, and the fluid squirted onto the dirt floor.

Lila snarled, "Bloody hell," and scurried back to turn the petcock off. She scolded the mother, wagging a finger, "We only have two or three of these left! What is *wrong* with you?" Lila summoned a checker. He yelled at the woman as well, but the mom turned away and shut her eyes even more tightly.

The naked little boy's fingers twitched, and his lips parted asking his mother for water. Sol was relieved, for now he might be resuscitated by mouth, but the checker glanced down, shook his head, and mumbled, "*Mat*," then nodded toward Lila and Sol, droning, "Dead."

Lila glared, "Yes, Muhammad, I know *mat* means dead in Arabic."

Sol asked Lila why the child had had a hypodermic needle sticking through his gut. "You draining an abscess?" Sol queried, "Irrigating?"

"No," she answered stiffly, controlling herself. "How do you reckon these little buggers have veins? They have no volume, no place to start IVs. We pump fluids into the abdomen—*some* of it gets absorbed. When they get rehydrated, if we can stand them up, sometimes we find a foot vein or two to start a proper IV. In the meantime, only a few kids live that long—very few, actually." Her voice trailed off, and her eyes drifted into a stare fixed on the thatched roof.

The woman sat for several minutes without a flicker then dragged the child to her breast. When he did not respond, she whispered, "*Mat*," though loud enough for the other parents to look up. She sprinkled a few drops of water on the child's forehead, and a peculiar hush descended over the hospital, the other moms turning away from the victim and lowering their eyes. A moment later, though, one chanted, "*Allahu Akbar*," and soon the other mothers wailed, perseverating that God is great, that God has willed it, and so it will be.

In a corner of the hut, four feet from the deceased little boy, another child lay curled on an encrusted grass mat. Lila lifted her chin. "Doctor," she intoned with a dollop of professional bearing, "our little Muhammad here has contracted what appears to be a spot of cerebral malaria. Still looks salvageable to me, but not for long. These kids do okay for a few hours, but they go downhill in a hurry when the time comes. He's still taking medicine by mouth, fading though. We've had him on Lariam, mefloquin, but it hasn't stopped the infection. Any brilliant ideas?"

Sol's face relaxed, and the corners of his mouth turned up slightly. "I think we can help Master Muhammad, but I need my bag. I'll go back and get it, and *I'll* drive, thank you."

She frowned. "That's double our petrol ration for the day. Won't do. We'll have to send the runners. Bloody hell. And that'll be an extra ten cups of *durra*, but I suppose we've more *durra* than petrol. It's extortion, really—one cup per runner."

"Ten cups of *durra* for what? And what is *durra*? You guys talk about it constantly."

"Oh, *durra*, sorry. It's millet, sorghum. Amazing grain, actually. Chinese ferment it for *maitai*. And don't get any ideas. Keep that lash in mind."

"I know, a hundred licks or something."

"I meant for alcohol—and it's only twenty. But I'm glad you remembered the other mortal sin as well. Don't let that slip your mind. You do talk about it rather repetitively, don't you?"

He drew a breath to answer, but she cut him off. "Anyway, when the weather's dry, the plant rolls its leaves to cut down on water loss. During a drought, it goes dormant but doesn't die."

Sol cut a tiny hole in one of the bags and pulled a fistful of the tiny, spherical grains free. He chewed on a few, screwed up his face, and was about to drop the remaining pellets on the ground when Lila hissed, "Don't waste that! It's a full meal!" Sol flinched and with great theater dropped the remaining specks back in the bag. "You'll see, mister." She went on. "The little girls grind it down, and the women boil it into mush. High vegetable protein. Complete. It's like kasha."

"How do *you* know about kasha?"

Lila stared at him. "Why do you ask?"

Sol drew back but managed a smile. "Okay, what about the ten cups? What are runners? And whatever it is they do for food, just tell 'em if they don't do it for free, their family gets shorted on market day."

"You don't understand. These kids are smarter than you and me combined. They've put together a relay team of sorts, ten boys. Anyone moves in on their territory, they squash them."

"They got scooters or something?"

"No, just long legs, and they're quite shrewd, you know. When we need something back at camp, we put out the word. A few of them appear out of the dust to get their marching orders. You see, the others have already left to form the relay team. Each has a specialized function. They gather in a flash and start out from the camp here.

Numbers one and two, maybe the slowest, but with the most endurance and brains, they start the lope back to our camp straight away and wait for orders. When they get there, number one, the kid with the most competence, that's Daud, he goes to work finding what we tell him to find while number two rests and drinks water. When number one finds the freight—takes a while because we always give him bollixed directions—he hands it to the second lad, who sprints just an eighth of a mile to the next boy, who runs a quarter of a mile, and so on until the final two chaps: one sprints two hundred meters, and the last one a hundred. He's flying so fast there's a cockscomb of dust kicked up behind him. Everyone thinks, because all they see are the last two, that the whole team's been moving like the *haboob*. Half the camp's waiting at the finish line cheering.

"There was another team who tried to compete. They marched around camp defaming Daud and his crew, but they were pathetic; twelve minutes late, so far behind, most of the spectators had already gone back to their huts when the final runner jogged into camp. Turns out they got lost on the trip back. Not a spot of competition since."

Sol pondered Lila's treatise for a moment. He shrugged, "If you say so. Anyway, if they bring my duffle bag, I've got some Artensuate, a *gift* from a pal at the Centers for Disease Control in Atlanta. Probably fix this kid up in a day or two."

For the first time in the twelve hours he had known Lila, her sad scowl slackened faintly. Slowly, her mouth twisted dubiously, but coyly, and her almond eyes brightened. Andre was right. She was enchanting. "Please, Doctor Solomon, if I may, tell me, are you saying the CDC *gave* you Artensuate? That was quite sporting of them."

"Well, Miss Lila, shall we say it was liberated from the CDC by one of their trusted scientists, who just happens to be a sweet little thing I dated for a while in residency. Didn't end all that well, I mean the relationship, and to be honest, I was surprised she even took my call. But when I told her I was headed to Darfur, she came up with the goods then flew out to Whitaker to deliver it herself. I think just to see if anything was still there. I hugged her and thanked her before I lied to her."

"You lied to her?"

"Well, I said it very quickly and in a whisper, so it doesn't count."

"What in God's name did you say?"

"I'm sorry, I'm married."

Lila stared at him for a moment, her gaze again involuntarily dropping to his left hand. She looked up quickly, hoping he hadn't seen, but he had, and she tensed. "I don't understand."

Sol paused, and Lila's mouth twisted, waiting for a smart reply, but his eyes turned away from hers as he went on in a monotone. "Maybe someday"

Lila turned to the checker who had been listening just inches from the conversation. "Muhammad, we need the runners. We have some special medicine. Can you fetch them?"

In minutes, Abdul Aziz Fudle, a lanky, sweet-faced, coal-black fourteen-year-old, sprung into the hospital toward Lila and, with a little bow, came to attention an inch in front of her. Through Muhammad, she told Abdul to get Dr. Sol's duffle bag inside the third hut to the left of the generator and bring it back to camp as fast as he could run. Sol, though, interrupted and reminded her the bag weighed fifty pounds. She thought for a moment and asked, "What does the package look like? Is there a name on it, and do you mind if he rifles through your things?"

"No problem. He can do whatever he wants. It says Artensuate in blue letters. There's two vials left. Have him bring one. I can draw a picture."

Lila interrupted. "Let's just write out 'ARTENSUATE' on a piece of paper. Daud's the captain. He's the one who makes the full trip; probably already there, and does the searching. If he were living in Great Britain, he'd be doing his 'O' levels and on his way to Cambridge. He'll find it. Not to worry."

"This I'd like to see. If I was fourteen years old, and someone wrote out a huge word in Arabic, there's no chance I'd recognize it."

"And you are not Daud, and he's only eleven."

Less than thirty minutes later, after Lila and Sol had gone on rounds through the hospital to witness two more skeletal children pass to the next plateau, thirteen-year-old Muhammad Hamed Idriss, the final sprinter, burst past the plastic curtains into the hospital. Sol's medicine was clutched in a diminutive, gaunt fist against his belly, the other hand covering the first. Though breathless, he threw his head back, jaw set to present the bottle to Checker Muhammad, who presented it to Lila, who presented it to Sol, who snapped off the cap and handed it back to Lila, who passed it to Muhammad, who drew up a few ccs into a used syringe.

As he moved forward to add it to the IV bag that drained into the child's foot, Sol held up his hand. "Wait a minute. We need to calculate the dose. So how old is the boy?"

Muhammad asked the mother, who answered eight-years-old, or maybe three or two. She was not sure.

"Ohhhhkay" Sol chuckled, "let's try this. So how much does our little friend here weigh?"

Muhammad lifted the child gently and carried him to a produce scale hanging from one of the tree branches that propped the roof. He settled the child into the filthy wicker basket strung below the scale. Muhammad stared at the dial marked in Chinese characters, counted on his fingers, and announced, "Ten kilo," but rolled his palm up and down several times.

Sol's face scrunched. "Wait a minute, ladies and gentlemen. He's, let's say, five-years-old, and only weighs twenty pounds? That's what a one-year-old weighs at home. I weighed that at birth. That's what we call failure to thrive back in the real world."

Lila ordered, "Get on with it, Doctor."

"Okay." Sol smiled. "Never mind. It's like 2.4 milligrams per kilogram, four times over three days, so that's a total of around 120 milligrams. I feel better already. At that rate, we'll have enough of this stuff to treat all of Darfur." Sol lifted his head confidently. "And when he's done with the Artensuate, we'll start Malerone."

Lila raised her head slightly. "Dr. Sol, if I may, and if I remember correctly, Artensuate is a life-saving drug, but it has a short half-life, and that's why you need to start the oral medication, Malerone, when the child is well enough to swallow pills. It's the most effective way to ensure all the parasites are killed. Am I right?"

Sol turned to Lila. "Whoa, young lady, so you know your stuff, don't you? There isn't a doctor at home who knows that, including me until my little sweetie showed up. I'm impressed."

She stared at him for a trice longer than he expected but caught herself, turned away quickly, and placed a cup of water to the child's lips. She mumbled, "Who knows what would happen if we actually got enough food here to feed these kids more than a quarter of what they should be eating? Anyway, come on."

As they emerged into the blinding sunlight, Lila put her arm in front of Sol to stop him. He slowly focused on two hundred children standing in a crescent twenty yards from the hospital. They were crowded along a frontier of curved, whitewashed rocks, as if constrained by an invisible electronic force radiating from the stones. Each child waved a red, green, or blue plastic cup. Sol was taken by their smiling, dark eyes, and he gently pushed past Lila with a smile he could not hide. A few of the younger ones, their eyes glazed by need, charged over the perimeter of rocks, grinding to a halt in a tight circle about him. These children tried to smile, but they were so jittery, they could not stand still.

When not a single of the intrepid children fell to the sand for having snubbed the stone gods, the rest of the kids slowly marshaled the daring to approach Sol. At once, they jammed plastic cups in his face with one hand, and banged on his canteens with the other.

He pulled the first of his two plastic water bottles from its army green canvas pouch. The growing mass pulsed, and Sol tried to take a step back, but his eyes locked onto those of a frail, irrelevant soul, a little girl who had been shoved to and fro in the crowd, tossed about like a stick of driftwood. As he reached forward into the mob to fill her cup, so many arms struck his and hers, the few teaspoons that reached the child spilled, water skittering across the fabric of her tattered, two-sizes-too-large, pink, princess dress. She caught a drop or two with her fingers and sucked in the fluid hungrily then thrust the cup back into Sol's face. He managed to aim a few more tablespoons of murky water into her plastic mug, which the little girl pulled protectively to her chest before she turned and pushed toward the perimeter, suddenly laughing ecstatically, not a single drop sloshing from her red cup.

With the furious rock-god of hospital perimeters clearly a paper tiger, the main contingent of children bolted into no man's land, a hundred tiny bodies pulling at the hair on Sol's arms, laughing hysterically, though another two hundred pushed their cups into his face chattering, "Just a little bit of water, Mr. New *Khawajii.*"

Sol's first canteen emptied in seconds, and he, laughing in resonance with the children, reached for his second, but Lila rammed her way to his side and pulled him powerfully into a fifty-square-foot grass-mat hut. She turned back toward the children and glared at them with a stare that sent most backing off beyond the white stones. A few extended their cups from beyond the crescent, but with Lila's glower, the majority shuffled off toward the camp center.

Lila scowled at Sol. After many seconds, she took another very deep breath to calm herself, though spoke bitterly, "Please don't give stuff to the kids. We're trying to discourage a begging mentality in this camp."

"It's just water," Sol reacted stiffly. "We do have water? Yes, Lila?"

"There's some. I just don't want these kids begging. Period. End of discussion." She shook her head and muttered, "Follow me, if you don't mind."

They marched two hundred yards up a hill to another dilapidated, grass-mat hut. "Anyway, this is your office for the day. We can use you to treat some children before you leave. Not to worry. Insurance—that's how you Yanks appraise your medical practices, isn't it? Kids here have, what is it, Blue Cross? The place is a diamond mine."

Sol considered answering but sealed his lips and inspected the ten-foot-by-eighteen-foot clinic. He ran his fingers along a peeling metal table and squinted at the few rusting folding chairs, the plastic cushions long since decomposed. The furnishings were identical to those in his *tuchel.* A large, moldy, cardboard box of medicine bottles, a pile of gauze, and a mound of assorted, loose tablets sat on sheets of yellowed newspaper lining the ground behind the table. Sol pulled a metal chair to the table and tugged the box to his feet to pick through the supplies. He selected several near-empty bottles, the contents of which he thought he recognized from the faded labels handwritten in German and Italian.

Lila sat next to him and began to catalogue the medicines. Within a minute, though, a commotion built outside the hut as a swarm of refugee women hurtled toward the clinic. A few jammed through the doorway, and Sol sprang to his feet. As three of the refugees settled on the floor inches from his chair, he retreated to a corner of the hut. But their eyes soon accustomed to the dark, and they were able to make out Lila. All motion ceased as she came to her feet, hands on hips. Their attention fixed on her blazing onyx eyes, and the three interlopers reversed to rush back into the neat, but wending, column of women aligned behind a row of whitewashed rocks. She turned to Sol. "You can sit down again. Thank you. Now, we're going to have to find some dye and paint the rocks a different color and then send out all sorts of threats that the gods now strike people dead if they cross, let's say, red rock lines. White no longer works, thank you very much. Not to worry. We'll just tell them accompanying you is a fresh set of nasty spirits."

Sol stuck his head out of the hut to witness hundreds of queued, hunkering, very young women, their infants tucked under washed-out *tobs*, which sheltered them from the scorching sun. Sol wondered what the temperature was under the robes, a hundred and twenty he guessed, but still cooler than in the direct sun, and certainly less than in the stifling clinic.

After a minute or two of calm, like little pistons, up popped a mom here, a mom there, rhythmically standing to redo *tobs*, occasionally shifting places, some inching closer to the clinic, most drifting further back as each measured her own doggedness against Lila's penetrating glare.

When Lila faded back into the clinic, three young ladies, kamikazes, eyes shut tightly, duck-walked to the front of the column. The trio paused, looked about surreptitiously, then crossed the line of rocks into the hut, never having risen out of a squat. With hands kept under *tobs* to drag their children along, they had no way to shoo the throbbing mass of flies hovering about them. Lila, inured to the pestilence of Umm Balla, pushed around Sol's table through the swarm, hissed at the women, and shoved them, though softly back out the doorway. The three retreated, but several more shuffled forward. As more and more women ignored the once-sacred Line of Stone, Lila pointed angrily at the markers, bolted stark upright, and commenced an invective which she commanded Muhammad translate. As the seconds passed, her feet and lower legs slowly disappeared, shrouded in a new accretion of sand blowing in from central Africa. She was being transformed in front of their eyes into an ethereal, colorless, suspended idol.

Muhammad, though, broke the spell, proffering his own version vociferously. "Cows, you may not cross this line until I tell you to do so. If I have to, I will order the spirits to make the stones red. Do you want that?" Most of the women stopped in their tracks, turned their faces away, and dropped their eyes.

Lila walked to the column and triaged. She guided the first patient to Sol's feet and began to drop into the seat next to him, but her attention was drawn away by shouting from a hut ten feet from the clinic. "Oh, bloody hell, not again! Excuse me, Doctor Sol, but court is apparently in session. There's about to be one of our daily cultural-religious eruptions. I need to go watch this."

"May I join you?"

"Yes, you may. Local juris prudence. May open your eyes a millimeter or two."

They walked toward an eight-foot-diameter *tuchel*. A woman was on her knees in the doorway, wailing, arms churning above her head. Lila whispered to Sol, "She's the plaintiff, I imagine, pleading her case. Let's see if we can reckon what she's being duped out of."

They peered into the dark center of the tiny hut. A grey-bearded, black skeleton sat cross-legged on a grass mat. He gesticulated with a scroll in his right hand. When he saw the foreigners watching, he poked the paper passionately toward the kneeling lady, mumbling incoherently. One of the checkers, who seemed to be attending the ancient man, nodded to Lila and whispered, "Madame, do you know what happen here?"

"No, Muhammad, please teach me. This is very important."

"Yes, important. The *qadis*, he say woman want blanket. Yes, she very cold, but she have no witness against man."

"Muhammad, I don't understand," she added goadingly as she turned toward Sol and rolled her eyes. "Watch this. Are you ready?"

The checker lowered his eyes and spoke to the judge in a whisper, asking for a moment to speak to the *jahiliyah khawajii*, the stupid foreigner. The *qadis* nodded irritably, and Muhammad continued in English. "You see, Ms. Lila, woman say man take blanket away. She blanket. Not man blanket. She say very cold night.

Man say he blanket yesterday night and yesterday, yesterday night. Man say no she blanket yesterday, yesterday night. She say have friend lady say she blanket, but friend lady scared come."

Lila smirked at Sol, "Ah ha, a he-say-the-ladies-say case. But wait *Doctori*, just wait until you hear this. Muhammad, sorry, carry on."

Sol raised his hand to interrupt. "Excuse me, but what did he say?"

"Hold on a sec, Muhammad. Okay, try to understand. He, Muhammad the checker, said the woman claims the blanket is hers, and she has a lady friend who will corroborate her story, but the woman is too afraid to come and look the *qadis* in the eye, so she sent a child with her testimony, but it was a female child, so the *qadis* refused to listen. Okay, the man says it's his, but he doesn't have anyone to back up his story. So now the judge is about to deliver his learned verdict."

"Now everything's crystal clear. Thank you so much. And why is she carrying on so much if he hasn't ruled yet?"

Lila punched him lightly in the shoulder. The judge's jaw dropped. "Because she already knows the verdict. I'll explain again. Evidently, the woman says this bloke pinched her blanket. She has a witness. He doesn't. But that's what I want you to see, so could you stop chatting for just a moment?"

Lila nodded to Muhammad, who nodded to the judge, who resumed court. The wagging scroll was now being jabbed at the lady as if he was punching her. An angry babble in nearly indecipherable Arabic became progressively vituperative, and Lila pulled Sol from the doorway. The man, though, abruptly terminated his tirade, and the woman rose and backed out of the courthouse, eyes cast down. She left for her hut crying aloud, "*Allah Akbar*," God is great, over and over, each repetition shriller than the last.

Lila nodded at Muhammad. "*Qadis* say two lady, one man word. One man one lady, give blanket to man. Lady happy because this word of Allah."

"See," Lila nodded, "what did I tell you?"

"Ms. Lila, I'm from New York City. Not the swiftest taxi on Fifth Avenue. If you don't mind, please translate?"

"Doctor, this lady loses her case because her word is worth only half of a man's. Now, the defendant, a *male* mind you, didn't have a single witness, but in *sharia*, that's Islamic law, the word of one man trumps that of a female. Actually, around here, it trumps two females, maybe more. It is very specifically spelled out in the Quran that women are flighty in their thinking, that they infect other women easily with their hysteria, and, therefore, the truth can't be taken from the word of a woman or women. It is 'so written in the Quran.' Nothing offensive about it. Well, not to them. Nothing wrong with women, mind you. It's just the way Allah made them, and Allah is infallible, and so there are laws to compensate for this natural tendency. And there you are.

"So, the man walks off with the blanket. Justice is served." She turned away from the courthouse sharply and tramped brusquely toward the clinic hut, but yelled over her shoulder, "Muhammad, you tell her I'll make sure she gets a new, clean blanket before tonight. No," she amended, holding up her index and middle fingers, "you tell her, she'll get two blankets and an extra cup of *durra*." She turned to Sol. "I wonder, though, if she'll take them now that Allah has spoken."

Sol followed, treading back to his medical office, picking through the now half-mile queue of supplicants, a thousand women frying in the African sun waiting to garner thirty seconds, if that, of his time. His feet had begun to burn, and he thought back to dawn, asking himself if he'd checked his shoes as André had recommended. Taking his seat, the prickly sensation abated a bit, and he nodded that he was, once again, ready to start seeing patients. But there were shouts from outside the hut that turned everyone's heads. Lila walked from the shanty back into the sun. She called out sharply, "Doctor Sol, may I see you?"

Sol exited to witness an old man prostrate on a makeshift grass-mat and tree-branch gurney. Several of the local elderly had carried him to the clinic. The men appeared to be praying for the fading patient over whom Lila was checking vital signs.

Sol asked, "What's the story?"

"They say he's had diarrhea for days, and they think he's dead. They want you to bring him back to life. I think they are saying he's the *qadis*' brother."

"You mean our friend the judge?"

"That's right."

"Okay, does he have a heartbeat? Is he breathing?"

"Yes, and yes. Thready, though, and labored, in that order."

"Let's put him in Trendelenberg and see if we can't get a vein."

Lila ordered the men to place the stretcher on the ground, but they hesitated and fussed that they would not take orders from a woman, particularly one whose arms were exposed and whose head was uncovered. Sol barked back that they were to put the cot on the ground, and when they did not budge, he pushed their hands toward the earth. There was a bit of resistance, but the stretcher found its way to the ground. The men lifted the gurney so the patient's head was thirty degrees in the air. Sol pushed it down, raised the other end twenty degrees, and kicked a carton of medicine under the foot end. The box, though, dissolved into a heap of black-mold powder, so Sol lifted his end again and motioned toward the holy rocks. The men gasped at the blasphemy. Sol dropped the stretcher, marched to the rocks, and picked the largest ones to lift the patient's legs. The attendants shut their eyes with great theater and blindly kicked at the rocks until a few found their way under the head end.

Checker Achmed translated that the men believed head-down was an unnatural and uncomfortable position in which to die, one in which only those going to *Jahannam*, Muslim hell, found themselves at the end. The oldest man stepped forward. "Since the colorless are actually the jinn in semi-human form, and since all the jinn are condemned to hell fire, the only way the colorless know how to die is backwards. Lower his legs, ugly bad spirit!"

Sol listened to the translation, grunted, "For Christ's sake," prodded the men aside, and again lifted the foot end of the bed, this time to nearly forty-five degrees. He stood in that position, holding tight to the stick rails despite the men jabbing and slapping at his hands. In thirty seconds, the deceased's head began to loll. Sol lowered his end a few degrees, smiled at the escorts, and kicked the stones back into position. The men dropped into a hunker, slack-jawed, as the patient grumbled angry demands to be left alone.

Lila smiled and hummed, "Guess what? We have a good vein in the arm. I'll get an IV going."

Sol breathed deeply and nodded to Lila, "Good work." With the saline flowing as fast as the tubing would allow, Sol advised, "He's really hypovolemic. Let's run in a few bags of normal saline, slowly though; we don't want to throw him into failure. And let's get him out of the sun." He looked about. "Put him in the back of the clinic until we can get him stabilized and down to the hospital."

He pointed to the corner of the clinic and told Achmed to stand guard. Achmed snapped at them, but the men refused to move, so Lila and Achmed placed the stretcher inside the hut. When Sol went back out, the rocks near the door had disappeared, their apparent consecrated status dissolved by the touch of a *khawajii*.

He ran to gather new rocks, but the sand had been picked clean of the stone—even the pebbles were gone. Lila came out of the clinic with Achmed. "You will replace the rocks, or there will be no clinic today and no meal when the sun is overhead." She jabbed an index finger above her head.

Sol piped, "Or tomorrow."

When Lila growled at Achmed, "Don't translate what he just said," Sol glared at her. "Doctor, they have no idea of what tomorrow means." If you wouldn't mind…"

She pointed to the inside of the clinic, and Achmed, Sol, and Lila went inside and closed the flap for two minutes, until the heat was unbearable and the carping from the old man's associates drowned out the grind of the building wind. Lila pulled the flap aside. The blast of broiling air was a relief.

When their eyes accustomed to the light, Lila hissed, "Bloody hell," and marched to one of a dozen scattered piles of whitewashed rock. The women, no longer in line, squatted in family groups pushed up against the walls of the clinic.

Sol gathered several of the larger rocks and heaped them under the far end of the litter. The men's squabbling rekindled and deepened until Lila ordered all but one man out of the clinic. There followed minutes of bickering followed by shouting, until she bullied all of them out into the sun, though yanked one docile, shriveled, old man back in and told him to sit by the patient and touch nothing.

As Sol took his seat, the women waddled into the hut and nearly surrounded him until Lila pushed them out into a jagged line. Sol was about to raise his hand and beckon the first supplicant, but his feet had begun to burn so badly, he held up his palms to stop the woman, took off his running shoes, and found streaks of blistered, angry, skin over the tops of both feet.

Lila glanced down. "Ah, the bastard beetle. Did anything crawl on your feet this morning?

"Everything crawled on my feet this morning."

"Well, Doctor Sol, if I may, it's no different than a second degree burn. Hurt for a few days, then it'll start to heal, and after six weeks, you'll be as good as new. We'll put a potion on it and keep it bandaged with death shroud."

"Miss Lila, where are we going to find a 'potion'?"

"Well, some mutton fat will do. Quite soothing, actually."

Woman number one had become impatient and shuffled past Lila, stopping so close to Sol's feet, he was looking straight down on the top of her head. Lila tried to pull the woman back, but the mom was distracted hauling the baby from under her gown. As the child appeared headfirst from the *tob*, Sol quipped, "Ah, the miracle of birth! Congratulations, Madame! You are the proud mum of a fifteen-pound, bouncing, five-year-old girl."

When the child began to revive in the relative cool, swirling air of the clinic, the woman smiled up at Sol. He smiled back. She lifted the toddler to her front, stopping a foot from Sol's crotch.

He leaned forward, hands extended, but the woman snatched her emaciated daughter back as if Sol's fingers were poison fangs. Having teethed in the inner-city hospitals of Manhattan and the Bronx, he smiled even more broadly at the woman, who beamed back cheerfully. Now confident of the human bond that had been confirmed by the universal sign of friendship and respect, he nodded slowly and reached forward again with his stethoscope. The young woman's eyes locked upon the tubes and metal. She gasped and shuffled backwards toward the door, at the same time stuffing her baby back into the airless oven.

Sol mumbled, "You got a sister in a village back up the road? Married to the police chief?"

A checker, one of several who had ambled in and out, snapped his fingers in the teen's face and yowled in Arabic, "*Abed*, let the doctor see the child, stupid cow." Without a change in expression, she extracted the baby but took two more wobbles backward toward the door.

Sol called to the woman, "Abed, come over here, please."

Lila jumped from the back of the clinic. "Don't call her that!"

Sol's jaw dropped. "I thought Abed was her name. That's what the checker called her."

"*Abed* means slave in Arabic. That's what most of the checkers call the refugees. But don't *you* use that word."

"Okay, I'll never do it again."

Now only six or seven feet from his first clinic patient, Sol inspected the toddler, starting at the top, focusing on the child's head, nearly bald—just wisps of patchy, no longer curly, reddish hair, a sure sign of advanced malnutrition and vitamin deficiency. The face was gaunt, skin as thin as parchment. Moving his eyes downward through the bare threads of a tee shirt, he focused on a potbelly so curved, the abdominal skin so tight, it seemed the baby was carrying an unborn twin. Further down, both feet were clubbed, bloated, and hung like a ragdoll's. He had never seen such edema in any patient, child or elderly, even with end-stage heart failure or cirrhosis of the liver. He thought back to medical school, to the kids in the Bronx who had found their way to his hospital, a few of whom were so poorly cared for, worms had co-opted their innards to the point they, too, appeared pregnant, even the little boys. But the South Bronx was kindergarten, and Darfur Province was graduate school, and he reeled in confusion, for he had missed the years of schooling in between.

Lila stared at Sol's blank face for a moment then opened another decomposing chair to sit by him. "I guess you don't see a lot of kwosh in the States, do you?" she asked gently. For a moment, Sol did not understand, but she quickly added, "Kwashiorkor."

Sol nodded. "Oh, yeah, no, not a whole lot of that in Whitaker. Most of us eat more than once every three or four days." Sol's head dropped a few degrees. "You wanna know what? To be honest, Ms. Lila, I've never seen it before."

"Well, to be honest, Soli, if I may, neither did I until I got here. Infants do okay until the mom's second child, when she has to nurse the new baby, and the first one's left to his own devices. That's where the word comes from, kwashiorkor, from West Africa, 'to be the first baby.' It's the lack of protein and vitamins that's killing these kids, not the lack of calories. Did my nursing final paper on kwosh, but I had no idea what it really meant until my first day in Africa, like yours. Look at her feet. So swollen. All the water we give them drains out of the bloodstream and collects under the skin. Worthless there, you know. They need the fluid *inside* the vessels to keep the blood flowing. It leaks out of the veins and arteries because there isn't enough protein *in* the bloodstream to trap the water inside. When it leaks out and gets under the skin, gravity pulls it down to their feet. So, these kids are full of water, and yet they're dying of dehydration. And the more fluids we give them, the sooner they die. That's what I think makes them so irritable when they show up here, so little blood to the brain because there's so little blood in the first place. And what blood *is* in the vessels is so thick, it can hardly flow. They get behind the power curve, and the more you do, the faster they die."

Sol queried, "Why not feed them mostly protein and just a little bit of carbohydrate, just enough to give them some calories for the digestion process? Some of the protein will get absorbed. Maybe they should be in a special unit or something."

Lila sighed, "We try to feed them protein, but one of the symptoms of kwosh is that they refuse to eat. I recommend you treat the ear infection, or the bronchitis, whatever, and get the mom to give the baby rehydration salts in water by mouth. Here." She handed Sol an aluminum foil packet. "You dump the crystals into half a liter of water. It's better than an IV. Getting these people to believe that is another matter, though. And getting them to actually give the kids the rehydration fluid is even harder. Sometimes they wash a pot in it." Sol looked away and bent forward to put his head between his knees. Lila tensed. "You okay?"

"Yeah. Just a little tired. Thank you."

The patient's mother had wriggled closer to Sol, her head cocked as if listening intently to the conversation. Lila stood and walked to the back of the tent to start another bag of fluids on the old man, who was trying to sit up, babbling angrily that he wanted to be left alone. Sol straightened himself and smiled again at the mother, using the ruse to lean forward and gently raise the baby from her hands. As his sweat-drenched body leaned back to start examining the waif, she lurched forward and grabbed the girl back to her bosom. A checker, Ishmael, who had been leaning against the doorway, snarled, "Hey, mama, let the doctor hold the baby. How is he going to cure the child, huh, huh?"

The woman's eyes dropped obediently, and she handed the limp creature back, but looked up with pleading eyes. Sol hugged the fifteen-pound three-year-old, gently kissing her cheek, and though the child smiled weakly, her head soon slumped. The mother gasped, as did Sol, but the child breathed deeply and turned her head to look up at her mother, who shut her eyes tightly and appealed in primitive Arabic, "Revolting, colorless man, save my baby."

Sol was trying to balance the patient in one arm and use his stethoscope in the other, but he nearly dropped the child. He motioned for the mother to sit in Lila's chair. She stared but did not move. "Ishmael, tell her to sit so she can hold the baby while I examine her."

He smirked, "*Doctori*, this stupid *abed*. Not ever sit in chair in life. *Abed* not know how sit. Only squat."

So, Sol held the baby and tugged lightly at the skin on the forearm, drawing it up until it tented, then let go rapidly. When the skin remained elevated, defying gravity, Sol muttered, "She's dry, and she's real sick. We need to hydrate this child fast." He turned to Lila, demanding, as if an arrogant, fuming surgeon, "Where's the IV fluid? And we need to give her some IV protein too."

Lila barely looked up, though spoke tersely. "There is no such thing as IV protein, and we've only got a spot of IV fluid left. That's what we were trying to tell you. What we have, we're trying to save."

"Save for what? Look, this baby needs it. She's real dry. Like you said, there's no chance of her eating anything in this condition. When she's rehydrated, she'll perk up and eat."

"Well, as I *also* said, we have these packets of rehydration salts from the UN. Just tell the mom to drip it down her throat. The baby'll be okay, or she won't. Plus, you've got a thousand people lined up out there."

"No! She's sick. She needs IV fluids. I want 'em started. We'll worry about running out later. I don't want to lose my first patient."

Lila hesitated and sat back down next to Sol, calming herself. She spoke slowly. "You are going to see this in nearly every child. We need to teach the moms that oral hydration will keep their kids alive. If we just hook her up to an IV, she learns nothing, and maybe the baby lives for the next few hours, but she dies of dehydration tonight after we're back in our compound. If we can get the mother to pour fluid down her throat, maybe she'll live for a few more days. And maybe one or two of the stronger kids will actually survive. Can't you see?"

Sol thought for a moment. "Humor me on this one. It's my first real patient. Let me err on the side of caution."

Lila nodded feebly and walked to the medicine chest, sorting around, and extracted a set of IV tubing and a bag of fluid. She mumbled, "We do kiddie IVs in the hospital. It's policy."

So, Sol gathered the child in his arms and took a step toward the door, but it struck him that the chattering from the back of the clinic had waned, and he turned to look at the old man on the stretcher. Three men were squatted next to him. Two had crawled under the thatch at the rear of the hut and shifted the pallet from feet up to head up. Their friend was again comatose. Sol placed the dying child on the sand and lifted the foot end of the cot, taking the stones from the head of the bed and shifting them to the other end. In seconds, the man lifted his head, grumbling that he wanted to go home.

Sol ignored the man and maneuvered the little girl past a snaking line of women squatted in the blistering sun, the column stretching down the hill far beyond the camp center. There was not a child in sight until Sol, heading in a straight line toward the hospital shed, cut the line several times, passing just inches from the queue of teens. Those who had the strength to look up vaulted away from the white phantasm, infants and reed-thin toddlers dropping from beneath their skirts. As Sol's pace increased, Lila fell behind, breathing heavily. Following uncertainly, a distant third, shuffled the mother, until Lila appealed breathlessly, "Doctor, please do slow down. She thinks you're stealing her baby."

Nearing the bottom of the hill, Sol eyed scores of refugees cowered in precious corners of shade outside the north wall of the the hospital. There they sat, hour after hour, numbly vaporizing the day. A few of the heartier walked aimlessly at a pace that made Sol think he was watching a slow-motion movie.

At the hospital, a pair of plastic door flaps cast darkened patches in which more leaden refugees took sanctuary. A pack of skeletal children milled about sluggishly, most carrying whittled sticks which they used to smack lined up pieces of gravel. The pebbles flew about like the swarms of bloated flies that plied the skies of Umm Balla, but when one of the stones hit an elderly man in the forehead, the kids fled fifty yards to the camp perimeter, dancing gingerly to avoid the piles of excrement.

Lila hissed, "They're off into the shit fields again, and mind you, one or two are going to trip and scrape a knee, and in forty-eight hours, we'll be fighting to save them with the last of the antibiotics we don't have."

Sol mumbled as he continued into the hospital, "They told me in London that they'd okayed hiring gangs of refugees to dig latrines. Said they were paying a good wage. No more defecation in the open. You should have seen them, sauntering around like they'd rescued an entire race of humans."

"We did start the project, but the checkers were extorting a finder's fee from the refugee men, which we ignored, but when the work got started, it wasn't three hours before there was a wildcat strike, organized by the checkers, demanding we pay the refugees a dollar a day on top of the extra food ration we promised for their labor. So, we raised the wage to twenty-five cents a day, but the men only got a dime of it, which we again ignored. Then work stopped later that afternoon when André showed them the plans for the latrine shacks to sit over the trenches they were supposed to be digging. The men refused to make houses in which they would sit and pass their bowels next to a neighbor not from his clan. This is not the sort of thing people do in public, well, not when you can look into your mate's eyes. They go off into a field and squat, facing away from everyone. *That* is their privacy. And anyway, the stuff would lie there for eternity, and they could not understand why we wanted to keep it. It's supposed to sit out in the open, in the sun, dry up, and blow away in the wind like everything else they have."

Sol settled the child on a vacant straw mat. Lila turned to look for the mother, but she was at the doorway on her knees praying. Lila clucked her tongue, ran back, took the woman's arm, and guided her gently into a hunker at the child's side. When Sol looked over his shoulder and smiled to reassure her, he noticed that the next mat on the dirt floor was empty, a hollowed ring of sheep bone cast off in the dust.

Lila called Muhammad and gave him Sol's order to start a fluid injection in the abdomen. He hovered over the Westerners for a moment before protesting gently, "Miss Lila, you speak in yesterday give tube water only children if soon *mat*. Here baby okay. Give ora rehy. It is enough."

The only part of the broken sentence that Sol understood was the "ora rehy," oral rehydration, and he shook his head no. "I want my initial patient to live through my first day here, at least until sunset."

Lila smiled at Muhammad. "Twenty-five ccs for one hour, twenty-five." She wrote the number "25" in the dirt in Arabic, and Muhammad nodded in submission."

Lila turned to Sol. "We need to get back to work. Muhammad can care for the child. He's quite good, you know."

"Are you sure? Does he know how to start an IV in a dehydrated kid? I mean, it's not a piece of cake. Took me years to learn."

"Doctor," Lila droned, "he knows better than you or anyone you ever met in your life. He's done it four or five hundred times in the past three weeks. We need to get clinic going."

"Well, I want to come back in an hour and check on this kid just to make sure."

"Doctor, we do not have time to check on every sick kid. They're all sick." Her face tightened as Sol took a deep breath to answer, but she cut him off. "Okay, fine, we'll trot on down here in an hour and examine every child."

"Look, Lila, it's a life, and this is one I can save with a quart of water. I'm coming back in an hour."

"Good, Doctor, come back in an hour, and every hour for as long as you're here, if that's what you want. But this is Africa, not the States. It's been here a very long time. You're going to have to trust others to do the routine work and then forget about it. What will be will be. You're going to exhaust yourself in a single bloody day."

Sol nodded, wheeled about, and headed crossly through the plastic flaps back toward the clinic. A hundred yards up the sand hill, he slowed and turned to see if Lila was following, but she had stopped, standing bent forward, hands on her knees, gasping for air. The minions of refugee women lined up to see the new doctor were still squatted in the open, though they turned as one toward Lila, staring impassively as she dropped to a knee. Sol ran back and tried to lift her, but she pulled her arm away and came to her feet on her own.

"I'm fine. You go on and get started. We are so far behind. I want to get done while it's still light. I have no intention of staying here after dark."

Sol retook his seat in the grass hut. The shanty was empty, the old man gone, and the interpreter down the hill at a feeding center, chatting up the ladies of the cooking detail. So, Sol called out with a laugh as he crooked his finger, "Next victim, please," and several women waddled through the opening to hunker in a crescent five feet to his front. Each pulled a baby from under her *tob*, first peeling muffin-sized crusts from the infant's eyes and nose before holding her child in the air as if for sale. Others stroked cheeks to quiet the fits of coughing provoked by having been moved a couple of feet. Though Sol's eyes settled on one of the mothers, and he leaned toward that child, the other women lifted their children higher, some over their heads, waiting for Sol to divine a diagnosis. The babies made feeble movements until they tired, gasped for air, and coughed weakly. When Sol leaned forward to take the first child, the woman jumped back, the signal for her mates to snatch their own progeny from the air and tuck them hurriedly back under their gowns.

So, Sol left his seat, dropped to his knees, and trundled forward. He approached mother number one palms up. With his reassuring, gentle smile, the young woman seemed to calm, but as the tips of Sol's grimy fingers arrived eight inches from her child, she sprang toward the doorway. That startled Sol, who tried to wobble backwards but lost his balance and tumbled onto his back. As a cloud of dust rose, the cluster of women jumped to their feet and sprinted from the hut, howling petitions for God's mercy.

That, he assumed, was the end of clinic for the day, but five more women shuffled in before he had dusted himself off. He pushed past the new group into the flaming day, searching for an interpreter. He spotted Achmed strutting about, making coy faces at the women who stood around a fire outside a mammoth grass mat structure. Sol bellowed over his shoulder into the hut, "Ladies, I'll be right back," and jogged down the hill.

As he approached what he now recognized as one of the four feeding centers, Lila came out of the flimsy, five-thousand-square-foot edifice and straightened, a look of confusion and disquiet on her delicate face. It was the first time he had seen her from a distance, the whole of her person at one time. He was able to appreciate the loveliness of her stature, the regal way in which she held herself. But he turned away quickly and spoke to the checker. "We can use you at the clinic, Mr. Achmed," adding with a mumble, "*if* you don't mind."

The man lifted his head slowly to glare at Sol. His nostrils flared before turning back to the ladies who were hunkered, laughing. Sol took a step forward, his fists taut, but Lila moved between them and spoke to the checker. "Achmed, would you mind helping *Doctori Soli*? Thank you." The man pursed his lips, straightened, and commenced a slow, arrogant swagger up the hill.

Lila turned to the women and spoke quietly. "Have the donkeys brought the water from the *wadi*?"

Sara, the oldest of the troupe, her figure somehow full, but with a face that was hardened and gaunt, looked away from Achmed and stood. She answered in Arabic, "*Naam*," yes.

"Is the gruel cooking?"

"*La*," no.

Lila called to the checker, who had only gotten a few paces back toward the clinic, "Achmed, please come back."

He turned and stared down his nose at her. "What is it?"

"Please ask Sara why the gruel for lunch isn't cooking yet. Is there something she needs? Firewood, oil?"

A conversation ensued in Sudanese Arabic, an exchange that consumed a good two minutes. "She say now start cook lunch, *Insha'Allah. Al hum de le la.*"

Lila nodded gently. "Good. I hope God does will it because we have a few thousand children to feed in a few minutes. Please thank Ms. Sara."

Sol took a hesitant step toward Lila and spoke softly. "I'm sorry, Lila. Could you come back up to the clinic and give me some direction? Things aren't going all that swimmingly."

She smiled weakly. "And *I'm* sorry for this morning. All the static. You go on. I'll be up straight away. But first, let me duck into the pedi hospital and take a peek at our latest patient."

Back in his chair, Sol nodded to Achmed, reached over, and touched his shoulder. "Thank you, my friend, for helping. You have a very difficult job. Without you, I cannot be a doctor. I am happy you are so good at speaking English."

Achmed looked up and nodded back. "*Doctori*, I am here to help the sad people of Umm Balla."

Sol winked. "And the ladies like you. I can tell," then whispered as if hiding the conversation from the moms. "You have to tell me your secret."

Achmed ground his lips together and let go the smile he had tried to stifle. "Maybe you come with Achmed night time. I show you Darfur girl. Very beautiful, but very worry trouble if catch with man. Other woman sew up pussy. But way to do. I show D*octori*."

"Okay! You're on, my friend." They shook hands heartily.

Achmed pointed toward the first woman in the crescent of five. She pulled the nearly comatose toddler from beneath her robes and held the jellied mass two feet in the air. Sol slid from his chair and kneeled, smiling, moving forward at a snail's pace. The woman snatched the child out of the ether and stuffed her back under her *tob*. "What is it with these people?" he asked Achmed.

"*Doctori*, to her, you are ghost—she stupid chicken. You just tell her what is sickness. Not touch."

"Okay, Achmed, I'll sit back down, and you tell her to let me look at the child. But first, let's start with a history. Ask her what's wrong with the baby."

Achmed spoke to the woman, but his gaze drifted out the door, eyes fixed indifferently into the sand-choked sky. The mother turned and looked out of the hovel toward whatever it was that had captured

Achmed's attention. Eventually, she answered blankly, "Fever, cough, and diarrhea."

The woman hesitated, lips slightly parted, as if waiting for an astonishing remedy. When Sol said nothing, she raised the baby a foot higher, though the upper half of the child's body crumpled forward. Sol placed his left index and middle fingers on his own forehead, pointed to the baby with a wagging right index finger, closed his eyes, and hummed an aboriginal incantation. He smiled, "Madame, do I look like Carnac the Magnificent?" When she turned her head in question, Sol laughed, "You know, Johnny Carson—*Late Show*. You don't get Channel 5 here?" Sol's eyes tightened. "Okay, that's enough. Shoot junior over here, lady."

The woman's face pivoted further, and she looked to the checker, but Achmed was staring at the ladies down the hill. The woman smiled faintly and stood to leave, assured a powerful cure had been bestowed. Achmed, though, brought his eyes into the hovel and grabbed her arm. He barked in Arabic, "Hey, *abed*, give him the baby. What's wrong with you?" He turned to Sol and added, "Dese people so stupid. Dey tink what you do is medicine man."

"Tell you what, Achmed, let her hold the baby, and I'll do an exam in less than a minute. It'll be over so fast, she won't know what hit her. Tell her that, please."

Achmed did as ordered, though the woman's expression curdled and she yelped, "*Allah kareem*," as she tucked the child back under the robes.

"Now what?"

"She say you no hit baby. And she not know what minute is."

"Can you tell her I just want to listen to the child? I promise not to hit her."

The conversation ponged back and forth until Sol lost patience, leaned forward, and placed his stethoscope on the child's back. "Now was that so hard?" he growled to himself, but his voice was sufficiently close to the baby's ears that the child responded with a spasm of screams and coughs. That drew Lila into the hut. She stepped over the crescent of four, not one of whom had moved a single muscle since they had wobbled in half-an-hour before. "Are you okay, Doctor Sol?"

"I'm peachy, but our patient here is unhappy. Her lungs are full of crud, and she's dehydrated, and she's coughing so…"

"Yes," Lila cut him off, "and she's crying loud enough to be heard in Cairo. Give her some rehydration fluid packets and let's take a look at the next patient. It's getting close to noon, time for the camp to shut down for a few hours while the temperature rises."

Sol sighed, "Rises?" and took a foil pack of rehydration salts from the cardboard medicine chest and handed it to Achmed. He asked him to tell the woman to add a half-a-liter of water and give it to the child over the next twenty-four hours. "Tell her the baby will be like new in the morning."

Again, Achmed did as was bid, and again the woman shrieked. The two Sudanese voices rose, rattling the grass walls until Achmed put up his hand to stop her. He declared to Sol, "She say no want new baby. Want baby she have now. Too much work when baby new."

"No problem, Achmed. Tell her if she gives the rehydration fluid, the baby will grow to be a beautiful woman, just like her."

As he translated, the mom's head tilted thirty degrees then lowered coquettishly. She slowly placed the baby back under her *tob*. When she looked up again, Sol was taken by her penetrating, black eyes. Her headscarf had become loosened and half her cornrows were exposed. "She's a cutie, isn't she?" Sol grinned to Achmed.

Achmed winked clumsily at Sol. "You like Sudan woman? Sudan woman like *Doctori*. Achmed to show you."

Sol smiled at the woman; she smiled back. Her teeth were white, perfect.

Sol waited for her to leave, but she did not move until Achmed barked at her to waddle backwards out of the hut. Achmed looked to the next woman, put an index finger an inch from her face, and spoke coarsely. They traded words for a bit, and when she finally reached under her *tob*, it took a while to extract the child, not because the woman was dallying, but because her son was very long and very skinny. Sol laughed to himself that she seemed to be delivering a serpent. He asked Ahmed, "How *old* is this kid?"

The interpreter asked the mom, launching another protracted conversation, the only word of which Sol recognized was *abed*. Finally, Achmed shrugged. "Maybe five years. Only Allah know."

"Does Allah know how much he weighs?"

The interpreter wrestled the child from the mother roughly and placed him in the reed basket hanging under an even more rusted supermarket scale than the one in the hospital. The child's legs and head spilled over the edge of the wicker, but he did not struggle when the corroded hand on the device rose in fits and starts to stop at 10.5 kilograms. "Shoot," Sol muttered, "that's twenty-three pounds and change, obese. Must be watching too much TV. Achmed, please ask the mom what is wrong with her son."

As they babbled back and forth, several men walked through the door carrying back the stretcher with the old man. They marched past Sol without a nod to the back of the hut. Lila followed.

Achmed returned to his conversation with the woman and honed the exchange to a condensed chief complaint of fever, cough, and diarrhea. Sol jumped forward, grabbed the child by the arm, listened to the lungs as the mother tried to pull away, and declared, "Now, this one really has pneumonia. No brainer—to the hospital with him."

"Doctor Soli, do you think we might treat him at home?" Lila asked quietly from behind.

"This one's real sick. He's not going to make it home."

She nodded, adding, "I don't think he's even going to make it to the hospital. We have to triage, I'm sorry to say." She hesitated and let her head droop as she whispered, "I'll take him down there if you wish."

"Yeah, I wish."

"I'll be back straightaway. But let's see if we can move along a bit faster. These moms are going to get sick if they sit out in the sun much longer." Lila looked down at the child and shook her head. "We have to speed up."

"Lila, I'm dancing as fast as I can. For today, I'm not going to save the masses...maybe just a few lives. It'll be okay for my one day in Umm Balla. Yes?"

Lila took a step closer to him. "Doctor, please listen to me. Perfect is the enemy of good. I love these people, but this is teamwork. We've got to do the best for the greatest number of kids." Her voice rose. "It is just not possible to do everything to perfection."

But she gently touched the mother's shoulder, gathered the child in her arms, and headed down the hill.

She was back in less than three minutes, and Sol crowed, "We're getting' this down to a science."

"Not quite, I'm afraid. The child expired fifty feet down the hill."

The next mom in the arc pulled a baby from her beneath her gown, but there was rustling outside the hut and the serpentine backlog of the waiting area stood, moving slowly away in the now one-hundred-and-twenty-eight-degree late morning. The ladies inside the hut, including the woman holding her child in the air, waddled backwards and dispersed like spokes on a wheel to disparate sections of the refugee camp.

"Not to worry," Lila mumbled, "they'll be back around three."

Sol asked, "So what do we do now?"

"Let's get the old man out of here. Send him home again. I'll have the checker tell his mates that if they put his head higher than the feet, I will tell the devil because I am part *jinn* myself. They'll believe that. And that ought to do it. Then we eat lunch." Lila smiled stiffly, "Or you can spend the time in the hospital and wear yourself down and become so pathetic, we'll have to admit you to the adult hospice as a patient, and André will be your doctor."

"So, where's lunch? I'll spring for Chinese or Italian, or maybe a good lamb curry. What do you suggest?"

"Well, in fact, we have several choices. Follow me."

At the camp center, they joined André in a small back room of the administrative center. Lila looked at him as he raised his index finger to speak but cut him off, advising, "I just don't want to know."

André nodded and pointed to a bench for Sol. "You are 'ere for ze treat. Midday meal at Umm Balla. Ze cuisine fit for ze emperor."

"It'll be better than on the bus."

"You 'ave not read our Spanish brozer Cervantes? Ze road is better zan ze inn. You see, here at ze inn we can offer to you ze menu of tin pea and carrot, or per'aps ze spinach." He opened a padlocked footlocker under the table and blindly chose a can, shaking it wildly, his face hardening as if a man sinking into madness. "East Europe finest gastronomic," he spit while percussing the tin with his middle finger as if testing the ripeness of a melon. He shrugged and laughed, "You see, it is ze Russian roulette I tell you about. Zis one say," he looked hard at the label, "ah *oui*, ze cabbage."

André jabbed at the top with a rusted can opener. Ragged holes punched, he poured the foaming contents into a glass bowl. Six mashed peas and a few shreds of carrot floated to the surface. "You see it is just green water bubbles. Ze idiots, zey put on ze wrong marque, and zen forget to put in ze pea and carrot. Ze bubbles? Zey forget to seal ze can. Sometime you get ze little vegetable, most times no. Ze roulette. *Mais*, it is better zey don't put any food in it. So, Madame Lila, perhaps ze doctor wishes ze crepe suzette. Zis is ze specialty of ze 'ouse—yesterday pita." He reached into a basket under the table and retrieved a three-inch disc of spotted dark plastic. "It is 'ard like ze rock, but it 'as ze delicious protein meal of bugs zat you turn away zis morning. We can offer you ze special soup du jour. Make croutons of ze pita and put 'em in ze green sewage from our communist brozers in Bulgarie, and you 'ave ze well-balanced meal for ze new doctor; all sree rancid food groups." André raised his arms into the air as if he had just won the Grand Prix. "You are 'appy you come to ze Umm Balla?"

Lila sighed. "Enough, André." She turned to Sol and shook her head. "I'm afraid he's not exaggerating. We do have some local yogurt, though."

"I haven't seen a single cow," Sol mumbled, almost as a question.

Lila paused. "Not from cows actually, and you don't really want to know; and a bottle of feta cheese. It's quite salty, but safe, I think. Eat the dairy with the bread. It's not that awful."

André tightened his lips for a moment but could not help himself. "It is ze poison, but, of course zer is also ze peanut. We 'ave bags and bags of ze raw peanut in ze store 'ouse. We are to be saving zem for ze end. Ze refugee 'ere do not care for zem at all, so we use up ze *durra* and dry okra first."

Sol asked, "Do you mind if I take a look at the storehouse? Just to get an idea of what's left. And would you mind if I ate some peanuts?"

Lila hesitated and exhaled slowly, "Okay, I suppose there's no harm in letting you see where we stand."

They ate a bit of pita and feta then walked to a colossal structure that dwarfed the feeding center and the hospital combined. Lila took a key from the rope lanyard around her neck and unlocked the twig-and-weed door. Inside was a vast, dark, earthen-floored warehouse, empty aside from woven nylon bags marked with the USAID logo. Sol asked Lila, "Is everything in this camp from the American government?"

"It is—the U.S. Agency for International Development. CIA actually, you know."

"So I heard at your headquarters in London. Don't see any bags from England. Was the English donation the *durra* that's used up?"

Lila answered, her mouth tightening, "The *durra* was USAID as well."

"And the soap and the powdered milk and the okra and the oil?"

"Yes, Doctor, all of it," Her head snapped back and her nostrils flared. "But a small price to further your government's vile foreign policy. We aren't fooled, you know."

"Then why do you accept the donations? You could take the high road and just say no. Or you could insist that your pals back in London petition Parliament or André's National Assembly back in Paris to contribute. Everybody knows you Europeans are pristine. No blood on *your* hands."

Lila's jaw tightened. "Your country is politically criminal. Period. And we British are not Europeans."

She began to turn to leave, but Sol barked, "Yeah, but you're in the EU and you use the Euro, and you haven't sent shit over here to feed or wash these people, have you?"

He stood glaring, waiting for her retort, but she strode away silently, leaving Sol to cross the warehouse in the dark to the mountain of peanuts. He chose a bag at eye level to slice open with his Swiss Army knife, but stopped to stare at the blade, a farewell gift his department had presented two days before he left for Africa, an epoch before, a few weeks before.

He cut into the nylon expecting a gush of raw peanuts, thinking back to the Ratskeller on 56th Street in Manhattan, and the nights he and his medical school cronies drank tankard after tankard of cheap beer and gobbled raw peanuts by the bushel, tossing the shells recklessly to the floor. It was the only act of impertinence he had allowed himself over the years as a medical student—perhaps ever.

A sudden sense of emptiness washed over him as he remembered the Saturday morning nearly twenty years before, the day the letter of admission to Einstein Medical School arrived by special delivery, the first time a mailman had ever climbed the stairs of the Forte's apartment building. "It is a gift from God," his pop, Jimmy, wept, not caring to veil his tears. "How can it be that an Italian Catholic goes to a Jewish medical school, and with a full scholarship? The Jews are good to us a second time? I don't know why."

That keyed the next memory, the night Sol took his father to the Ratskeller, to introduce him to his new friends. Sol weakened, recollecting how they had embraced his father, literally, arms around his shoulders, demanding he accept their offers of rotten beer and peanuts. But Jimmy didn't drink, and hadn't since the night in the Korean War that a GI had saved his life.

"Tell us," one of the women students asked softly, putting a hand on his beefy forearm, "why you named Sol, Sol."

So, Jimmy took a deep breath and told the students that he no longer drank or smoked, or even cursed, "…all because of a man, just another jarhead private. His name was Solomon Jaffe. They shot 'im twice, the commies did, at the Choson Reservoir. You heard of it. The worst battle of the Korean War they say. Somehow that guy crawled out, I don't know how, there was lead everywhere, like mosquitos. I been shot twice, and this guy comes out on his belly from behind a chunk of ice, must a been same size as this room. And this Marine, Solomon, he pulls me back, I mean I don't know how. I weigh two times what this guy does. But he gets me back behind the ice cube, away from the Chicom machine guns. All of a sudden, them medics crawl over and stop the bleeding. So, I named my son Solomon."

Another student asked, "Excuse me, sir, but what's Chicom?"

Jimmy stared at the kid for a moment but smiled gently, "That's Chinese Communist soldiers. The worst nightmare I pray none a youse ever gotta see."

Someone else asked, "Mr. Forte, so why did you stop drinking? What happened?"

"Ya know, we guys, him and me, we was next to each other in the hospital. They come through with a bottle of beer once a week, and we look at each other and I says, 'Hey, I'm givin' mine to that poor jerk over there in the corner. He needs it more than me, don't he?' And Solomon, next to me, he says the same thing. Then he says, 'Ya know, Jimmy, I ain't gonna drink or smoke no more until I get home outta this hole.' So I says, 'Me neither.' And here we are in the Ratskeller, and I ain't had a drink since. Helps me remember."

Now, many, many years later, and many, many thousands of miles from Jimmy's grave, Sol's eyes reddened. He asked God to let his pop know what he'd become and how much Jimmy had shaped him.

* * *

Sol stood paralyzed for a moment in the stinking, musty storehouse but finally looked at the sack he had slashed. Though he had anticipated a gush of crisp, fresh, salted Ratskeller peanuts, there flowed instead an ooze saturated with a stench more powerful than the operating rooms where patients with perforated bowels were treated. One putrefied rodent carcass, crawling with maggots, squeezed out and tumbled to the dirt floor, then another, and Sol sprang backward. He gathered himself and slit open another bag. It, too, dribbled a semi-liquid, semi-solid sludge that trolled to the dirt floor, soiling his running shoes. He climbed the mountain of nylon, slicing into bag after bag, seeking a single peanut, but he reached the crest, a good ten feet off the ground, and still there was not one kernel to be salvaged for his lunch, or for the lives of the refugees of Umm Balla. Every bag he tested was stuffed with the remains of vermin that had departed this life cramming themselves on the last of Lila's hopes.

Sol left the warehouse to find her but slowed for a moment when he noticed the shimmer of the roiling air lifting off the plastic sheets of the hospital roof. He detoured into the building, bumping into the nurse at the doorway. "Muhammad, how is that little girl we brought down here this morning?"

"Which one?"

"You know, the dehydrated kid."

"Which one? Please you show."

Sol took the man by the wrist and very gently guided him a dozen yards into the massive structure, wending his way around motionless pediatric patients, some on mats, some on the dust. Several were new, not there an hour before when Sol and Lila had last gone on rounds. Sol asked, "Where did these kids come from? Is there another clinic in camp?"

"Oh, *Doctori*, sometime mama come beg have baby live here. Very stupid, very afraid white skin of you. Miss Lila say can do."

"Right. Free admission. Anyone who wants to be admitted, no problem, find 'em a bed. Sort of like University Hospital back in New York. That was a real hit. Mayor got reelected on that insanity. So, let me get this straight. I get shit for admitting a dying kid, but a teenage mom pops in and says she needs a bed, and that's okay? Whatever, so where's our little girl?"

Sol looked across the dank structure and pointed, "Ah, there she is. And guess who's sitting up?" He dropped to a knee and pinched the child's skin. It snapped back, no longer tenting. He listened to her lungs—a bit clearer. "Great work," he smiled up at Muhammad. "Lila said you were very good. Best in Sudan." The dark-skinned, young Sudanese man blushed when Sol stood and put his arm around him and smiled, "She was right. Do you know where Lila is?"

"Miss Lila go to feed kid. I show."

Muhammad grasped Sol's fingers tightly, and the two walked hand in hand out of the hospital toward the feeding center. As they passed the cooks, Sol tried to pull his hand free, but Muhammad tightened his grip, and they stopped for a moment, still holding hands, to watch the women work. They were brewing the gruel that the Western world supposed held the promise of life for a full generation of Darfurian children, the salve that allowed the eating world to eat.

The ladies were all scrupulously wrapped from the tops of their heads to their ankles in once-colorful, flower-patterned gowns of flowing cotton. Some were arranging sticks of wood in tepee shapes under half-55 gallon oil drums. Others were out combing the shit fields, scrounging more firewood and dried dung for fuel, and yet another clutch hovered around a herd of diseased donkeys that had clopped up from the *wadi*. The undersized creatures stood, heads drooped, foaming at the mouth. They swayed near collapse under distended cow-stomach bladders. The women drained murky, khaki water from the bursting animal skins into gourds, which they emptied into the oil drums. A commission of particularly ragged ladies arrived to massage the last drops of fluid from the bladders, half-filling plastic buckets, which they carried to the other side of the feeding center.

The head cook at this feeding center, Howwa, nodded to a hunkered, ancient woman, who carefully, reverently, struck a match under the first barrel. The straw tinder ignited. Two more women fanned the embers madly with little squares of discarded grass mat until the fire burned brightly. That was the signal for the first woman to walk submissively to Howwa, hand her the matches, and return to the barrels to light the other three fires with a burning stick from the first. More women bent over to fan. When Howwa was satisfied the engines of life were glowing, she rang a hand bell, drawing a wave of chattering women from within the wind-protected feeding center, each laden with a fifty-pound bag of milk powder, a cask of vegetable oil, or a sack of white sugar. She ordered them to stop beside one of the four slowly heating oil drums. Another woman with a scimitar came up from behind and slashed at the bags, allowing some of the contents to stream into the now-tepid water. A new contingent of ladies appeared from the ether carrying tree branches which they speared into the concoction, stirring until the slurry thickened. Howwa, the oldest of the work force, the least smiling, and like her colleague at the other feeding center, somehow still rotund, poked her gnarled finger into the mash, tasted it, screwed her face in revulsion, and nodded. Her eyes lifted to the heavens, and her lips formed a prayer.

Sol smiled at her, raised his thumb, and purred, "*Al dente!*"

He drifted over to the other side of the structure, to watch the particularly ragged women toting the dregs of the donkeys' water bladders pour the near-mud into plastic five-gallon pails. Three more women opened the gate of twigs, allowing a line of skeletal children into an eight-foot-by-eight-foot paddock, a sign over which read in English, SANITZATION CENTER. He had entered the handwashing zone.

The women checked the plastic bracelets on each child's wrist, insuring the color jibed with that feeding center's shade, and that there was a name and age on each. Sol walked up to one of the kids and gazed at the wristlet, laughing that engraved in the plastic was the logo of a grand hotel chain he had never had the money to patronize.

He glanced at several male adolescents who had both wrists wrapped in plastic bracelets—each band a different primary color. The boys sought admission to the feeding center by flashing the strips arrogantly in the face of the woman at the gate. The bracelets were held together with wisps of nylon thread nicked from the bags of *durra*. The string had been threaded through holes where plastic rivets on the bracelets had been torn out. One of the bands bore a female name and an age of three.

The female workers plucked the interlopers from line, admonishing that the impostors had bought themselves a heap of trouble. One woman called Sol over to administer a punishment commensurate with the felony of sneaking into lunch. Sol shook his head theatrically at the gallery of miscreants then waved an index finger indignantly, but when it became too hard to veil his laughter, he headed into the feeding center to find Lila or André.

Lila was talking with the cooks, informing them that roasted peanuts were soon to be the fare, and that when that came to pass she would have to fire most of them. There was a bit of wailing, but Lila put her arm around the shoulders of several of the women and hugged them tightly, rubbing her forearm across her eyes as she looked up toward Sol. "Is there a problem, *Doctori?*"

With the one word they understood, the women straightened a bit and took steps backward, lowering their eyes. Sol spoke softly, "They want me to discipline the kids or something. How do you do that?"

Lila turned to the women and mumbled through the interpreter, "Not to worry, maybe a fresh supply of stale provisions will appear before it's too late." There was a round of "*Bookera Insha'Allah*s" and "*Al hum de le la*s," tomorrow if God wills it, thank God, then more hugging and crying.

Lila walked toward the kids' intake chute, Achmed following at a distance, ambling slowly, busy polishing his teeth with a tree twig as he ogled the kitchen ladies. At the Sanitation Center, Lila turned to look for him, but he had dropped out as they passed the hospital. He was chatting with a friend, both sliding twigs in and out of their mouths with intensifying ferocity as the conversation heated.

Lila listened closely to one of the women, who stooped in mid-sentence to redo her *tob* before pointing excitedly at the teens who had dared access Feeding Center 1 while bearing Feeding Centers 2, 3, and 4 bracelets. Several more women arrived to point angrily at the tallest of the teenaged boys they had captured and made squat in a corner. When they were sure they had Lila's attention, they took her by the hand to the delinquent, jabbing fingers at a blue bracelet that was several sizes too small.

"We know we are the best feeding center, but we can't save all the tribes, Miss Lila," Howwa barked as she stomped over from the now scorching oil drums.

"Look at this, *Doctori*," Lila demanded, "these teenage boys are cheating. Typical, isn't it? They get a meal at the other feeding center, bully the little kids and pinch their bracelets, then sally over here for dessert. Not cricket, you know."

"No, we can't have that," Sol nodded weakly. "Men are the worst creatures on God's Earth. Pond scum at best. Same everywhere you go. You're right. We won't have it, period."

Lila's jaw tightened. She ripped the bracelet from the tallest boy's wrist, waved it in his face, then jammed it into her scrub suit as the teens were herded out of the paddock. She called after them in English, warning that if they came back, the lot would be sent to dig latrines for the rest of their lives.

She marched over to the line of urchins nearing entry, supervising as they dipped their hands into the bucket of water dregs, taking the filthy bar of raw soap tossed from the child to their front, scarcely sliding it over their hands before passing it back to the next ragamuffin. By the third or fourth customer, the water was as black as the Sudanese nights, and the foam curling off the soap like tar. The children wiped their washed hands on a towel of death shroud proffered by a lady at the door to the center, but some looked at the towel and just dried themselves on their filth-caked shorts. The woman inspected palms closely, sending an occasional waif back to the end of the line.

At the portal, each of those who passed muster took a red or green or yellow plastic bowl from a pile, held it out with two hands, and accepted a ladleful of the milk powder, cooking oil, and sugar gruel before entering the feeding center. They dropped to the earthen floor and squeezed, elbow to elbow, with the next refugee child, rows as far as the eye could see of cachectic waifs leaning back against the grass mat walls.

Lila bristled from the handwashing corral into the main compound, eying the teen she had summarily dismissed. He had taken up reconnaissance behind a donkey, but when Lila saw him glaring at her, she strutted up to the teen, put a finger up into his face, and sent him swaggering off.

She called to Sol and bade him follow the eighth of a mile to Feeding Center 2. It was a grass mat monstrosity reserved for babies and toddlers; their moms, hundreds and hundreds of sapped teenagers, hunkered in the musty dark, occasionally pulling their progeny from under *tobs* to offer sips of scorched gruel. Less than a foot into the door, Lila's face hardened to a prison guard's façade. She marched the lines scowling at the women directly to her front, though she was actually scrutinizing the unsuspecting ladies on the other side of a three-foot-high grass mat partition. When Lila spied one of those women stealing a long draw of the gruel for herself, she lifted the divider, ducked under, and halted dramatically to wag a finger in that mom's face. She instructed the interpreter to ask if there was an excuse for the breech of procedure, and when the young woman dropped her eyes, Lila ordered her to spend one hour hauling water from the *wadi* back up to the cooking pots, "Just like the donkeys, and you tell her I said that."

When the mother asked, as did each of the convicted, who would watch the baby while she served her sentence, Lila hissed, "Tell her she should have thought of that before she ate the baby's food."

After she punished five or six of the girls, Sol called Lila aside. "I think we need to talk for a minute."

"I know what I'm doing. I don't need any advice on how to run this feeding center."

"No, no," Sol dropped back a foot or two, "it's not that. There's something else."

Lila stared at him guardedly as she asked, "Do we need to do this in private?" Sol began slowly, but Lila snapped, "To the point please. I have two more feeding centers to visit. They don't run themselves, you know."

"Ms. Lila, please listen to me for a minute. You need to be strong and quiet for just thirty seconds. Okay?" When she didn't answer, he went on. "There are no peanuts. Every bag is mush, rodent shit, if you please. The rats got to the whole supply. There's *nothing* left."

Lila stood quietly. Eventually, without acknowledging Sol, she ordered one of the checkers to the food distribution center to fetch André. As he arrived in front of Lila, smiling condescendingly, she put her hand up to stop him, nearly cuffing his face. "And ze catastrophe *du jour*?"

Lila's eyes reddened. "I don't need your pomposity at the moment. She jabbed a thumb toward Sol. "He says the peanuts are gone—eaten by vermin."

André rolled his eyes. "And now you are ze George Washington Carver? Come on, we see."

At the warehouse, Sol stopped at the entrance, more to avoid the stench of the decomposing animals than the coming tsunami. Lila cried out, "Oh, my God. This is the end. We need to make plans to leave right now."

André nodded but turned quietly to Sol. "Doctor, well, you are correct zis time. *Mais*, do you 'ave ze advice?"

Sol dropped his head for a moment then looked up. "May I respectfully request we go back to the compound? We'll sit and drink tea and talk, quietly, and if we try hard, we'll come up with a solution."

André thought for a minute before fuming, "Zis time, Doctor, zer is no choice. We must leave."

"André, please, if I may, there is always a choice, always an alternative. *Mon ami*, I do not know you well, but I do know you and Lila are fine people. You've been thrown into the worst circumstances on Earth, and you're still fighting. Please, let's go back to the compound. We'll figure something out."

Lila brewed tea, André placed his pack of Gauloise on the table, and Sol brought a pad from his hut. André pushed the pack toward Sol, who hesitated but drew a cigarette from the pack and lit it with André's matches. He pretended to smoke. "Okay, my friends, you know far better than I how long we can hold on. From what you say, the day the food runs out, *we're* to blame, and the consequences will not be pretty. So, André, how much is left in the distribution center? I mean in days."

"*Mais*, it is not ze days, but ze type of supplies we can provide. We must give ze soap and ze…"

"André, my friend, how many days of *food* do we have left for the refugees?"

André snatched a sheet of paper from Sol's pad, grabbed Sol's pen, and wrote figures. He added, subtracted, and wrung his hands until they blanched, finally lifting his head and declaring, "I say zer are eight days to ze end."

Sol asked, "Lila, is that your assessment?" She thought for a minute and nodded.

"So be it." He stood and declared, "I will be back in five days with enough food to keep us going for a few weeks. If there is no food in five days, I mean if I'm not back in five days, leave camp on the sixth day, meet me in El Fasher at the UN office, and I'll pay for all of us to stay there until we can get a flight to Khartoum. I will provide money for you to fly home to England, France, or wherever you want to go. I will settle accounts with the home office after this is all over. Can you stay here for that long?"

"*Mais*, zer are too many of ze problem. It will take two day to get to Nyala, and sree more to El Fasher. Zen what if ze Janjaweed attack?"

"Have they attacked yet?"

"*Mais non*, but zey can come at any time."

"They don't know we are out of food. So why would they bother just yet?"

"For ze slave. For ze woman. You do not know zem."

"I do not but, of course, if you really believe they are about to attack, you must leave immediately. But from what I understand, they have not attacked a single Western-run camp."

"Not yet," André hissed.

"Look, if you have evidence that they are changing tactics, then leave right away, for sure. I'm just asking that you not leave based on the projected lack of food. Give me a few days. I think my money'll talk real loud in El Fasher."

Sol agreed to take the Land Rover, though it had not been moved in a month. The wheels were so consumed by drifts of sand, it looked more hovercraft than jeep. He dug for half-an-hour freeing the tires only to find the battery with as little life as most of their patients. The battery had fallen victim to André's scheme to start the engine once a week but shut it down immediately, before even a molecule of the oil could circulate, to say nothing of a single electron pushed into the battery for recharge.

As Sol used a lamp cord to jump the Rover from the Cruiser, André fretted, "Maybe ze battery is so dead. it would never 'ave ze recharge. Maybe ze engine will melt, and you are left in ze desert to die by ze vulture. And zen I am ze one for ze blame."

CHAPTER THREE

Sol left a thousand dollars for them and bumped out of the camp an hour later, mid-afternoon, the air so stifling, he did not have the energy to turn back for a last look. As he wove along the single-track road through the village of Umm Balla, not a soul was visible. He rolled past Mighty Joe Young, who was at the base of his wall curled in a thimble-sized disk of shade. Sol laughed, stopped the jeep, tore a piece of pita, and walked toward the monkey, clicking his tongue to wake him. When the screeching began, the lady darted out of her *tuchel*. Several toddlers crawled about, and neighbors poured from their huts rubbing sleepy eyes. The woman cracked at Sol in a local dialect several linguistic time zones away from proper Arabic. When he didn't react, she took a step toward him and grabbed for the bread. Sol jerked the pita away and handed it up to Mighty Joe, who had scampered up the wall and puffed himself into a defensive posture. The woman tried to snatch the bread from the monkey, but he had already hunched his body over the prize, bared his sharp yellow teeth, and growled menacingly.

Mighty Joe wolfed the crust ferociously then hissed again, more at the lady than Sol. She ignored the creature, though, and tramped toward Sol, who jogged to the jeep, ducked in, and snatched a full round of pita from his sack. He turned and offered it to her with two hands just as she arrived at the vehicle. That sent the neighbors into a frenzy, several dozen bodies closing in on him with hands outstretched, the younger ones pulling at his DARE tee shirt and scrub pants. Sol recognized the peculiar scent, the same one clinging to the camp refugees and the passengers on the bus. It calmed him, and as his face relaxed, so did those of the villagers, whose shoulders he patted gently.

He smiled and called out, pointing at himself and then into the desert, "I'm going to El Fasher to buy food." Met with silence, he thought for a moment, rubbed his fingers together as if handling money, and mimicked purchasing pita and trucking it back to Umm Balla to feed this lady, the next child, and Mighty Joe Young. A wave of chatter built, and they came up to him and patted his shoulders awkwardly, looking to each other to make sure they had gotten the gesture right. Sol tapped back, the smiles broadened, and a path opened to his jeep.

The backseat of the Rover was piled with packets of Russian oatmeal and donated Namibian whole milk powder. There was a jar of donated cocoa from the Netherlands; six cans of Bulgarian food product, each with a smudged sketch of tired peas and carrots; and several more rounds of speckled pita. It was stuffed into crevices between the NATO jerry cans of fuel and water and the four spare tires, the maximum the laws of the Sudan allowed any one vehicle to carry.

He struck out across the desert he had passed through less than twenty-four hours before. To save fuel, he did not use the air conditioner, though he was so mesmerized by the moonscape, he did not sense heat or cold or fatigue.

After he had been on the sand for a few hours, he spied a dried riverbed in the distance that seemed to parallel the path east toward Nyala. He drove to the edge of the *wadi*, a bone-dry gash in the earth, eight feet deep and fifteen feet wide. He got out of the jeep and stumbled down the sheer bank to test the floor, whacking his heel against the smooth surface. It was rock-hard and went on for miles. As he climbed out of the riverbed, he peered as far as he could in all four directions, distinguishing nothing but ruddy sand and seared undergrowth. Not a hut, a road, a telegraph pole, or a creature, nothing beside his dark memories and the jeep suggested that life had ever crawled upon Earth. He became lightheaded and slouched against a scorching boulder until a wave of nausea passed, followed by a swell of despair. His eyes reddened, and he stood rigidly, finally slapping his thighs as the decision was made. He would turn back to

Umm Balla, admit defeat, gather his colleagues and drive, safer in numbers, to El Fasher. The deal would remain the same; he would pay the way back to the Western world for his colleagues and then fly home to face whatever Please Help the Children in London, and the State Medical Abuse Commission in Whitaker, resolved to do with him. He needed to know if he had a future in medicine.

He restarted the Rover, hands frozen to the wheel, his mind numb, until the tires rolled slowly down the embankment into the *wadi*, away from Umm Balla and the setting sun. He cursed at himself, "Well, shit, when you die out here in an hour or two, don't complain. You got no one to blame but yourself."

He kept one eye on his compass and one peering into the distance, a line of ancient telegraph poles eventually materializing on the horizon. Every few minutes, he added a bit of speed, and for the next hour-and-a-half, he neared thirty miles per hour.

Drugged by the heat and the absolute barrenness of the proto highway, he lost track of time, just staring into the future, on and on until his head dropped, fighting sleep. When he lost his battle, his eyes sagged, and he fell into a dream, this time about being, yet again, unprepared for an exam in medical school.

A thump startled him awake. At first, he thought it was a nun cracking his knuckles with a ruler, but he saw the jeep skidding wildly toward the *wadi's* bank. The driver's side of the vehicle lifted so abruptly, his horizon rolled counterclockwise as if he were being twisted in an explosion. His heart clutched, and he spun the wheel madly, though he gained no purchase, neither of the front wheels in contact with the desert. It had happened so fast, he did not have time to worry that his life was ending, and even if he had had the time, it would not have mattered to him.

The right front wheel, though, found an elevated crook in the *wadi*, one fashioned by the Creator several million years before. The Rover leveled and lugged to a mushy stop with the *wadi* bank outside his door and a boulder an inch from the passenger door. Though Sol was shaking furiously, he managed to free himself through the rear hatch and spent the next minutes kicking at the exploded left front tire. When his foot began to throb, he ran up the side of the *wadi* and scrutinized the perimeter of his new world—endless red sand, red hillocks, a bit of red-dust-enveloped, long-dead scrub thistle, and a red haze that did little to block the glowering red sun.

He rambled back into the dry riverbed, built a tiny fire from blowing twigs, crouched in the shadow cast by the jeep, and cooked a bowl of cocoa oatmeal. He ate slowly, his mind locked in thoughts of André and Lila, wondering if he would ever see them again. After his new friends, he imagined the boy with the mutton bone talisman; the dying old man who eventually lifted himself off the cot and died again, but was resurrected when Sol came to his hut and lifted his legs for three minutes; the fifteen-year-old mother who had sipped a tablespoon of gruel; and Lila's summary justice that had shipped the girl off to do donkey's work. He laughed at himself, feeling better knowing that it was all just a dream and that he would soon awake, safely ensconced in the center of the bus.

* * *

By sunset, Sol had gone eighty or ninety miles, changed tires twice, and was down to a single spare, as one of the standbys was already flat, the valve having blown out of the rubber during the crash in the *wadi*. He was still dozens of miles from Nyala, the first settlement on his vague itinerary, and while that was only halfway, a semi-paved road ran north to El Fasher from there. As he drove, he spotted lights, balls of orange flashing in the distance—the *jinn*. He thought of making for them, perhaps coming upon a village and people with whom he could share his humanity. But he remembered the dread his fellow travelers suffered when they spotted the Devil's lights bouncing across the sands, so he drove on, satisfied to keep his own company. He stopped an hour later and whisked up another bowl of chocolate oatmeal, this time eating the porridge cold, unwilling to surrender his position with a fire whose light would stretch miles over the blackened desert.

As the temperature plunged, he wrapped himself in the double length of death shroud André had cut as Sol packed the jeep. "It will keep you warm...or it will take you to ze next plane." When Sol eyed him askance, André laughed, "Oh, Soli, I am joe-keeing wis you only." André hemmed and hawed as he approached Sol to hand him a pack of Gauloises. "For you, Doctor, number sree of ze packet left. I souvenir you to remember me."

Sol promised André a carton of the pungent cigarettes when he returned in a few days, but the young French doctor demanded, "'Ow can I be sure you will ever come back to ze Umm Balla Resort?"

Sol handed him another hundred US dollars. "As a deposit, my friend."

He slept for an hour until the biting cold percolated through the shroud, and he covered himself with his change of clothes. That worked for barely three minutes, after which he slipped into a big black garbage bag Lila had given him in which to place his food at night to fool the animals. Though Sol knew the futility of trying to hide food from starving predators, he accepted the bag with thanks, and now put it to work as another layer against the cold. That bought him fifteen minutes until the vapor from his breath and sweat condensed on the inside of the plastic, dribbling in freezing beads, first onto his face, then soaking into his clothes. Now he was wet, and he shivered and cursed until he got out of the jeep and walked for a few hundred yards.

In the distance, he saw the *jinn* bounding closer, orange fire skittering along the sand. The glow allowed him to make out the silhouettes of mounted horses galloping across the desert, a platoon of cavalry hurtling west toward Umm Balla. But he rubbed his eyes, and the apparition dissolved, as did the lights, his perimeter once again secure.

Sol started the engine, turned the heater to full, took a couple of Tylenol, pretending they were sleeping pills, and lay back down, scrunched on the front seats. He promised himself he would get up in a few minutes and turn off the motor, but he did not wake for several hours. When he jumped up, he was soaked with warm sweat. The engine was still idling, and the fuel gauge neared empty. He had a single jerry can left, and he forced himself to keep his hands off of it until morning.

When he arose, folded in a rigid, fetal ball, the sun was just a thin crescent in the far horizon. He unfurled slowly, each joint stiffer even than on the bus. He pried himself from the jeep to answer nature's call, though when he turned back, he saw the front left tire flat on the ground. Desperate to convince himself it was an illusion, just a small mound of sand that had blown against the tire, he kicked at the dirt, but his shoe struck the squashed bulge of dead rubber. He replaced the flat with his final spare, washed, ate a bowl of chocolate oatmeal, and headed off slowly, stopping to clear the *wadi* of suspicious, thorned brush every few hundred yards.

As the desert deepened, all the burnable debris had been picked clean centuries before, leaving nothing to destroy the last of Sol's tires. He increased speed, sailing north, confidence boiling as he plotted his position just twenty miles from Nyala. Though the fuel gauge was drifting left at an alarming rate, he was convinced of his skill to conserve fuel and make it to the outskirts of Nyala within two hours. He turned up the volume on the tape deck and sang along with the music, each track, one way or the other, celebrating the America he had learned to love from his immigrant mother and father. A sense of well-being swathed him, and he nodded proudly that he would soon negotiate to save the lives of the dispossessed refugees camped in Umm Balla. It was the reason he had been placed on Earth.

As *We Are the World* began, he spun the volume to full, opened the windows, and sang so brashly, he did not hear the pop, but he soon felt the Land Rover pulling to the left again, and he let the vehicle climb out of the riverbed to sit as high as it could on the horizon. He had not used the air conditioner that morning, saving fuel by relying on the breeze, but just seconds after coming to a halt, the temperature inside the cab rose to 118 degrees. He closed the windows and started the engine to suck a few breaths of tepid air from the air conditioner. When the engine temperature gauge rose faster than the fuel gauge sank, Sol shut the motor down before it seized.

He examined the three flat spares in the backseat, as if one of them might have come back to life, sealed and reflated by the laws of quantum mechanics, where things that could not happen did. But they were as flat as they had been the day before; the jerry cans were still bone dry.

He did have water, and chocolate, and oatmeal, so he dumped a double portion into his red plastic bowl and tried to find a spot of shade outside the jeep, but as noon approached, the best he could do was place the death shroud over the open door to fashion a tent under which he ate slowly, licking the bowl at the end to save the water he would have squandered rinsing. He laughed, thinking of his long-gone father, and how Papa had licked his plate at dinner, winking at Marie, assuring his family with all the bluster of a New York City concrete truck driver that it was socially acceptable, for he had rotated the plate clockwise.

Sol searched the horizon for hours, waiting for any soul, even a nomad, to hail and pay to gallop up to Nyala and hire a tire mechanic. But when the sun crashed below the horizon, Sol removed the shroud from the door, draped it over his shoulders, cooked another bowl of chocolate oatmeal, and cursed at the end of the meal as he licked the bowl counterclockwise. As the first stars appeared through the desert haze, he wrapped himself in all of his clothing, and then the shroud.

He dreamt of medical school and residency, the decade of sleepless nights. Every time he closed his eyes, most often at two A.M., there was an angry, controlling nurse ready to page him back to the floor to place a suppository in an old man's behind. Without fail, she'd call him back in an hour and berate him for his therapeutic failure, demanding he disimpact the ancient soul by hand. He was often surprised that the sad years of his residency still lurked so close to the surface.

* * *

Hours later a grinding sensation woke him, and he broke free from his cocoon to see a vehicle in the distance lumbering westward. Soon, he could make out a truck, then that it had metal sides, and eventually that there were stick figures on the roof. By the time he was sure it was the bus, and though he ran after it shouting, waving his arms in the pitch black, the vehicle had pushed too far across the desert to catch on foot.

At dawn, Sol sacrificed the tire and rim and drove toward the telegraph poles to wait for the bus on its return trip east. By mid-afternoon, when the shimmering silhouette rose above the southern horizon, Sol's water ration was down to a few mouthfuls, and he jumped up waving his arms maniacally in the path of the coach. Eventually, he could make out the driver, neck craned forward, straining to focus on his next ordeal. As the man rolled closer, he seemed to recognize Sol and turned the truck into the looser sands, willing to chance the mire to avoid the pallid devil. When the lorry's bald tires failed, the bus jammed to an abrupt halt.

Passengers poured from the tailgate to claim tiny patches of sand on which they unfurled prayer rugs. Sol approached the driver slowly, rolling a flattened spare, his other hand waving the pack of André's Gauloises. The knobby little man shrugged his shoulders and lifted his hands to snatch the gift, but also snapped in Arabic, "You again? Evil white spirit! You are like the *jinn*. Yeah, the *jinn*. The Jew. A curse. That's what you are. And what the hell do you want now?" He waited a moment, shook his head, spit on the sand, and ordered Sol to lift the tire onto the roof. The boys were so excited to see him, they followed Sol into the desert to fetch the other flats, two of the jerry cans, and a duffle bag of oatmeal. They refused to allow Sol to carry even his personal paper bag of clothing.

As they loaded the new freight carefully on top of the cardboard luggage, Sol stuck his head into the cab and wrote down the bus's odometer reading. Pulled up by the passengers, he climbed over the tailgate and pressed forward to his former seat in the middle of the morass. Almost before he had settled in, one of the patrons motioned for a glass of cool water for their guest. That began a period of grousing from the old man, but a full penny shuffled across the bench, and Sol was soon greedily sucking down the muddy water.

Two hours later, the bus jounced into Nyala. Sol handed the driver a five-dollar bill and the boys a buck each, the latter patting him on the shoulder, grinning, promising they would never forget him. Sol stuck his head back into the cab to record the new odometer reading, but the numbers had not budged.

Sol hailed a cab, piled the tires into the backseat, and gestured with his hands for a fixit shop. "Ah," the driver nodded and smiled, screeching through the streets at breakneck speed. He plowed into back alleys, through piles of trash, and onto a rutted thoroughfare, the main street of Nyala, and dropped Sol off in the front of the Hotel Finest Africa.

Sol, his paper bag of clothes, three tires, and jerry cans were hauled up to a room on the third floor by a team of desperately thin porters, all of whom stood by the door until Sol dropped a dollar into the tallest man's outstretched palm. Sol motioned for him to divide it equally. The man bowed his head obsequiously and took off down the stairs. The other porters remained at attention outside the door until Sol pressed a dollar into each of their extended hands. As the men descended the stairs, Sol smiled at the whoops of joy and the beating of drums outside his window.

Accepting it would not be his to see the tires repaired that day, he undressed and went into the bathroom to wash. The shower stall, which was the entire bathroom, aside from the hole in the floor at the other end, was flooded with murky green water, more viscous and forbidding than that on the bus, or the fluid at the Umm Balla feeding center upon which the future of that generation of Darfurian children hung.

Sol worked the drain for a minute until he pulled what he was sure was a rancid pork chop from the pipes, but he imagined that particular species of meat an unlikely find in the strictly *halal* thousand square miles that surrounded the hotel. The putrid water gurgled away slowly but stopped flowing with still an inch left. He stood in his flipflops and activated the one faucet—cold—to release a dribble no stronger than the shower in Umm Balla.

He stretched out on the bed after the shower but was soaked in sweat within seconds, so he rose and jiggled the wires sticking out of the wall to turn on the overhead fan. It twisted a few revolutions per minute, barely stirring the air, but quite sufficient to sluff years of accumulated dust on him. At 6:30, he walked the two flights of stairs and left the hotel to find dinner. The one local restaurant's door was lashed closed with a bit of ancient rope, and though he rapped several times, and could see figures moving in the shadows, no one came forward to greet him.

Sol went back to his room, fixed a bowl of tepid chocolate oatmeal, and read for a few minutes until the electricity seeped away volt by volt, taking with it the light and the meager puffs of air from the ceiling fan. He fell into an uneasy sleep for an hour until the heat built, and he had no choice but to open the windows, allowing in both the din of irritated camels from the courtyard and battalions of anopheles mosquitos. He closed the window. Some of the attack squads of mosquitos were thwarted, but the heat rose to a point where he began to hallucinate. He stumbled back down to the desk to beg for a new room. The clerk was asleep, without a pillow, but covered in a threadbare blanket on the tile floor behind the desk. He smiled warmly as he explained that the power was off for the night, and that there were no other rooms.

At 6 A.M., Sol showered, though the drain was again clogged, this time with the accrual Sol had washed off himself the night before. He rolled one tire down the stairs, but in the lobby, the clerk jumped up from the floor mortified, loudly hailing the gang of porters, who flowed in from the courtyard, where they had passed the night on the pounded earth, without pillows or blankets. They had shared their patch of land with a dozen Darfur camels corralled each evening by their *jamali* and tied to the ground for safekeeping. By dawn, however, several of the beasts had already worked through their bindings and clopped into the street to pick at piles of garbage; the rest of them blocked the front door of the hotel, growling and nipping at each other.

When Sol tried to leave, the porters flapped their arms and made grunting noises to clear a path, though all they were able to open was a narrow lane. Sol tried to sneak past the herd, but the animals appropriated his alien scent and set about kicking and spitting wildly, scaring him back inside.

Twenty minutes later, when the camels had drifted away into an adjoining neighborhood, the porters jumped up from the lobby floor, tugged at Sol's shirt, and led him into an alley where three teens snatched the tires. Without a word, they began to pry the rubber from the rims. But the work ceased suddenly, and one of the boys ran from the alley to fetch a fifteen-year-old, who considered the matter with great concentration, finally explaining to Sol that, because there were tubes in the tires, an unexpected obstacle, the total charge would be substantially higher.

"Okay, and how much will *that* be, seven hundred dollars?"

There was a protracted discussion punctuated with commentaries that sent the boys into rolls of laughter until the fifteen-year-old held up his hand to stop the badinage. "Fifteen cents?"

"Well, okay. Just make sure it doesn't get any more than that."

When it was over, the boys sprinted off through the streets of Nyala, jumping and twirling, hollering to pedestrians and taxis that they possessed a dollar. Sol made his way to the bus depot and found the driver, bribing him with a pack of local cigarettes. The bent, little man lifted his nose as if insulted, though took them and nodded crossly toward the tailgate. Sol was again nudged into the heart of the human cargo, where he passed an hour before insisting he be allowed to sit in the cab to search for the jeep.

After another hour, with no sign of the Land Rover, Sol's legs began to thump, and he asked the driver if he was sure they were on the same route as the day before. The man just lifted his nose and pushed harder on the gas. When the bottom rim of the sun touched the horizon, the man waved his index finger in Sol's face and his thumb into the back of the truck.

At midnight, the bus pulled up to the gates of the compound in Umm Balla. The generator was silent, but Lila and André were reading by candlelight. They looked up as neutrally as they had three nights before, staring at Sol as if they had never before laid eyes on him.

Sol started the conversation. "Good news and bad news. We have three good spare tires but no Land Rover. It got stolen on the desert."

* * *

He left on the bus for Nyala the next morning without the spares but with a fresh supply of oatmeal, powdered milk, and cocoa. When the bus stopped at the various settlements along the route, he hunkered on the floor and slept until the village in which he had crushed the old lady's bird eggs. He snuck off the bus wrapped in his death shroud and walked deep into the desert to pee. When he re-tied his scrub pants and turned back toward the bus, a gaggle of Bedouin approached—AK-47s pointed toward the pale man. They surrounded him and demanded money for soiling their patch of desert with infidel water. He removed the portion of the shroud covering his face, sure they would recognize the nice doctor who had treated one of their own, but hands just tightened on the weapons. Sol handed over an inch-thick wad of quarter-penny notes.

As he lifted himself aboard the bus, he spotted a rectangular, black object on the other side of the primitive town. Not having expected any object with squared lines, he stared harder, and through his squint discerned a Land Rover, all its tires inflated. Two men sat in the front smoking, drinking tea, and swaying to Arabic music, the engine at idle with the air conditioner on high, puffing lukewarm air.

Sol ripped the shroud away, threw it into the back of the bus, and bristled past an old lady. Her basket of three eggs tumbled in front of his feet, and though he danced over them, she hit one with her fist and curdled the marketplace with her screams. Without stopping, he flung a few notes onto the egg mash and continued toward the Rover. Though he saw the AK-47s in the back, he yanked the front door open and motioned irately with his thumb. "Get out, both of you!"

The two froze, but just for an instant. They reached into the back for their weapons then charged out of the vehicle so harshly, the door banged into Sol and knocked him off his feet. The men jogged away but stopped and turned back to stare at him, their black faces reddening to the tint of the ferrous earth.

He jumped in and threw the vehicle into gear, but as the clutch came up, very little happened at the back wheels. He tried second gear, and the clutch slipped even more harshly. Back in first, he slammed the gas pedal to the floor and wheels abruptly gained purchase. The vehicle shot forward, fishtailing through the sand. He stopped at the bus for his death shroud and duffel bag. When he popped the clutch and waited for the tires to grab, the two men and their reinforcements marched toward Sol, AK-47s pumping above their heads. With the wheels barely turning, he let a five-inch stack of quarter-cent notes flutter from the driver's window to mix with the rank smoke from the burning clutch.

The gang of nomads threw their weapons aside and converged on the wafting money. As the tires engaged, the rubber generated a tornado of hot sand which peppered and blinded the men, but did nothing to stop their mad groping for the tiny bills.

* * *

In Nyala, Sol found a merchant with new tires and jerry cans. After his screams of disbelief at the inflated estimates and threats of death proffered by the salesman who brandished a corroded AK-47, they settled for nearly ninety percent less than the original quote. Sol paid the sixteen dollars with a scowl, but the storekeeper smiled, took Sol's hand, and shook it warmly. Sol gave him four more dollars.

He went to the restaurant near the hotel, and while it was noon, and the staff was clearly visible crawling in and out of the kitchen, the doors were still lashed shut. He went back to his hotel to eat a bowl of chocolate oatmeal in the barely air-conditioned lobby. He studiously ignored the stares of locals who were being charged half-a-penny admission by the desk clerk to watch the foreigner take his lunch. It was not until late in the afternoon that the clutch had been repaired, and he left for El Fasher.

Nearing midnight, Sol found a hostel in El Fasher that accepted foreigners but not Americans. So, he showed his Umm Balla Feeding Team papers and the address of the home office in London. He was given a bunk in the open dormitory. The dinner of spaghetti and meatballs was hours past, but the cook heated water for a bowl of chocolate oatmeal. The bathroom was also communal and had only a tub, one crusted with an oily sludge so thick, he returned to his cot to wait for darkness. At nine, he filled a plastic bag with the cold, green water from the tap, hung it from a low tree limb in the rear of the pension, punched a few holes with a bent nail, and showered in the drizzle for thirty seconds.

At first light, he drove to the El Fasher UN office to collect his funds. The secretary's head was bowed as she shuffled papers from the left side of her desk to the right. When she looked up, though, Sol gasped. The woman was magnificent, Norwegian, her hair the brightest blond, eyes sapphire blue. Sol felt he was staring at a ghost. When he gathered himself and asked for entry to the safe to withdraw money for an emergency food purchase, she asked in very meager English for his passport.

"Well, Miss," he gestured, moving his index finger in steps, "my passport's in the safe with the money."

She shook her head briskly, and her eyes dropped back to the papers.

"Ma'am, I need that money."

She huffed, "You do not have your passport. I cannot permit."

"Lady, look, don't screw around with me, okay? I'm not particularly in the mood. We've got a day or so left before our people start to die of starvation. I need into the safe."

"I will not screw with you," she shouted and jumped from her chair to sprint from the office.

An instant later, a large Scandinavian man pushed his way into the room and stood toe to toe with Sol. "What is the meaning of your sexual assault? This is not little America, you know."

By the time the various levels of UN administrators had weighed in, it was nearing noon and the office closed for lunch. They advised nothing could be done until mid-afternoon, and that when he returned, he needed to follow a strict protocol of sexually appropriate etiquette, as defined by the UN.

Sol agreed solemnly and walked to a *suq*, where he bought a few rounds of pita, comforted by the dearth of dark particulate matter. He paid a few pennies for a hunk of brine-soaked feta cheese, worried about his blood pressure for a moment, and paid two cents for a paper bag of dates. At the periphery of the market, he parked himself in the shade of a palm tree near a herd of camels being loaded with bags of grain. The camel drivers tied raw sacks over the animals' sore-covered backs. With each hundred-pound burlap bag thrown carelessly upon the last, the beasts screamed and spit in deeper and deeper defiance until Sol yowled at the *jamali* in English. His protests brought only the cessation of work. When they dropped their bags and started toward him, he turned and jogged back to the hostel.

At a roundabout in the middle of a barely paved intersection, he passed a circle of teenagers sleeping amongst the weeds. One of the boys awoke and looked up at Sol. He smiled, and Sol handed him the paper bag of dates. The boy took Sol's hand gently and shook it.

At three in the afternoon, the UN workers returned sluggishly to their duty stations, a steady patois of accented English reviling the heat and the bugs, but mostly the Africans. Sol went back to the office. The Norwegian had been replaced by a portly Bulgarian woman with a moustache. She glared at Sol as he dug through his cardboard cache. He withdrew twenty-thousand US in tens and twenties, placed it in three Zip Lock bags, tied them with a length of tooth floss, undid the cord belt on his scrub pants, dropped the bags into his underwear, tied the floss to the belt, and swaggered, nose high, from the room.

He went across the dirt road to the office of the UN High Commissioner for Refugees and asked where he could buy twenty-thousand pounds of food. The American woman at the desk stared at Sol for a moment. "We're not going to have any trouble with you, are we?"

"No, Ma'am, none whatsoever. Just tell me where I can purchase the food I need to feed the people we're supposed to be out here saving, and I promise you will *never* see me again."

She looked away and lifted the phone but dropped it harshly. "Same damn thing every day." She rose and brushed past him. Sol, thinking he had been dismissed, stepped into the hallway to leave, but the woman rounded a corner with a diminutive Icelandic man on her heels. He spoke with an accent so thick, Sol did not understand a word. The man wrote instructions on a slip of mildewed paper and pointed to the door. At a warehouse that had a number similar to that on the scrap of paper, Sol knocked at the wooden doors and waited. When there was no response after a third try, he went back to the UNHCR office. The American woman looked up and mumbled, "I thought you said you were leaving."

She fetched the Icelander, who whistled between his teeth. "Follow me," or that was what Sol thought he'd said. They marched back to the warehouse—the doors were wide open. An Asian man emerged into the blistering sun and invited them into an endless cavern of bagged grain. There was a somber discussion weighing the propriety of selling food to a non-UN agency, and Sol stood silently as the analysis went on, neither man speaking sufficient English to communicate.

A fire bell suddenly chimed at the UNHCR office, and the foreign staff retreated en masse to a larger building. The Asian man invited Sol to join them for tea, but when they got to the break room, the tiny Icelander greeted Sol with a glare, and Sol excused himself. He walked slowly through the broiling streets of El Fasher, nodding and smiling at the populace, who nodded and smiled back. He came to a *suq*, where he bought several freezing liters of Evian, found a bench in the shade, and laughed when the citizens stopped a few inches from him to point at his azure eyes.

A parade of teenaged girls in private school uniforms skipped by. Sol was struck by the starched white blouses, spotless after a day at the El Fasher Girls' Preparatory Academy. The navy skirts were neatly pleated, and the knee-high white stockings were still knee-high. They gawked at him as well, but coyly. He offered an unopened bottled of Evian, and they chattered at him. A comely seventeen-year-old stared at Sol with eyes so intense, his chest tightened. When he offered her a mint from a little tin, her comrades jumped back, though she took the candy. The girls stared then broke into a torrent of excited laughter that brightened the scalding air of the desert city. They soon drifted off, though most waved back at Sol, giggling and covering their faces.

A few minutes later, the first girl reappeared, her mother and father in tow. Dad pressed a plastic bag into Sol's hands. Inside, he felt a soft, warm round of pita, and Sol reached into his pocket to give the father a few pennies, but the family refused in unison. The father shook Sol's hand and blessed him with the grace of Allah.

At 4 P.M., he returned to the UN High Commission for Refugees, the UNHCR, building. The Asian man from the warehouse, now alone, introduced himself as the station director. He brought Sol into the storage building. The man pulled a small paper bag from his desk and asked if he would like tea. Sol noticed the lettering on the bag of loose tea and asked the man if he was Korean.

"How come do you ask?"

"I recognize the *Hangul* script."

"*Hangul*. No one know this word." He stared into Sol's eyes then stood. "I make tea."

Five minutes later they sat in the shadow of hundreds of tons of bagged food, crates of blue sheeting, plastic cups, bowels, and pails. The man smiled warmly. "Yes, I Korean. Impress you know *Hangul*.

"My father was a Marine infantryman in Korea during the war. Got shot twice. Why am I telling you all this?" Sol laughed sadly, adding, "He loved it there. We used to listen to Korean music on Sunday mornings in New York when we were kids, *nongak* and *pungmul*…"

The man's chin dropped, and he interrupted. "Oh, my God. You know *nongak, pungmul*?"

"Of course. I grew up on it. Even have some on my CD in the Rover. Anyway, he never forgot the Korean nurses or the local men who came into the hospital at night to light candles for the wounded. He said the Korean women were the most beautiful on Earth, and the men the toughest, even tougher than the Marines."

The man grasped Sol's hand, shaking it warmly with both of his. He muttered with eyes lowered, "You family sacrifice for my country Korea. Now you and family sacrifice for Africa. I thank you family and you. My name Chun Sae Il. Now, we fix for you."

He stood and beckoned, palm down, for Sol to follow deeper into the warehouse. They stopped at a tiny office. Chun worked at the primitive computer and produced a bill of lading granting 10 tons of *durra*, vegetable oil, dried okra, soap, sugar, coffee, powdered milk, and tinned *halal* meat to the refugee camp in Umm Balla.

He asked, "When you need supply?"

Sol thought for a moment and shook his head. "Probably too late to save the weakest. I was supposed to have the emergency supplies there by tomorrow. It's going to be three or four days until I can get the food down there, *if* I can find trucks and crews, and *if* we're not attacked."

"You think about fly supply?"

Sol sniggered but caught himself. "I don't mean to be rude Mr. Chun, but there's no airfield closer than Nyala, and that one is like a moonscape. Even if we got in there, I'd still have to hire trucks to cross the desert between Nyala and Umm Balla. I suppose we could drive around the clock and get the supplies there in a day if everything went perfectly, but it'll probably take days and days. Camp'll be closed by then. And where, my friend, are those people going to go?"

The man laughed again. "How you know to call me Chun, not Mr. Il like all American people?"

"Chun is your family name. Everybody knows that."

Chun shook his head and made a call on his cell phone. A white United Nations Land Cruiser rolled to the front of the warehouse. They jolted along the quasi streets of El Fasher to the airport, rolling up to a cinderblock structure not much larger than a walk-in closet, the chunks of hollow concrete forming the wall balanced at the amusement of gravity, no mortar having been expended in the bunker's construction. Signage was smeared in faded red letters on the raw concrete blocks near the corrugated metal roof.

CALCUTTA HELICOPTER
SERVING WORLD

A beturbaned South Asian man sat sleeping at his desk in the torpor of the afternoon. When Chun cleared his throat, the man jumped to his feet, nearly losing his balance. As he stuck a hand out to Chun, he knocked his ebony nameplate—**MISTER SINGH**—off the desk, and it landed face up on the floor.

"Mr. Il, so good to see you. Sit, please." The man pulled two chairs from the wall and introductions proceeded as he took two paces into the far corner to brew fragrant tea.

Mr. Singh sat facing his guests, snapping his very long, yellow fingernails. Finally, he announced, "Mr. Il, Doctor, have you noticed vind is dying? So, now our helicopters are ready to serve. Ve have new pilots, fresh from all over vorld, so much good fuel. Maintenance? Best in Sudan. So, vhat brings you here today?"

"Mr. Singh, Dr. Forte has large consignment UN food deliver Umm Balla. He want to use truck save fee for fly, but UN make sure your business good, so he listen *if* you good offer."

"Mr. Il, you know our price lowest in Sudan. And how much ve are to move?"

"Fifteen ton."

Before Chun's lips stopped moving, Singh's complexion transmuted from deep brown to red, his pupils narrowing into pinpoints. "And how far to go to Umm Balla?"

Chun looked to Sol, who answered, "Three hundred kilometers."

Singh's body shuddered and wavered as if he were about to lose consciousness. He sucked a deep breath of the boiling air. "Oh, no, it is no problem," his voice cracked like a teenager's. "Ve do dat all time." He rubbed his hands together. "So vhen you to go?" he asked brightly as he snatched a cell phone out of the desk drawer and punched in numbers. He held his palm up to Sol and Chun as he put the phone to his ear. He spoke in Hindi for some time, raising his voice occasionally, spit flying from his mouth in outrage, but he also mellowed and winked to his guests every few seconds as he listened. Occasionally, he nodded assuredly while he was speaking but ended the conversation abruptly, in midsentence, and flipped the phone back into the drawer. "Ve can do for sure, gentlemen. So ve vill go in morning, yes? Now, Doctor, how you to pay for service, if I may ask?"

Chun nodded to Sol, who spoke cautiously, "Cash. American dollars. But you need to give me a figure."

Singh sucked air through his teeth. "Oh, sir, dat very difficult until flight over. You see, you must leave certain amount, and ve vill refund vhat ve do not use. It is vay is done in Africa."

Sol laughed coldly, "Well, sir, it's not my money, so I can't really agree until I have a price and, of course, I still have to call my boss in London. He's such a stickler, that one."

"Oh, it is so hard. You know bring helicopter to Africa vas such expense, and aviation fuel so dear. And government. So many rule and regulation. Dis not old days, you know. Dey control everyting. So many license fee. Who knows vhat price to be tomorrow? And pilots. Oh, da pilots. Dey have awful union. Dey just vorking class, you know. Very low kind. It so hard make dem to understand economy and helping human being. Dey can fly, but not so very intelligent as doctor or UN man."

"Yeah, well, my father was working class and a union man, so I know what you mean." Sol looked at Chun and shook his head, then back at Singh. "Sorry we couldn't do business with you, but I can't just hand over piles of money. I'm sure you understand."

Sol rose and headed the three steps toward the door, waiting for Singh to stop him. Instead, Chun called out, "Doctor, let see if Mr. Singh come up with price in hour. Is okay?"

Sol paused, pretending to gather his patience. "Yes, sir, it would be okay."

"Very well. Mr. Singh, we come back in hour you have firm price?"

"A firm price, my friend, it impossible."

"A firm price, sir. Can you do?"

"I vill do best."

"Of course, do best, Mr. Singh," Chun smiled thinly.

Chun and Sol retired to a hotel in town to drink tea and do the arithmetic to come up with a bid of their own. At first, Sol calculated the price for the entire fifteen tons, three or so weeks of supplies, but Chun suggested they get enough to Umm Balla to last a week and truck the rest down. They could load five tons that night, take off at dawn, and have the first supplies in Umm Balla by early morning, when the air was still cool and the helicopters' rotors could work efficiently. Hopefully, they would still be able to take off from Umm Balla after offloading, and the sun had broiled the earth for an hour. The second sortie of two helicopters would have to wait until late afternoon to leave El Fasher, when the temperature had dropped below that of the surface of the sun. The pilots would spend the night in Umm Balla and return in the cool of the morning. Singh would hire, but the UN would pay for, laborers and trucks to get the food to the airport and onto the helicopter.

Chun was quiet for a moment then spoke softly, "Doctor, I must tell you something. I was ROK soldier Viet Nam—crew chief Huey helicopter. Are you angry at Chun?"

"Sir?"

"We hear many American hate soldier Viet Nam. Maybe I not tell you Chun soldier."

Sol shook his head slowly. "You, sir, are a hero. This American's father almost died for Korea, and you almost died to support us in return. My pop used to say the Republic of Korea soldiers, the ROK, were the toughest warriors on the planet. He loved you."

Chun brightened. "Doctor, Chun tell you money for Huey. Chun know HUEY like back hand.

"UH-1H carry maybe ten soldier. Soldier, gun, pack, radio, maybe one hundred kilo." Chun took a sheet of paper from his pocket and smiled comfortably as he scribbled numbers up and down the margins. "So, maybe one thousand kilo one helicopter. Two helicopter, two trip, four thousand kilo, one more helicopter, that more ten thousand pound. Good?"

"It's a lot more than we have now. It'll buy time."

"Okay, Chun tell you. Singh helicopter old. Weak. Maybe one hundred fifty kilometer one hour, maybe only one hundred thirty kilometer." Chun stared toward the heavens, thinking, churning numbers in his head. "Six hundred kilometer go Umm Balla come back El Fasher. Four-and-half hour go come back, give time load off food. One hour five hundred dollah. Maybe two thousand-four-hundred dollah one helicopter, one thousand kilo, give Singh few dollah to keep happy. Two helicopter go Umm Balla two time, then one more helicopter go, almost twelve thousand dollar. If Janjaweed see, helicopter go more high in sky, more fly time, more dollah. You have fifteen thousand dollah?"

When Chun and Sol pulled back up in front of Calcutta Helicopter, Mr. Singh was waiting outside, drenched in sweat. Chun looked at him and turned to Sol laughing. "He snap fingernail like a brick of firecracker on August Ten. That India day of independence from English."

Singh bade his new friends into the office with a broad smile and a nod. He brewed tea and pulled the rotting wicker chairs away from the wall.

There were smiles as the Darjeeling steeped. Singh lectured, "Ve must vait full two minute for flavor be released." He went on about the difference in the caffeine in tea and coffee, ending the treatise, "Coffee lower class. Pilots drink."

With the cups full, Singh took a seat and produced a pad of paper covered in delicate Devanagari. He began quietly. "My friends,

I have cut to bone. There is nothing more Calcutta Helicopter do to help UN and doctor. Mission to serve, but there bills and awful pilot union. I am only being realistic. Ve normally call for one tousand US dollars for hour, probably lowest in vorld, but for you, ve cut so much to nine hundred."

Sol's teeth clinched, but he locked and held Singh's eyes. "Okay, sir. Thank you. And how many hours are we talking about?"

"Now for entire twenty ton, ve…"

Sol interrupted. "Sir, we are going to deliver five tons now, and if that works out well, we will consider the whole load, and that was fifteen tons anyway. So how many hours are we talking about?"

"Well, this is new situation, yes? My calculation based on twenty ton. I need several hours to reanalyze situation, even den…"

"Mr. Singh," Chun interrupted, "we need helicopter very early tomorrow morning, and price need much better. You have two Huey, and only two Huey. Aircraft old, not carry many ton. You helicopter slow, dangerous. We not have time, so please give final price five minute."

Singh's shirt dripped with garlic-scented sweat, and he wiped his brow with the tail of his turban. "Give Calcutta Helicopter one minute, my esteem colleague." He pulled his chair up to the desk and took out the cell phone and a calculator, turning both on at the same time. He made a call, raised his voice, then quieted, and finally winked and nodded at his guests. He slapped the phone closed and smiled as if the deal had already been finalized. He tossed the phone toward the desk drawer, though his hands were trembling so, the phone missed its mark and slid along the floor, coming to rest at Sol's feet. The doctor picked it up gently, though he accidently touched the redial button—the last call had been made the day before.

Singh calculated furiously, finally drawing a deep breath, stuttering, "Now you please, cost fuel, union, cost bring airplane helicopter Sudan."

"So you say," Chun smiled.

"Okay, dis such low price. Give every consideration."

"What is it Mr. Singh?"

"Okay, for five sortie, six hundred kilometer, that five hour one sortie." He sucked in a grand gulp of fetid air, "At *only* eight-hundred-and-fifty dollar for hour, dat just twenty-one-tousand-two-hundred-fifty, and ve lose money, for sure, but ve here to serve poor people."

Sol stood and wiped his right hand on his filthy pants as he turned to the door. He called over his shoulder, "Mr. Singh, thank you for your time. You are a true humanitarian."

Chun followed and caught up to Sol. "Doctor, not to worry. Bastard drop price half, and he still make killing. We stand by here thirty second."

And when Singh ran from his bunker, Chun winked at Sol. "Mr. Singh, you had mellow of heart?"

"Vell, Calcutta Helicopter, ve here to serve poor, not profit. Come, come back to office. Ve find vay."

Sol smiled directly at Singh and nodded. The anxious little man's shoulders dropped in relief. He filled the kettle to brew more tea and defended over his shoulder, "Oh, but do you know, sir, expense of rebuilding, and fuel, and pilots, and union? Dere is no money in aviation here. Just service to people."

Sol asked abruptly, "What is your final offer Mr. Singh?"

"I must do more calculation. You see, tomorrow, but I hear fuel price go sky high."

"Sol sighed, "Enough. I'll give you thirteen-thousand. Cash money right now. Yes or no?"

"Oh, Doctor, you do not understand…"

Sol rose. Chun shook his head at Singh and walked out. As they got into to the UN jeep, Singh ran to Chun's window. "Okay, eighteen-tousand."

"I said thirteen," Sol spat, leaning across his new UN colleague.

Singh waved his head back and forth, the sweat dripping in cascades. "Okay, sixteen."

"Good." Sol smiled. "Fifteen. You have a deal."

Sol emerged from the jeep with his right hand extended. Singh muttered aloud to himself that he couldn't fathom how he was going to meet that price and stay in business, but nodded toward the office and shook Sol's hand halfheartedly. Once inside, he pulled reams of documents printed on Sudanese government, tissue-grade paper from a desk drawer. Singh started to write, though paused and looked away from his guests. "Oh, dere is one more issue, you know. It is very important. And, of course, I have no control over dis ting. Dere is da matter of da Minister of Aviation, Muhammad Ibin Ibin's personal fees, and dose of Airport Director Muhammad Ali Ahmed Yahia al-Quarish, and den da fire chief and fuel merchants. So, you see, da bill, he is back to twenty-five tousand."

A wave of nausea clutched Sol's gut. He became lightheaded, sat down, and dropped his head between his knees. Singh eyed his customer wearily, though droned on adding per diem fees for the pilots who would have to spend the night in Umm Balla after the second sortie, the air far too hot for the ships to take off in the late afternoon and fly back to El Fasher, even if they were empty. "Oh, Doctor, you must pay hotel cost, taxi, meal, tip, laundry."

Chun laughed sarcastically. "Mr. Singh, there not hotel or taxi in Umm Balla since creation. Doctor, you so kind provide place to stay night for crew...and meal?"

Sol looked up, pale and confused. "Do you think they'll eat chocolate oatmeal?"

"Excuse me, Doctor?"

"Well, we have no food. It's Umm Balla. They need to bring their own, and blankets, toiletries, and water. They knew that when they signed on to fly at the end of the Earth, or should have. Any other questions?"

Sol reached into his underwear and pulled one of the clear baggies of money free. He proffered it to Singh, who hesitated for an instant, his nostrils flaring, until his eyes fixed on the wad of green inside. His hand shot forward, fingernails tearing at the bag and pulling the cash out with a sigh. He fanned the bills vehemently, then again, and a third time. "Dat is only ten tousand, Doctor."

Sol nodded. "You get the other five when all the food's on the ground, intact, in Umm Balla, and that has to be within the next forty-eight hours. Deal?"

Singh hemmed and hawed, his hands shaking so, Sol could feel the breeze churning from the bills.

"Chun grunted, "Deal?"

A nearly inaudible, "Deal," was moaned, a single signature appended, and the covenant was ratified.

William Stuart Gould, M.D.

CHAPTER FOUR

A t eight that evening, in the roasting Sudanese dusk, laborers and trucks rolled toward Calcutta Helicopter, though one had a blowout and pulled onto the active runway to change the tire. *Jellabiya*-begowned men loaded the two helicopters quickly, tossing in bags helter-skelter, leaving several hanging halfway out the door, and a few piled on the pilots' seats, leaning against the controls. When Singh drove up in a brand-new Land Rover, he became apoplectic, ordering the gang to offload the shipment and place the bags in cargo nets.

Sol held up his hand to stop the work and hissed at Singh, "Wait a minute. This burlap is worthless." He pulled a scrap of the rotted material easily from one of the bags. "What if the bags break during the flight? What happened to the nylon bags it was originally sent in from the US?"

"Ve change bags to burlap at varehouse. Sell nylon bag. Save money for you."

"You mean I owe less than five more thousand?"

"No, it mean you not owe more dan eight tousand."

Sol carped, "This stuff is crap. These bags won't last five miles, especially if they're riding in that cargo net. The grain'll drop out onto the desert. What good is that? This is beginning to piss me off."

"Doctor, you do not have to punch me vit profanity. And vhat if der is problem during the flight, and ve have to lighten ship? Did you vant pilot climb over seat to trow out bag? Dis vay, ve just push cargo release pedal, drop load. Save ship, yes? And anyvay, ve need to send along fuel barrel. No room inside for *durra*. Not to vorry, Doctor, ve know vhat ve doing."

At four the next morning, Chun and his driver were waiting in front of Sol's hotel. They drove the silent alleys of El Fasher, suffering but a single flat tire. When they met the pilots, four of them, in the tiny office, the seven men were squeezed so tightly, there was no need to plug in the space heater, which would not have worked, the generators of the City of El Fasher still hours from rebirth. The men poured over the sectional maps by flashlight, though Sol noted, despite Singh's palm flattened over the legend, the charts were many years old.

When the bickering ceased and a flight plan agreed upon, the two sets of pilots departed to preflight their ships. Sol walked with them and asked where they came from. The two captains were Filipino, one silver-haired, one quite young; one first officer was Indonesian, the other British, an older, pasty-faced man who reeked of stale alcohol and whose hands trembled as if he were already in flight.

When it was time to take off, the pilots belted themselves in, did the pre-start checks, then sat, hands folded on their laps staring at Sol. He had, though, backed away from the helicopters, worried that as soon as the engine lit, the Englishman's breath would set off a fireball. But they did not push the buttons to start the engine, and Singh drove his Land Rover to Sol and asked, "Doctor, is dere problem?"

"No, sir. Just waiting to watch the supplies go."

"Doctor, dey cannot take off until you go aboard."

"Me?"

"Doctor, how vill dey find Umm Balla if you not go?"

There was no seat for Sol, nor a piece of metal, rubber, or cloth left aboard to clutch, the ships' guts having been stripped of every ounce of original material that did not make money for Calcutta Helicopter. So, he wedged himself between the leaking barrels of aviation fuel and grunted several extra Hail Marys.

The ship shuddered as the tow rope became taut, and the elderly pilot cursed loud enough to be heard over the racket of the prehistoric jet engine. The man lowered the collective, allowing the ship to settle a bit, but suddenly pulled hard and got a head start going straight up. This time the cargo net popped off the ground, swung a few arcs, and set the ship undulating in a resonance that caused it to rock faster and faster, until the pilot dropped the collective and landed. He jumped out of the ship, swore at Singh, went to the net, offloaded three bags by himself, jumped back in, and pulled full power all at once. The aircraft vaulted from the ground, entering a sort of stable hover taxi, dragging the cargo net along the packed, orange earth. Kernels of grain soon popped free to shoot about in the rotor wash, thrashing the sides of the aircraft like pellets of sand in the haboob. When there was enough airspeed to transition from a hover to actual flight, the silver-haired pilot crossed himself, dropped the helicopter's nose, mumbled his own string of Hail Marys, and pulled up hard on the collective lever. At an altitude of five hundred feet, the ship's oscillations began again, but the pilot just cursed and kept them headed southwest. During the entire operation, the British first officer remained in his right seat, head back, perhaps asleep, body unflinching, save trembling hands the captain refused let touch the controls.

As they gained altitude very slowly, a vast, hazy expanse of reddish desert opened before them, and the air aboard the ship cooled. Sol leaned against one of the exposed structural ribs, shivering, but eventually drifted off into a troubled sleep. He awoke to find the helicopter had reached three thousand feet, cruising at nearly a hundred miles per hour over the desert, the compass never budging from the southwesterly course the captain had set.

The other ship flew low and to the right, off less than a hundred feet. Sol waved to the captain below; the younger Filipino pilot saluted and smiled broadly. When Sol gave him a thumbs up, the pilot lifted his ship and drew closer, and then closer still, until the main rotors overlapped and the swinging loads of *durra* nearly bounced into each other. They flew like that for a few minutes until a bit of turbulence jugged them around, and the blades came within inches of striking. The other helicopter dropped off and retook its place on the flank. Sol, with hands quivering as uncontrollably as the first officer's, dropped to the floor to lie flat on his stomach, head protruding from the open rear hatch, watching the desert go by. As Nyala passed to the left, Sol searched for the desert track, the telephone poles, and the *wadi*. When he finally spotted his landmarks, he could make out the bus in the distance, surrounded by tiny dots on prayer mats facing Mecca.

The captain yelled to get Sol's attention, pointing out the other door, and Sol crawled across the floor to see a massive mountain looming just miles to the right of their flight path. The pilot yelled out, "Mount Mara. They say Jebel Mara! Ten thousand feet!"

A few miles further into the flight, Sol noticed a cloud near the surface moving southwest in a straight line. He guessed it was a meteorological phenomenon, perhaps a desert cyclone, and he thought about the thermodynamics of the air being heated so ferociously, and how privileged he was to be witnessing nature in the raw. All of it made scientific sense until he saw, out of the corner of his eye, the pilot's hand yank on the collective so hard, the ship hurtled upward, jamming Sol into the floor as if the seventeen bags of the *durra* had been dropped on his back. The aircraft's nose rotated up, and the ship climbed frantically for a few more seconds. As the helicopter leveled, Sol noticed it had slowed to a near stop, but was much further above the desert floor. The captain had traded all of his airspeed for altitude, but Sol did not know why.

The pilot turned to Sol and shouted, "Five thousand! No sweat!" His thumb flew up into the air, and he reached across to shake the first officer's shoulder in congratulations. The latter barely nodded and settled his head back against the seat.

The captain worked the controls, inching the helicopter forward, mile-per-hour by mile-per-hour, until they were cruising again at ninety knots, though they soon began to jink left and right as if avoiding airborne obstacles that only he could see. Despite the rocking, Sol's pilot was able to keep the cargo from swinging, but the other helicopter's load was banging around like an out-of-control pendulum. Sol's empty stomach growled and soured, and his head was soon back out the door retching up the meals he had not eaten in weeks. When the helicopter settled back into a steady course toward the southwest, Sol crawled forward, roaring to the helmeted pilot, "What's going on? I'm dying back here."

The man pointed down, hollering over the engine noise. "Doctor, the Janjaweed." His finger jabbed at Dr. Forte's low altitude weather system, now a band of mounted riders, all of whom had stopped and were firing rifles at the helicopters. Green tracers arced back to Earth a thousand feet below them, and the two aviators laughed derisively, the captain staring blankly at the riders and uttering in Tagalog, "*Pasyensya na lang po, ako ay kulang-kulang.*"

Sol shouted, "What does that mean?"

"Same as that," the pilot laughed, nodding at the co-pilot, who had come back to life, his index and little fingers extended out of the window, pumping up and down at the horsemen. "He calls it, 'The old two-finger.'"

A few miles past the Janjaweed, the helicopters settled back down to three thousand feet, and in half-an-hour, the Umm Balla camp came into sight, a smudge of blue-black interrupting the orange wasteland of western Sudan. Sol stood between the pilots' seats and pointed excitedly toward the blemish on the horizon. "That's it!"

The pilot smiled and yelled, "Sounds to me, Doctor, that you can't wait to get back to your home in the desert. That takes a special man."

They made a slow, sand-enveloped approach toward the shit fields, churning the clouds of flies in the main rotor. The more of them they minced, the more they sucked up from the acres of drying feces. Sol directed them to the other side of the camp, to an open area that was devoid of squatting figures. As the cargo nets touched the ground, waves of refugees rushed toward the food, and Sol felt a wave of gratification he had never before sensed. His life had finally earned meaning—innocent souls would live because he had dared to act. But the masses of tattered, bone-thin humans ran forward, arms madly waving off the helicopters, throwing stones and wads of scorched earth at the aircraft. The checkers amongst them pointed wildly toward the other side of the camp.

Sol's captain lifted off, barely, and flew, dragging the cargo gradually along the sand, hovering over a patch of earth back in the realm of the shit fields. Suffering no obvious opposition to dropping the food there, the captain looked to Sol, who shrugged. The pilot hit the little red DROP LOAD pedal, and the cargo net tumbled six feet to the ground. The helicopter did not gain or lose an inch of altitude. When the other ship pulled into position, it burst a hundred feet higher as its cargo was released. Sol's captain laughed and turned to his co-pilot. "That's something we need to work on, isn't it, First Officer?" but the man was barely awake. The two aircraft hover taxied closer to camp, blowing the plastic from the tops of a quarter mile of huts.

André was the first to greet them. "*Mais*, Doctor, why do you land first time in ze graveyard? And now you break zer house. Ze people are very mad, you know."

Sol started to answer, but turned to the four crew members, calling out, "Welcome to the gem of the Sahel, Umm Balla Refugee Camp, where fifty people a day died of starvation each day until you brought food. God bless you for your work."

He shook his head and strode past André to the mob of checkers standing beside their foreman, Muhammad. "Mr. Muhammad, please tell the people of Umm Balla that we are sorry to land in the graveyard, but that we have brought food from the UN to give them so that they and their children can live."

The man turned to the crowd and, eyes down, spoke in an embarrassed whisper, the assemblage quiet at first until an old man called out loudly in Arabic, "Very well, but why do they desecrate our dead? *Al hum de le la*."

"Because we don't want any more dead," a shrill, angry voice spat in English from the back of the throng as Lila pushed her way through the masses. She stopped in the center, inches from Muhammad's face, repeating her dictum. "Tell them, Muhammad. Loud. Tell them."

So, the slender, handsome man took a deep breath and tried again. This time, several of the men came forward and shook Lila's hand, bowing faintly. She waved them forward, toward the largess that had dropped from the sky, and bid them open the nets and carry the sacks to the distribution center.

As they turned to do Lila's bidding, the older pilot tapped Sol on the shoulder. "Sir, we must be on our way. Are you coming?"

"No, I'll stay here until you bring the second load this afternoon, and then I'll go back with you tomorrow morning to pick up the jeep and settle up with Mr. Singh. You be careful on the way back. Fly high and fast." The Filipino captain shook Sol's hand warmly, as did the young captain of the other ship. By the time they had removed the kids from the pilots' seats and pulled another two dozen from their crawl over the fuselage, another fifteen minutes had evaporated. The aircraft jumped into the climb before the heating air denied flight, then sped off into the sun.

At dusk, the two helicopters cruised back into camp, another cloud of flies blended in the rotors, specks of what appeared to be volcanic ash settling over Umm Balla. The gang of porters who emerged from the black fog to offload the helicopters studied the grains of descending pepper; several of them tasted the cinders they plucked from the patina on their forearms. Their faces remained neutral, and that way for the next thirty minutes as the complexities of lifting a sack and carrying it to the storehouse were hashed and rehashed with the checkers and the men.

As the labor force began hauling bags of *durra*; shrink-wrapped, four-packs of plastic, one-gallon vegetable oil bottles; and boxes of salt, pepper, dried okra, milk powder, sugar, and soap from the cargo nets, the British first officer sidled over smiling, carefully eyeing the procession, particularly absorbed in the transfer of the vegetable oil. When one old man lifted a bundle of oil bottles and rested it on his shoulder, the Englishman lunged toward him, an open pocket knife aimed at the porter.

Lila gasped and ran toward the copilot as he sliced, but the blade was directed at the plastic wrap, not the man. He pulled free a single container, one a slightly different shade than the others. He folded his arms over it, hurried back to his duffle bag in the back of the helicopter, and placed it inside as gently as if laying a baby in a bassinette.

He made his way to the Land Cruiser, where he crawled into the backseat and drifted off to sleep. The bags were loaded, and the jeep lurched off toward the foreigners' camp. It struggled under the weight of the seven bodies, and André was forced to drive just a couple of miles per hour. There was little conversation until Sol muttered, "I'm glad to be back. Umm Balla's bad, the road's worse."

"Ah, our old friend Cervantes again," André snipped.

"Whatever. We have one more shipment tomorrow, so I think we'll be okay for a week or so. I'll go back to El Fasher in the morning and get some trucks to bring the rest of the food. That's a month's worth. We can relax for a while."

André asked harshly. "How do you know ze rest will get srew?"

"Same as I knew ze first load would get *srew*."

In the common hut, the party fell into seats silently, exhausted. The British co-pilot, though, dug through his bag and drew out the plastic bottle of "cooking oil." While he held it high jubilantly, the other airmen rolled their eyes until the man asked for several cups, filled them, and passed the mugs around. The Indonesian first officer winced, shook his head, and turned his back to the Brit. André opened his meager store of powdered Tang, added a teaspoon to his drink, and downed his cocktail in less than thirty seconds. Lila's drink was also gone quickly, and though everyone expected her compatriot to guzzle his, the man sat quietly for a bit, staring through the cloudy fluid at the flickering candles, his lips vibrating subtly as if in prayer. Sol and the two Filipino captains shrugged and sipped their drinks quietly. The British flier suddenly howled an incantation, pulled the cup roughly to his lips, poured it down his throat, then whispered behind his hand, nodding toward the Indonesian co-pilot, "A Mohammedan, you know."

Lila kicked off her sandals, leaned back, and stared at the plastic jug. The host refilled her glass. Lila giggled, "André, my good man,'ow 'bout you pour a little sugar on me, sugar?" André scooped out a larger teaspoon of the Tang than he had taken for himself, and Lila's second round was gone in a single swallow.

After the third, Sol stood, stretched, and mumbled, "Well, time to get everyone bedded down. We need to be up really early. Captain, why don't you bunk in my hut. It's tiny—barely holds one, but we'll be okay."

He suggested the other men divide themselves between André's shed and the common room, but the Englishman looked at Lila and slurred, "And why not the British fight the night together, eh what?"

Both André and Sol glared at the man, but she laughed, "Not to worry, gentlemen. I can care for myself, and anyway, my mate, here, he couldn't you know what…"

Sol nodded and put his arm around André's shoulder. "Our lady's just fine. See you in the A.M., my brother."

The British pilot tried to stand, fell back onto the couch, tried again, failed again, unhitched his belt, pried off his boots precisely, placed them on the ground with great care, and bunched one of the cushions into a pillow. He rolled onto his side and was snoring before the older captain opened the first officer's bag to pull out a blanket and cover the man. The two Filipino men hugged each other and spoke a few words in Tagalog.

In Sol's hut, the captain pulled out an inflatable air mattress and a mosquito net, but Sol insisted he take the cot. They washed and brushed their teeth alongside Lila and André at a pot of water propped on a stool in the moonlight.

When Sol blew out the candle, he asked, "Captain, what brings you here, and you know, sir, I am embarrassed, but I don't even know your name."

"Doctor, I don't know yours either. It is wrong. We are very important to each other, yes?"

"Indeed, we are. I am Sol Forte."

"And I am Romeo Luzon. But everyone calls me Romey."

"Do you live up to your name?"

"Oh, I did many years ago. Great memories, every one of them." He was silent for a moment before adding, "But now I leave that to my son."

"Where is your son, sir? In the Philippines?"

"Philippines? Doctor, no. He is the other pilot! You didn't know?"

"Oh, my God! What a kick, flying with your son—in Africa! Where did you learn to fly?"

"In the Army, the US Army. I was a pilot in Viet Nam, a warrant officer. Three tours. Where do you think I learned to curse so well?"

"What are you doing here?"

"Like you, I hope doing something, Doctor."

"You could be making a lot more in the Philippines, I imagine."

"Oh, I retired years ago. Twenty-three thousand hours. It was enough, but my son told me about this job, and I love him so much. I thought what the hell, as long as we could be together."

"How much is that guy Singh paying you?"

"Twenty-six an hour."

"Oh, my God. What a bastard."

"Well, Doctor, he wagered his whole life on these two helicopters. He has a family, too, back in Tanzania. He's losing everything right now. If you hadn't come along, he was done. He was going to go back to Tanzania, a failure in front of his family, especially his two boys. That is very painful for them, you know. He wasn't even going to be able to pay to have the aircraft sent home. He was going to donate them to the Sudanese government. He was sick at the thought. Do you have children, Doctor?"

"No, I lost my wife and sister on…" He stopped short and looked down. "It isn't such a big deal after you see Umm Balla for a while."

"So, you understand."

Sol nodded and asked, "And your first officer?"

"Malcolm? Another tragedy. The worst drunk I ever met, and I knew many back in the army. He flew attack helicopters in the Royal Air Force, in the Argentine War. Shot down, captured, mutilated…"

"I'm sorry, I don't know what you mean."

"Well, Doctor, let us say that he would not have been much of a threat to your Ms. Lila. RAF discharged him immediately after he was released from the POW camp. Gave him a few hundred pounds and showed him the door, claimed he would be a distraction if he remained in the forces. Yet he still wears his RAF boots. Can't understand that. Keeps them shined, too, just like in flight school."

In the morning, the crew brought out the food they had carried. Malcolm roasted bangers over an oily kerosene lantern. The Filipino men opened tins of *baboy adobo*, while the Indonesian first officer fished from his duffle bag balls of glutinous rice spiced with bits of beef, onion, and garlic, all wrapped compactly in banana leaves."

"Where did you get all of this?" Sol laughed as the spoils were passed around.

"We have our contacts in Khartoum, and they sneak this out to us on the relief flights. Beer, too, but our friend Jati here doesn't know about that, do you?" Captain Luzon jibbed.

Jati ignored the teasing but finally stammered. "And when they catch you, it is one hundred lashes, *each*! And I am the one they choose to deliver the blows, for sure." He laughed and sputtered, "And I will be captain of both ships in those days!" He put his hand on Captain Luzon's shoulder and grasped it warmly, pulling away slowly to scoop a heap of his rice onto the Captain's plate.

When they took off in the cool of the morning, the light ships sprang off the desert like gazelles and sprinted back to El Fasher at 6,000 feet. Captain Luzon had Sol sit on the left, in the co-pilot's seat, while Malcolm snuggled up between the oil drums and drifted off, snoring so loudly it swamped the din of the jet engine. Passing over Nyala, Luzon croaked into the intercom, "Take the controls, Doctor. I need a rest and a beer."

Sol placed his right hand gently on the cyclic, the stick that turned the helicopter left and right, nose up, nose down. Romey leaned back, pretending to close his eyes, but every time there was a hiccup, Romey's hand snapped to the controls. No matter how many times Captain Luzon redressed the ship, after a few seconds, the helicopter began to swing like a crooked pendulum, up/down, back/forth, left/right, until the first officer called from between his barrels, "Cap'n, what the 'ell's up? You got a maize cob up your arse or somethin'?"

In El Fasher, one ship was loaded quickly with the remaining freight, and Sol hugged Romey, who had volunteered to fly the sortie back down to Umm Balla. Perhaps he would see the captain and the first officer again, if Sol had trouble hiring trucks and had to stay the night, but Chun drove up and told Sol that he had a caravan loaded, ready to head out. Romey saluted Sol, hugged him again, and whispered, "Thank you for your work." The captain jumped aboard the ship and was gone.

William Stuart Gould, M.D.

CHAPTER FIVE

It took twelve hours for the trucks to work their way a hundred miles down the paved highway toward Nyala. Between prayers, smoke breaks, and flat tires, the convoy pulled off the road into the desert every few miles. Late that night, they drove into the sands surrounding Nyala. After the men prayed, they boiled water for tea before crawling under their rigs to sleep. Sol spent the night in the jeep, having gathered a half-dozen burlap bags from the UN warehouse as insulation. After a bowl of chocolate oatmeal, he fell into a comfortable sleep.

They set out at dawn after prayers, and one of the early-teen tire-changers begged Sol to let him ride in the jeep. He said through the interpreter that he wanted to see what air conditioning was like and listen to CDs. Each time they stopped, the boys traded places, and by the village with the lady selling eggs, all of them had had a turn. Sol remained out of the settlement, but the men went to the *suq* for tea and cigarettes. They came back mumbling amongst themselves, small cells of drivers and mechanics pacing in circles, grumbling more vociferously each time they completed an orbit around their trucks. The interpreter came to Sol. "Worker disturb. Very angry. Big fighting desert south. Many green tracer fly to sky. Many fire smoke. More money."

Sol laughed, explaining, "Tell them that was just the Janjaweed shooting at the helicopters, but their bullets do not go high enough to harm the airplanes. Not to worry. Everything's fine."

Sol considered upping the pay from a dollar to a dollar-fifty a day and allocating the bonus from his own funds. But he thought about Chun, who had ventured so perilously close to being sacked in order to get the supplies to Umm Balla. He had asked nothing from Sol, cooking the books to make it appear he had determined the need in Umm Balla was so urgent, the UN was justified in paying twenty cents over the normal eighty-cents-a-day for truck men. When word of that largess leaked, the queue of men who had lined up in El Fasher for the jobs was a mile long. The contract was simple and foolproof: not a cent was to be paid until the food was offloaded in Umm Balla and the trucks safely back in El Fasher. As added surety, Chun had had all the men swear on the *Quran* to Allah that they would not quit until they completed their mission.

But there was André's tale about the workers in the Umm Balla camp striking on the first day, and Sol realized Chun's contract, or any pact made in Darfur, had milk teeth at best. He spit hard, walked to his jeep, cranked up, blew the horn a few blasts, and let a few bills blow out of his window. Wind spread the money, and the truckers drove off frantically after it. Sol sprinted off west, leaving a riot of sand in his wake. When that settled, he glanced in the rearview mirror and laughed at the cloud of filth enveloping the convoy that was chasing him. Sol slowed but stayed a hundred yards to the front, as if still running to get away.

He drifted southwest until the *wadi* came into view, then dropped into the trench, spinning up to nearly twenty miles per hour. The trucks, though they had followed Sol's vehicle to the edge of the dried riverbed, refused to roll down into it. Sol stopped, drove back to the main contingent, and asked the interpreter why the convoy remained in the soft sands. He shook his head, "Mister, truck if go in *wadi* not come out. Man unload carry load. No money enough." He rubbed his fingers together expectantly, but Sol spit again and took off in his jeep with the trucks moving parallel to the *wadi*, bumping at ten or twelve miles per hour in the loose silt.

After several more kilometers, Sol was far to the front of the lead truck, and he slowed to let them catch up. When the caravan came within a hundred meters, the lorries stopped abruptly, and the drivers jumped from their cabs to run into the desert. Sol lost sight of them as they sprinted, and he imagined they had been spooked by the *jinn*, so he pulled out of the *wadi* to chase and persuade them to come back. To hell with the money, he cursed. They were close, so close.

As Sol's Rover pulled up to desert level, he saw the men, dirty white *jellabiyas* blowing in the wind, gathered around a black, smoking ball in the distance. They might have, he speculated, actually found the *jinn*, and that would be an opportunity to show them that the devil was but a paper tiger, a toothless mirage. As he drove closer, however, he realized the smoldering mass was not a spirit, but a twisted heap of metal, a truck, one of their friend's rigs, he imagined. He stopped the jeep and pushed through the mob. His heart clutched when he saw the wreckage for what it was, an aircraft. He could barely breathe.

The gang of trembling men opened a passage to what was left of the cockpit. There were a few small holes through the metal on the right side of the fuselage, and two in the transmission housing under the intact, but charred, rotor. The left seat was empty, the door open, slamming rhythmically in the ceaseless wind. Though the seat cushion was somewhat charred, there was no burned-in silhouette of a former occupant. Sol was confused and lifted his eyes to lock on a compact, scorched mass in the right seat. He gasped, and his field of vision darkened as he walked to the other side of the ship. He barely noticed skid marks that came from a hundred meters back in the desert right up to the helicopter. He did not know what they meant but didn't stop to think about it. He continued on to the co-pilot's side and wrenched the door open, his eyes drawn down to the dangling pair of blackened poles below the remains in the seat. Sol was not shocked to find a pair of blistered, leather RAF flying boots welded to the floor. Despite the charring, there were scraps of unburned blue cotton pants, the uniform of the men who flew in the Sudan.

Sol's gut contracted, and he turned away, so lightheaded and nauseated, he was barely able to struggle back to the jeep. With his head hung, he could not help but notice the ground was covered with a veneer of black, unctuous soot under which sat a troop of hoof marks spread around the circumference of the wreckage. He started the Rover's engine, turned the air conditioning to full, and sucked in globs of lukewarm air until the nausea passed.

The drivers and helpers jabbered for a bit, lit cigarettes, and drifted back toward their trucks, pointing at the debris and then at Sol.

And there they sat, staring at their employer, waiting. When his blood pressure rose adequately, he lifted himself slowly from the driver's seat and approached the men. He mumbled for them to mount their trucks, spread out, and find the pilot. He took the interpreter by the sleeve. "Tell them he can't be far. Tell them to yell, 'Romey, Romey.'"

The man shouted at the drivers, but they pointed at the ground and shook their heads vehemently. The interpreter squawked, "Horse foot here. Many, many Janjaweed. Take man. Money you give truck man. Driver 'fraid Janjaweed. No go."

"Tell them fifty dollars for the truck that finds him and brings him back alive. Do you understand me?"

The man's forehead broke into a glaze of sweat, the toothbrush twig falling from his mouth. When he spoke, the men's eyes blazed as fiercely as the *jinn*, and Sol's shoulder's relaxed faintly, but they did not move. Sol kicked the sand angrily. "Okay, tell them one hundred dollars. And that's it. If they don't get moving, I'll find the man myself, and they'll get nothing."

When the interpreter calmed himself, he spoke tremulously, "Sir, you can no do. You no know desert."

"Watch me now." With not a flicker of movement from the hunkered troops, Sol roared, "Screw it." He started toward his jeep, but the men shot in a mad dash back to their trucks, pushing, shoving, and hollering at the slower of their colleagues to move aside. The vehicles belched gusts of greasy smoke that enveloped the dozen helpers who had not yet reached their lorries. The latter lunged aboard the nearest vehicle, but most tumbled onto the desert floor as the trucks sprinted off in first gear, tires chucking funnel clouds of sand over them. In seconds, a half-dozen antique jalopies jockeyed for position as they crawled away from the wreck, waiting for tires to gain purchase. A blue, smoky fog soon billowed from the trucks as the drivers burned away the last of the rubber. Two of the lorries dropped out when their tires burst. The remaining four ground on, in line, following the hoofprints. They drove for several miles until two more rolled to a stop with flats. Another stalled with a radiator that gushed a stream of rusty water onto the sands. The last truck sailed off across the Sahel weaving left and right, avoiding the thorn bushes until it ran out of gas. Sol rode up, gave the driver a jerry can of fuel, and screamed, "Murphy's fuckin' law," and made hand signals, sending the man back to the helicopter.

When all the trucks gathered again at the wreck, Sol had the interpreter go to each of the drivers and get an assessment of how long it would take to repair the vehicles: two days, maybe three, and only if they dragged the one with the damaged radiator. Sol ordered the men to remove it from the truck and throw it into the back of his jeep, the last rivulets of rusty water dripping onto his dwindling cache of oatmeal. He triangulated the map position of the trucks, drew a diagram of the local features, told the interpreter that he would be back within two days, and headed east toward Nyala.

Sol was out of spares when he rolled up to the Hotel Finest Africa. The porters tripped over each other to grab his bags and shook their heads when they saw the accumulation of flats in the rear. "Didn't we just get these fixed, *Doctori?*"

He spent the night in the same room. The shower drain was clogged, and he rasped at it with the end of a hanger until he pulled a lump of toilet paper free. The municipal electric services were again terminated just shy of 8 P.M., as the sun set, and a column of mosquitos filed in through a tiny crack in the window. He fashioned a tent of the bed sheets, suspending them from the fan with lengths of dental floss. It served to lock out a few of the less aggressive parasites. At dawn, he had the tires repaired, bought a used radiator that looked only remotely like the one he had traded in, cooked a bowl of chocolate oatmeal, and assured himself that the rusty aftertaste meant he was recharging his body with the minerals his diet had lacked for so many weeks. By the calendar, it was well into the 21st Century. Surely, he would find a telephone to call Singh and the UN in El Fasher to get word back about what had happened.

When Singh answered, he did not understand who was on the other end, so he cursed aloud and closed his cell phone. On the third try, in between Singh's ranting, Sol yelled for him to shut up and listen, then hurriedly related the catastrophe. Singh remained quiet for several moments before breaking into a fit of enraged yelping, first in Hindi, then English. In between the man's gasps, Sol spoke softly, soothingly, but Singh plummeted into an unintelligible sob. Sol assured Mr. Singh he would help Calcutta Helicopter in any way he could, but the line went dead just as Singh had calmed sufficiently to ask how.

Sol called Mr. Chun. After a few tries, there was a ring tone on the other end, but the secretary, hearing the name Dr. Sol Forte, lost the call. Sol called back, changing his voice and claiming to be United States Senator Edward Kennedy.

As Sol told the story, Chun remained speechless, though after a few seconds, commented, "Romey Luzon—he good man. Singh never replace pilot like that. Damn Africa."

Sol interrupted. "Mr. Chun, wait. I don't believe he's dead. I think they took him for ransom. It looked to me as though the helicopter may have been hit with bullets, but it didn't crash. I'm sure. One of the pilots had to be very alive and alert to land it so gently. Thinking back, there was a track in the sand where they slid to a stop. It was a hundred meters long. It had to be a soft stop, not a crash. I'm betting Captain Luzon put it down, saw the co-pilot was already dead, and was out the door before it burned. There wasn't any structural damage except where the fire melted strips of plastic. There was definitely no explosion. The fuel tanks were intact, with fuel still inside, but the cap on one was open. I don't understand that.

"And there were hoof prints all around the wreckage, horses, but the charring on the sand was on top of them. That's it! The fire was set by hand to make it look like the helicopter had crashed. The charring happened *after* the horsemen left. So, they took Captain Luzon for ransom. That's the only explanation.

"This was well planned. The Janjaweed are not stupid. Well, maybe they are, but the people in Khartoum who are calling the shots are not."

Chun whispered into the phone, "Doctor, you not talk that. Government," he hissed, "not control militia. Please careful what you say."

Sol muttered, "Thank you, sir, for the warning. But here we are, and we have to do something with the first officer's remains. We can't leave him out there. And we need to find Captain Luzon. What do you suggest?"

"Doctor, right now, you need to get supply Umm Balla before Janjaweed capture food, kidnap you, kill driver. Then you come back El Fasher. I meet you here with Singh. And Doctor, again, please very careful what you say. You not in New York."

* * *

The trucks and drivers were where Sol had left them. A few of the tires had been patched, the remaining flats sat in the sand, untouched, next to a pack of camels hobbled in a circle. Nomads hunkered next to the drivers and raucously hawked goods, none of which Sol recognized. The migrants shoved a good portion of their wares back into nylon bags marked with the USAID logo when they saw Sol. Several of the local men charged their AK-47s, but Sol walked past, ignored them, and dumped the new radiator in front of the disabled truck. The *jamali* glowered at Sol, and a few recharged their rifles, calling loudly to each other in mocking, guttural Arabic, pointing at the jeep, then at two of their number, back to Sol, and then at the AK-47s, which they recharged again, though not one of the rifles had a magazine in it.

Sol's eyes narrowed, and he walked to the interpreter and grunted, "If these men want to be paid, they will fix the radiator, get the tires on the lorries, and be ready to move in thirty minutes, because that's when I'm leaving with the money."

Sol spun to his jeep, turned on the air conditioner, the CD player, mashed oatmeal, cocoa, and milk powder into a tepid slurry, licked the bowl clean, repacked it, and opened the door of his jeep. "Now it's fifteen minutes. You tell 'em." He held his hands up, flashing fifteen with his fingers "I'm leaving in fifteen minutes and then no pay. No goddamn pay!"

Though the radiator was dropped into place, the men sat back down on the ground. The interpreter explained that the bolts had disappeared in the sand, and there was nothing to be done, though "*Bookera Insha'Allah*," tomorrow, if God wills it, the screws will reappear." Sol went to his jeep, took out the tool kit, went to three of the other trucks, took one radiator bolt from each, climbed into the engine compartment of the broken vehicle, and attached the radiator well enough for the trip. He jumped down and made for his jeep, brushing past the nomad merchants so closely, a vapor of fine dust settled on the men and their USAID cache. When he was inside the Rover, the drifters raised their fists and rifles. Sol rolled the window down and raised his middle finger. The men's eyes relaxed, and they smiled and waved good-by with their middle fingers.

In Umm Balla, neither Lila nor André were in camp when the trucks arrived at dusk. Sol gathered a dozen men to offload the supplies, promising an extra cup of *durra* to any refugee who carried three of the hundred-pound bags into the warehouse. A high-pitched humming of Arabic radiated from the center of the circle that had gathered around him, and before the first sack was pulled from the back of the first truck, a line of laborers had formed, stretching from the warehouse, winding around the hospital, up to the clinic, and back down to the warehouse. Sol calculated in his head the amount of *durra* in each bag: two-hundred cups, and he called together the checkers, who agreed to open a couple of bags and dish out to each porter his bonus.

When the battalion of men ran home with their windfall, Sol paid the drivers and helpers, slipping each an extra dollar for the unexpected days and nights on the road. The men danced wildly, and a team of refugees hurried over to beat drums. The drivers tipped the musicians a penny or two.

Sol drove out of town in the dark, feeling his way along the road toward the foreigners' camp. He took a wrong turn at the confluence of several four-foot paths. As he leaned forward to search the darkness, the vehicle abruptly dropped from under him into a *wadi*. A tire exploded. Out of spares, he left the jeep in the dry riverbed and walked back toward the foreigners' camp, stumbling in at eleven. It was dark in the common hut, and he went to André's and rapped on the door, though there was no answer. At Lila's, he knocked gently, but with no reply, he called out softly, "Miss Lila, it's Doctor Sol."

She unlatched the door, the towel she had hurriedly wrapped around herself bathed in the bare moonlight. "Oh, my. Dr. Soli, you're back!"

"Are you surprised?"

"Actually, I am. We heard there was fighting west of Nyala. We worried about you. The government was flying fighter jets against anything that moved on the ground. Did you see any of it?"

"Just a bit, but it wasn't government planes. It was," he paused, "it's not important. We brought a load of *durra*, and it's in the storehouse. We need to talk. Is it too late for tonight?"

"I'm afraid André's a bit under the weather. Looks to me like a touch of malaria."

"Malaria? I thought the pills were working."

She shook her head. "You know the Frogs as well as I do. Wouldn't take them. He's quite ill. You might want to look in and see if you have any ideas." Sol turned away as the towel dropped, and Lila slipped into scrub pants and a tee shirt. She nodded, "Come on."

Lila marched into André's hut without knocking, though it made little difference; the young French medical student was supine on his cot, head lolling. He groaned in French, though Sol understood only a few words. "I want to die. I cannot live. Mother, let me die."

Sol kneeled at his cot and shook him gently. "*Mon ami*, it's Doctor Sol. Do you remember me?" André quaked so violently, the droplets of sweat tore from his head as if from a dog shaking after the rain. "André, listen to me," Sol snapped, "you need to get ahold of yourself. We need you. We have a lot of new food. The camp is going to stay open."

But André just moaned, even more vociferously, that the world had come to an end, that his life had been cursed by Africa, and that everyone in the hotel would soon die. Sol was about to try again, but Lila whispered, "I treated him with some of your Artensuate, a large dose, most of what was left, but that was just a few hours ago. I'm frightened that it may have gotten into the central nervous system, the malaria. We see a lot of it here."

"Well, we won't allow it to go any farther. I have one more vial of the Artensuate in my bag. Won't hurt to give it to him IV, no matter how much you gave him. And then we'll keep his temperature down with cool towels all night. We'll take turns, yes?"

"Of course. But you must be terribly worn. Go get the meds. I'll inject them, and you rest. I'll wake you in a couple of hours. And Soli, thank you for the food and thank you. I'm really quite sorry for the way I've treated you."

At 2 A.M., Lila shook Sol and whispered, "Would you mind taking a shift?" Sol followed her back to André's hut. Instead of retiring to her shelter, she sat on the ground and leaned against the mud-straw wall. "Soli, if you stay out here long enough, you will become like us, you know. When I first met André half-a-year ago, he was a happy man. Well, maybe not chipper, but not like now. He used to talk about medical school at the Sorbonne. He was one of the great pranksters. Found himself on probation for a full year for taking a foot out of anatomy laboratory."

"A foot. What'd he want with a foot? I can think of other more useful things to steal for a prank." He paused and grinned. "No, no lashes, please. Okay, I can't imagine. Please go ahead."

"He and his mates took it to *Au Pied De Cochon*, the Foot of the Pig, the fanciest restaurant in all of Pigalle. They truly have the nicest French onion soup on Earth, which the boys ordered as the last course, and naturally, the foot found its way into the bowl, poking through the grilled cheese. The pack of them demanded free meals, or they would go to the newspapers. The maître d' agreed. He told them he'd be right back with the cancelled bill. Instead, he rang up the police. Cost them all a night in jail, and the next morning, a visit to the dean's office."

"I can still think of something funnier to pop into the soup. Dopes." Sol paused, wiping André with a wet towel, fanning to let the water cool. He went on very softly, "Lila…I want to know something…"

She interrupted, "Let me guess. You want to know if I am having an affair with André; number two: what happened in my childhood to make me so difficult; and number three: if I'm a lesbian, and if not, could we spend the night together because why not, we may not be here tomorrow? The answer is…" and now she hesitated and laughed gently. "I shall give you an answer to number three: not on your life. But someday I might tell you about the other two, though keep in mind number three is not a clue to numbers one and two. Now, what was it you wanted to ask?"

Sol was speechless but rebounded quickly. "No, no, young lady. What I wanted to know was if you were planning to stay here alone if I have to take André up to El Fasher to get him on a plane home."

She laughed again and lay back on the earthen floor. "You're quite nimble, you know. And we'll cross that bridge when we come to it." Her head dropped, and she was asleep.

By dawn, André's temperature had risen to 105 degrees, and Sol wasn't able to wake him. Sol shook Lila gently. "We need to get him to a hospital. But we can't move him now. He won't last a mile on the backseat. I need to get the helicopter down here."

She rubbed her bloodshot eyes and stood behind Sol. With her hand on his shoulder she sighed, "Soli, why didn't you wake me? It was my turn."

"Because you've done enough—enough for a lifetime." He searched her eyes and saw them soften. "Lila, would you mind making tea? Let's eat something and talk."

They opened the door of the hut, the air still cool and unusually calm. While Lila brewed the tea, Sol dashed into the shower. It had been several days, and when he peeled off his clothes, he understood why Lila had been so adamant about number three. He laughed so brashly, she called out, "Have you gone mad?"

He thought about shaving, but the water ran out, so he dressed in a fresh pair of scrubs and took his place at the table. The tea was fragrant and sweet, the pita and jam peculiarly edible. Sol began by relating how he had found the downed helicopter. Lila's eyes reddened, but her expression did not change.

"There's no time left," he warned. "You're a nurse. We need to make some tough decisions. You know where we are with André. He's going to expire, or at best live with permanent brain damage, if he doesn't get expert care. I checked my PDA on malaria in central Africa. Post three days of these fevers, he's toast. I'm not going to sit by and watch that happen."

"Soli, my father was a leftenant general in the British forces. I think you say lieutenant, but we British are loathe to pronounce anything the way it is spelled...anyway, he always told us, '...if you come to me with a problem, you better have a solution.'"

"A general! A hah! What was that, number two?"

"You just mind your manners."

"Okay, here's my thinking. He can't be transported by Rover. Not a consideration. But he can be air-evaced. There's still one helicopter left. They can bring him to the hospital in El Fasher. Docs there know how to handle malaria better than me, certainly. We'll give them the meds and pay them."

"And where is this money coming from?"

"The money I have. Problem is, and that's what we need to decide, if we spend it on the helicopter and the hospital, we won't have a lot left for supplies. I used a chunk of change just to fly the stores down here."

Lila nodded, her eyes now moist. "You really were a godsend, Doctor Soli. Even André said that. And you won't be hearing that from me again, at least in the near future, so enjoy it. Grand. How do we get word to the helicopter people?"

"I'll drive back to Nyala. You need to stay here and safeguard André. And when the helicopter comes, you need to go with him to El Fasher. He'll need an advocate, and if I needed something in this world, you'd be the one I'd want on my side."

Lila scowled. "What you really mean is that I can't stay here alone; that *you* won't allow it."

"André needs support. The checkers can run the camp until we get back. It's their country."

The air temperature had risen several dozen degrees during the meeting. They stopped talking and sat silently, tensely, drinking tea. Lila refilled the cups, gave Sol another tiny round of pita, and wiped the surface of the marmalade to spoon out a dollop with fewer green threads. He stole several peeks at her face. It left him breathless. He pushed the bread into his mouth simply for something to do.

He thought he sensed Lila stealing glances at his cobalt eyes as well, but decided it was only his imagination. Once, though, they both gazed up at the same instant. Sol flushed, and Lila laughed. "You look like you've eaten a chili pepper!"

But this time she did not avert her eyes, and a sense of pleasant tautness grasped his chest. He opened his mouth to speak, but there was a bellow from one of the huts, and they both jumped off the picnic bench. André stood at the door of his shed in his drawers, searching the compound with his eyes.

"So zere you are you two. Making ze plot against me, *oui*?"

A single tear dropped from each of Lila's eyes. As they rolled along her perfect cheeks, she quickly wiped them away and hardened her mien. Sol ran toward the weaving Frenchman. "André, you need to get back into bed. You are sick. Very sick."

"No, Doctor, I am fine and 'ungry."

"Angry? Angry about what?"

"No, no. 'Ungry, 'ungry, not 'ungry. I must eat ze food."

Lila sprang into the common hut and emerged in seconds with cup, a plate, and a very small bottle with a teaspoon of brown powder at the bottom. She lifted it and waved it toward André. "I've been saving this, you know, for a special occasion. Belgian coffee *avec* your precious chicory."

André staggered toward Lila, his arms outstretched as if to embrace her, but lost his balance and fell forward. His face slammed against the corner of the picnic bench. He groaned, slumped to the ground, and curled into a ball, blood squirting from his nostrils. It stained Sol's running shoes, and he dropped to his knees to see a new crook in the bridge of André's nose.

"Shit," Sol hissed, "you broke your nose. Lila, gimme a hand. Let's get him to the table here. I need to fix it before the swelling sets in."

They helped him onto the wooden bench. Sol spoke loudly. "André, do you understand that I need to reduce the fracture?"

"*Oui*, Doctor. I am very sorry to make you ze extra work."

Sol called to Lila, "Are there *any* surgical supplies, like instruments?"

"We have a few IV needles left, but no hemostats. Wait. There is a suture kit, though. It's got a needle driver, but it's only half-an-inch long."

Sol stared at André's nose. "And our patient's generous, but classic, Gallic beak is somewhat more extensive than a single centimeter." Sol thought about the implements in the Rover, a tire iron, a jack, and a screwdriver. "What about tools for the generator?"

"There's a kit in the shed, but I've never opened it."

She rushed into the generator hut, exiting with a green, fishing tackle box. Sol grabbed a spoon from the table to pry open the rusted clamp. The tools were as tarnished as the case, but he found needle-nose pliers, wiped off some of the superficial rust by rubbing them on his scrub pants, and held them up to the light. "This is what we need." He pointed the pliers at Lila and asked her to boil water to disinfect it, but stopped her with his open palm when she actually stood. "Just kidding," he laughed. "In this case, Nurse, we must sterilize our instruments *after* the procedure."

She took the device into the common hut, scraped it with a fragment of aluminum foil from inside a pack of LIFE cigarettes, and put a pot on the kerosene stove to boil. Sol went to his *tuchel* to load a syringe with lidocaine. He fit it with the smallest needle he could find—22 gauge. He mumbled to himself, "This thing is going to feel like a steel pipe going in. Sorry, André."

He approached his patient and asked, "*Mon ami*, are you ready? Let's go to your *tuchel* and get this done. Be over in a flash."

André grunted, "Go ahead, kill me in my own bed. No one care." As Sol took a breath to explain, André laughed, "Doctor, it is fine, *et merci*."

Lila led him back to the hut, but the sheet was soaking, and she had him sit on the edge while she ran for a couple of yards of fresh death shroud. He looked at the material and sighed, "And you, too?"

She made his bed, smoothed the sheet, squared the corners, then settled him onto his back and wiped the jelly-like blood delicately from his face. Sol got on his knees, Lila next to him, playing a flashlight up the nostrils. Sol unsheathed the needle. "Sorry, André, this is the most painful part. While André did not speak, his jaw tightened, and his eyes closed rigidly. Sol asked, "Are you still with us?"

"I am fine. Please, you do not worry about me."

Sol waited a couple of minutes for the lidocaine to numb the nerves, though he knew the injection was more placebo than anesthesia, there being little chance, he told himself, that he had gotten the medicine into the tissues immediately surrounding the broken bone. But he had no choice, and he guided the pliers up André's nostrils, moving slowly, gently, until he could sense the lopsided bone between the jaws of the device. He drew the handles together, harder and harder, pulling back, twisting his wrist and working the fragments until he felt the pieces grind into place. After a final pop, he withdrew the pliers quickly and jumped back before his patient exploded. André, though, had not shuddered.

Sol asked Lila for the flashlight and played it along the outside of André's nose, checking the alignment.

"'Ow does 'ee look, Doctor?" André queried with a forced smile.

"Better than before."

"*Mais*, it is not possible."

Sol grasped the young student's shoulder. "André, you are back from the dead. We were so worried."

"I am fine now, but to be honest, I do not remember ze last few days. What happened 'ere?"

Sol laughed, "You can thank Lila. She treated you. Gave you Artensuate. Apparently, it worked. But now we need to keep you on Malerone."

"I did not know we 'ad Artensuate."

Sol took a breath to remind him but smiled instead. "Yep, a friend at the CDC gave it to me, but I had to agree to make love to her first."

Lila wagged her finger, "Short-term memory deficit, I see. The lashes, eh what. Keep it up." She pushed a chair to the bed and explained that a full shipment of food had gotten through, and that they had a three-week reprieve.

As she spoke, Sol suddenly jumped up, smacking his forehead with his palm. "I forgot. The Rover's sitting in a ditch somewhere down the road. It's got a flat. Lila, can you drive me out there? As soon as we find the thing, you can come back. I don't want André alone for too long."

"Soli, I'd love to, but I do not drive."

André lifted himself into a sitting position. "Come on, Doctor. I weel drive ze car. It is not ze problem." He stood and weaved about for a second until Sol shot forward and caught him just as he was on his way down, nose first.

"Well, I guess that answers that, my friend." Sol rubbed his hands together. "So, here's what we can do. I'll put a spare in the Cruiser, drive out, find the Rover, change the tire, drive it back here, then walk out again and bring the Cruiser home."

Lila shook her head. "We can leave it out there. No one's going to touch it. It has a flat anyway."

"Nah, somehow they'll figure out a way. Fool me once, shame on you, fool me twice, shame on me." He stopped and groaned, "Another day pissed away on a road in darkest Africa. I'll be back, but don't wait up."

The jeep was sitting in the ditch, a platoon of local kids crawling over, under, and inside it. A fifty-pound, twelve-year-old squatted in the driver's seat, swinging the wheel left and right. Two boys were stuffed on the floor, one pumping the gas pedal, the other, most of his bony lower half outside the door, working the brake pedal with his right hand and the clutch with his left. Another of the boys was in the passenger seat pushing radio and air conditioning buttons; next to him a child pulled the parking brake up and down. The fifth had wedged himself between the seats, jamming the gear lever from first to second and back as fast as his arms could move, as if the rover was a railroad handcar.

When they saw Sol drive up, they exploded from the vehicle back toward the village of Umm Balla, a cloud of dirt higher than the tallest of the local trees sucked along behind them. Sol shouted in fractured Arabic for them to come back, and when the boy from the driver's seat stopped, the others turned to watch him. Sol waved his arms, and the little boy approached slowly, a few of his playmates following cautiously. When Sol handed the first boy the jack handle, a few more drifted over. Though this was surely the first time they had ever been close to a car, or any device more complex than prayer beads, or had ever touched a metal tool, as Sol showed them how to operate the jack and remove lug nuts, they pushed him away softly, took charge, and had the spare in place in minutes.

Sol started the engine, pulled the vehicle out of the ditch, then allowed the boys, one by one, to sit in the passenger's seat and steer. As they crawled toward the foreigner's camp, first the backseat, then the front and rear fenders, and finally the roof became encrusted with boys waiting their turn. On the tiny path through the village, their laughter brought mothers from huts, each boy yelling to his that he had driven a car. At the gates of the foreigner's compound, though, the cook, Zahra, waddled out of the kitchen hut, wooden spoon whacking at the air. The boys peeled from the jeep and raced off toward their village, leaping about as if gazelles.

André was asleep in his *tuchel*, his temperature back to normal and the shocking sweats gone. It was time for the next dose of Malerone, and Lila woke him gently. He grasped her arm warmly, whispering, "I will never forget you."

She brushed his forehead with a kiss. He moaned and fell to sleep.

Lila and Sol met in the common hut. She spoke first. "Doctor Sol, I want to apologize for what I said last night."

"Which part one, two, three?"

"Three, the part about accusing you of wanting to spend the night with me. You have been a perfect gentleman. It was rude, and I am sorry."

"Miss Lila, please understand. We are out here at the end of the Earth. You know very well that you are an exquisite woman. You've heard that all your life. Any man would want you. But I was married, and she was the love of my life. And she's gone, and then they took away my passion for medicine. So, I'm a burned-out shell. I should never have let her out of my sight, but I did, and here I am, and for all I care, really, I will be gone very soon. Tonight would be fine.

"On the other hand, I really want to get this done, and I don't want to hurt anyone along the way, especially an innocent woman like you. Would I turn you down? Probably not. Would I push it? Never. It's too late."

She let her head drop, eventually asking in a whisper, "Doctor Soli, please tell me what happened. I will never tell another soul."

He paused and looked away. "Someday. Maybe."

Lila was silent again for a long time. "Okay, when you're ready." She looked away for a moment. "I am so sorry for the way we spoke to you when you first descended upon us. How could you have known what had just happened..." She paused, the air of Umm Balla suddenly vibrating and thumping as if a cyclone was scudding through the Sahel toward them.

They went into the open and searched the sky, fixing on a helicopter toting a swinging load as it made a steep approach into the refugee camp. Sol turned to Lila. "I need to see what's going on. We didn't order any more supplies." Sol jumped in the jeep and started off to camp.

Lila yelled, "See if you can bring it back in one piece this time... Oops, sorry again."

Sol sped to the ship, which had landed on the edge of the shit fields, the cargo net already open, hundreds of old men queued to carry the bags. When Pilot Romeo's son, Crisanto, saw Sol, he ran to him and threw his arms around the doctor. "Mr. Chun paid for another load. He said to find the helicopter and take the co-pilot back to El Fasher. But first, I need to find my father. Singh said you knew where he is."

Sol gave the man the same explanation he had Chun. "I am sure the Janjaweed have him."

"Then I need to get out there and look for him. We'll climb to fifteen thousand feet. That will give us a good view of the desert. We have an M-79 grenade launcher."

"Crisanto, I guess you can look, but there are too many places for the bastards to hide. And as soon as they hear the rotors, they'll find a cave, or better, shoot you down as well. It's been at least forty-eight hours. They can move twenty miles a day, easy, so that's over sixteen hundred square miles by now. One helicopter, no chance. Even if you got high enough, it would take days, and they might be even further than I'm guessing. Now you've got three or four thousand square miles. And if you did spot them, you would never know if your father was with that band. If you turn on them and come down to look, they'll kill you. If you fire on them, they'll torture your father, but not kill him. He's of no value as a slave if he's dead. We need to wait for them to contact us. They'll find a way to get word to Singh.

"Right now, you need to get Malcolm back. It's the right thing to do. Let me fly up there with you and help. I'll pay for the trip back down here when we're done. Maybe we'll talk Mr. Chun out of another load, stock the place up, and then leave. Our André is not doing so well."

Crisanto agreed but warned they had to leave right away before the temperature climbed, and they wouldn't get the lift needed to haul the fuselage back to El Fasher. Sol called one of the checkers, told him where he was going, and gave the man a dollar to hire the runners to tell Lila.

Sol stood just behind the pilots' seats guiding Crisanto along the *wadi* between Umm Balla and Nyala. They passed over the tiny settlements, and Sol was sure he could see a tiny box on the sand, the police station, and Officer Muhammad squatted outside. Sol steered them in a fairly straight line, having become nearly as familiar with the territory as he was with the alleys of Little Italy. When they spotted the wreckage, Crisanto headed directly for it, making an approach as fast as the ship could fly, but when they could see many new footprints in the sand, the pilot slowed the helicopter and hovered cautiously as he called to Sol, "My father told me the enemy rigs these wrecks with explosives. I'm going to go slow, Doc."

Sol recommended they go back up and do a reconnaissance of several square miles to make sure there were no horsemen in the vicinity. Crisanto nodded.

At the ship, Malcolm's remains sat untouched, but gone were the jet fuel barrels and the pilot's seat. The instrument panel was missing the airspeed indicator and altimeter, though the other gauges were still in place, their glass faces gouged from the daggers with which the looters had apparently tried to pry them free. The surviving instruments had not been press fit, but attached with small screws, a technology far beyond the ken of the souls loping across the desert on camelback. The remaining dials sat indifferently, needles at zero, more evidence that the helicopter had auto-rotated and landed softly.

Crisanto examined the hull and called to Sol. "Look, Doc, the holes in the transmission cowling didn't pierce the gear box." He pointed to the rotors and the hub. "A couple of rounds in the blades, maybe a rough ride, but my father flew with a lot worse in Viet Nam. The only way he would have landed was to help Malcolm. The bullet holes were on Malcolm's side of the ship. He got hit. No way my father would have let him bleed to death in the air. My father knows all about taking care of his crew. He got the DFC in Viet Nam for saving his crew chief when they got shot down. Kept him alive hiding in a bomb crater all night, a million VC sniffing around for them.

Took over 24 hours until the medivacs could get in and rescue them. Maybe someday he will tell you the story."

The co-pilot, Jati, keened, "*Allah Kareem.*"

Sol asked, "Crisanto, what's a DFC?"

"Distinguished Flying Cross. They didn't just give them out to little Filipino warrants, you know. He earned it. My father would never have let Malcolm die in his seat, no way."

Crisanto turned to Jati. "What's the temperature, First Officer?"

The slight Indonesian man peeked into the helicopter and yelled to Crisanto, "Thirty-eight C. Freezing."

Crisanto thought for a moment and nodded. "Doc, that's only about a hundred degrees. Nothing. Even with you aboard, I think we can lift the whole ship. Ours is a newer H-model. Singh put the best engine in it. The other one's an old B-model, ten years older. We'll drain the fuel and oil, get a running start for a few miles, and see if we are able to climb out. If can get a couple thousand feet, we'll skim along and probably not bump into anything between here and El Fasher. I think we can do it."

"What's the difference between the B and H type that you said?"

"B's old. No power. Singh didn't even know the difference."

"Then why did your father take the weaker helicopter?"

"Because when you're flying, Doc, he who has the highest energy wins every time. If there was ever a problem, he wanted me to have the advantage. He always said he could get a water buffalo into the air. Those Viet Nam guys…" Crisanto's head dropped, and Sol took a step back. "Okay, Doc. Here we go. Jati," he yelled, "let's rig the ship and get the hell out of here."

Jati howled back, "You do not need to speak so, Captain. God is listening, my friend."

"I hope he is."

The two men opened half-a-dozen plugs in the hull of the downed helicopter and stood in the burning sun while all manner of oily liquids dribbled onto the sand. They crawled aboard the burned hull, ripping and tossing out every particle of debris they could get pull loose. Finally, Crisanto rigged a hawser around the main rotor hub of the downed aircraft and yelled for Sol to come aboard the main ship. As the helicopter lifted to a hover and pulled on the load, Sol could feel the floor puckering under his feet, and the sides of the helicopter inching in. Crisanto cursed and added even more power than he knew was prudent, as if a *jamali* overloading his camels. He jammed the stick roughly. The skids of the downed aircraft dug into the sand as they tried to inch forward, so Crisanto pulled back on the cyclic. With a bit of reverse movement, he pushed the cyclic forward and bought a foot of creep into the wind, then two feet backward, and four forward, the load rocking as if a car mired in snow. Soon, they were crawling a few miles per hour into the wind, though every few yards the engine groaned, the ship dropped, and the skids of the towed aircraft banged back into the desert. Crisanto beeped up the power to max, cursing more loudly as the ship jerked about, gathering forward momentum slowly, until the airspeed indicator read twenty knots. At that instant, it lifted smoothly into the sand-choked winds of the Sahel. Crisanto and Jati grasped hands, and the young captain turned to Sol to give him a thumbs up. Sol returned the gesture, smiled broadly, and settled between the fuel barrels for the flight north.

* * *

When they reached El Fasher, the outside air temperature had risen to 115 degrees, and Crisanto told Jati over the intercom that they would have to make a running landing over the main runway and hit the cargo release pedal at about thirty miles per hour. The towed helicopter would slide along the runway for a few hundred feet and, if the Creator so willed, not roll and ignite the lingering fumes in the mostly empty fuel tanks.

Jati warned that they were chancing the wrath of the El Fasher Airport's government officials, especially Airport Director Muhammad Ali Abdul Yasir al-Shaloob. "What if the ship explode," the diminutive first officer asked, "blast hole in they have just paved runway? He is Muslim, yes, full of compassion, yes, but we go to jail if we hurt runway."

Crisanto spat back, "Full of compassion, my ass. To hell with him."

Crisanto noticed Jati grimace as forcefully as if Crisanto had had called the first officer's mother a whore. Crisanto sighed and changed course to line up with 36, the older of the two runways. He released the load when he got his helicopter as slow as it could go and still stay airborne. Their ship lanced upward as the freight fell away, the ascent so violent, it pinned Sol against the floor, head outside the rear door. Before he could draw himself inside, he watched the burned hulk slide along the tarmac, hit a runway light and yaw left before careening toward the passenger lounge, a sand-brick shack not far from Calcutta Helicopter.

By the time the mass hit the lounge, nearly all of its energy had been dissipated, much of the momentum having been spent tearing a gash in the fresh macadam of the new runway where it crossed 36. Sol relaxed in relief that the collision had done little more than dent the door of the waiting room. Crisanto, who had been watching over his shoulder, stopped the helicopter in mid-flight and hovered back toward the wreckage.

Three Sudanese flew from the lounge, fists raised. Crisanto flipped them off as he flew circles at ten feet, blasting them with his rotor wash.

Singh darted from his steaming lair, fist raised as well, screaming and maniacally flashing hand signals, ordering the helicopter to land. The skids had barely touched the crumbling concrete abeam the Calcutta Helicopter—Serving World sign when he ran to Crisanto's door, pulled it open in a rage, grabbed him by his white shirt, and tried to haul his now chief pilot from the aircraft. Crisanto, firmly belted in, grabbed the collective and lifted the ship into a hover, the rotor wash gusting his boss to the ground. He hover-taxied fifty yards away and set the ship down. When Singh got within a few feet, Crisanto lifted up just over the man's head and crept back to the office. Singh chased, gesturing madly.

Sol crawled forward and spoke gently. "Captain, let me talk to Singh. I'll make him understand what happened." Crisanto thought for a moment and looked to Jati, who nodded in agreement.

Sol jumped from the ship and trotted toward the breathless man, though Singh loped around the helicopter, dove into the shack, and locked the door. Sol knocked gently, "Mr. Singh, please, we need to talk. Everything is going to be okay. Please open the door." There was no movement. "Mr. Singh, don't forget, I've got a lot of money I still owe you." The lock clicked, and the door opened a crack. "Mr. Singh, excuse me, sir, but we need to work together to solve some problems, and then we can move forward and rebuild. I'm here to help you. Please."

The door opened another few inches, and Sol saw the scarlet and the moisture in Singh's eyes. The man nodded, bidding Sol in. He put the tea kettle on the electric plate, stepped outside, and numbly hailed his remaining crew.

The four men sat quietly for several minutes until Sol muttered, "Mr. Singh, have you heard from the men who took Crisanto's father?"

"No. Vhy vould dey contact to me?"

"Because we believe they are holding him for ransom. You know that. And who else would they call?"

"Now I am to pay ransom?" Singh broke into an even deeper sweat, the fluid wicking into the few dry rings left in his soiled turban, the helix of cloth a physiologic chronicle of the man's worldly struggles. "I am not made of gold, you know. I have to pay for broken helicopter, and now passenger lounge because…"

Sol's hand came up to stop him. "Mr. Singh, we did not say you had to pay a ransom. Captain Luzon, and First Officer Jati, and I just want to know if you had heard from the people who might have Romey. It is his father, after all."

"Doctor, I have not heard from anyone, but I vill hearing from government about crash. Vhat is to be done? I vill not pay for dis damage caused by you and Luzon."

"Mr. Singh," Sol lectured in a near monotone, "I did not cause the damage, and Captain Luzon had no choice. It was too hot to land. Now, let's go take a look at the lounge. Didn't seem too bad from the air."

The four joined several dozen Sudanese men who stood smoking and inspecting the scratched front door and the single pane of broken glass. The men wrapped and unwrapped their *immahs* as they discussed reparation. One of the onlookers expressed caution and reminded the men of the day Muhammad Hamed Idris, an airport maintenance man, generated an international incident that led to the withdrawal of European humanitarian relief in 1985.

He recounted for the younger men how Muhammad had been sent out to dig a hole for the first electric landing light on an airport in central Africa. His labor, though, coincided with the arrival of a German Air Force C-123 loaded with eighteen tons of relief supplies. Muhammad had been ordered to dig a hole, and he wasn't going to lose his job, he later explained, by running away from an airplane. The freighter zoomed just feet over his head, a signal, the air crew believed, that would indicate their intention to land. Despite a second pass, the man continued picking away at the rock-hard earth with an ancient shovel. On the third fly-by, the pilot aimed his landing gear at the man's head, though the warning served only to blow the man's *immah* into the desert. Still he picked at the dirt.

So, the mercy ship had to divert to El Geniena, where an air reconnaissance of that runway revealed it to be no more promising than any of the mud-soaked alleys that crisscrossed the town.

The German pilot cursed and turned the plane east to fly the six hours back to their starting point in Khartoum. He knew there was no airstrip in the thousand miles between that was adequate to handle the C-123, a plane designed specifically to land on very short, poorly maintained, third world runways. The German government was so dispirited with the futility of their humanitarian efforts, they pulled their mission, which resulted in an official complaint lodged with the United Nations High Commissioner for Refugees by the Sudanese government. That led to the sanctioning of Germany and Israel by the Security Council.

The Zionists had become implicated for having demanded reparations from Germany after World War II, some forty years before. The restitution granted the Israelis came in the form of Mercedes cars sold at ridiculously low prices in Tel Aviv. That served to drain the *Bundesbank*, leaving little for Germany's suddenly-conceived moral obligation to build the modern airports demanded by African governments from Cairo to Johannesburg. The final pronouncement from the UN found both Germany and Israel complicit in the Western blueprint to let the African people starve. Israel, though, was assigned a majority of the blame.

* * *

Singh moaned and swore to his God, so Sol put his arm around the man's shoulder and announced he would pay for the damage. An obese Sudanese man with a pockmarked face stepped forward and declared in perfect English, "You have caused thousands of dollars of damage to my airport. Thousands."

Sol turned his head in confusion. "Sir, all I see is a dent in a wooden door and broken pane of glass."

"The man's lips pursed and his eyes hardened. "Why, just look at those damaged airplanes over there." He pointed to three aircraft sitting in front of a maintenance hangar, each missing a body part. There was a small piece of the helicopter sitting on the ground several meters from the first airplane. Sol started to walk toward the piece, but the man stopped him. "That is a secure area of the airport. You may not go there."

Sol spoke quietly. "Sir, I am about to open my billfold. What I hand you will be my first and last offer. If you refuse it, I will be on my satellite phone to the American Embassy in Khartoum before the wallet is back in my pocket. I will tell them you are threatening an American citizen. Are we clear?"

The man huffed, "I am Airport Director Muhammad Ali Abdul Yasir al-Shaloob. Just who, young man, do you think you are addressing?"

"Are we clear?" Sol took an American hundred from his wallet, waved it in the eyes of all present, crumpled the bill, and placed it in the man's hand. "Are we clear, sir?" Sol turned, nodded his head toward Calcutta Helicopter's hut, and walked away. The three foreigners followed.

Inside, Sol waited for thanks. There was, however, only silence until Captain Luzon sighed, "Doctor, we should contact the UN for help. This is bigger than we can do."

Sol answered, "Captain, you are right, but first we have to take care of Malcolm. He's still out there in the helicopter."

Sol asked Singh to call the police. They arrived in great numbers with lights and sirens blasting. By the time Sol was finished paying for the investigation, several more hundreds of dollars had passed from his hands into those of a dozen Sudanese officials. The police chief ordered Sol to recompense a holy man to purify the area surrounding the body and the ground over which the remains were wheeled on a gurney. He went on to blame Sol for the sacred earth of Darfur that had been sullied by the presence of a deceased *kafir*. The fine was an additional fifty dollars.

Sol balked at the next hundred-dollar fee, one levied by the local medical examiner. "You see, *Doctori*, he was not only one who tried to hide from the truth of Allah's teachings, a *kafir*, he was also," the man declared behind his hand in a distressed whisper, "I do not want to say in loud, but this was woman who walk around like man. And do you know, *Doctori*, what is in woman pocket?"

Sol shrugged, "A rabbit's foot? I have no idea."

"A metal bottle! Inside police report alcohol."

Sol grumbled, "Hundred lashes for him," but stuck his hand in his pocket and paid.

Singh, the two pilots, and Sol drove to the UN compound to meet with Chun, who had been contacted by the Secretary General in New York via the satellite phone. The weary Korean diplomat warned that the situation was so complicated, it might take weeks for a resolution.

Sol screwed up his face and shrugged, "Excuse me, Mr. Chun, it's no big deal. I've already paid for the door, the window, and a few shovelfuls of tar. It'll be done in twenty-four hours and forgotten in three days."

Chun looked at him askance. "What door? What window?"

Singh sat in the corner of Chun's office groaning and clutching his abdomen as if it was on fire. The howling was so loud, Sol had to move his chair closer to Chun's desk.

"Doctor, no one care El Fasher Airport. I am talk about secure release Pilot Luzon. I tell you, government in Khartoum no connection with Janjaweed. Must be patient, let word filter down. Do not become involve any more. It is way we do here."

* * *

Very early the next morning, Mr. Chun split the cost of another load of food with Sol, and the helicopter was on the ground in Umm Balla by 9 A.M. With the sound of the approaching ship, Sol could see the swirl of dust and the flash of off-white *jellabiyas* dashing into a queue that snaked across the entire camp. He set out to look for Lila and André, but the checkers told him they had not been to work for a couple of days, so the helicopter dumped its cargo, hauled Sol the two minutes to the foreigners' camp, and said good-by quickly. The ship headed back without shutting down.

Sol found Lila in André's hut placing cool towels on his head. "Not good. Is the radio working? I'll call the helicopter back and get him to El Fasher."

But André looked up and groaned, "*Mais*, Doctor, I am fine. It is only ze surgery you do zat is ze problem."

Lila shook her head. "No, it's the malaria. But it's not cerebral. The antibiotics worked at least for that, but the fevers are back."

"How far apart?"

"Six to eight hours. But nowhere near as bad as they've been. He's on the mend. I heard the helicopter. Did you bring more supplies?"

"We did. We've got enough for over a month. It's a reprieve. And I've got some money left. It'll buy a few more loads, so say two months altogether. I brought a couple of cartons of rat poison, and one of the UN guys told me how to use it. We'll be okay."

Lila leaned back. "Jolly good. But we need to get back to doing clinics. That was why we came here, isn't it? And will you stay, Soli? Please."

"I'm not going anywhere until I am sure you and André' are safe."

"*Mais*, Doctor, I am zhust ze fine one. You do not 'ave ze worry."

"André, I do worry. You're not out of the woods. But, believe it or not, you're better off here than on the road, or even in the helicopter. Let's be smart. You take your meds when Miss Lila says so, rest a few days, and you'll be fine. And you can thank her.

"So, here's what we can do. Let's hire the running team and leave half of them here during the day, and we'll have Zahra the cook look in on André every thirty minutes. If there's a problem, she'll send the runners, and we'll dash back. How does that sound?"

"Brilliant," Lila nodded, "and we can put the boys to work here cleaning up. Zahra can oversee their labor and make sure they get a meal."

Sol rushed to his hut, brushed his teeth and washed his face, but realized his spoor was so rank, he splashed on a bit of aftershave. At the jeep, Sol stopped Lila as she began to climb into the passenger's side. "It's time, young lady. Hop in the pilot's seat. We'll get you your wings in three days, if that."

Lila's body bolted straight. She whispered, "I suppose you're right. I haven't been of much use, have I? And are you going to be wearing that cologne often?"

Sol shrugged his shoulders. "I don't know. You like it?"

She did not answer as they bumped and jerked the few miles to the refugee camp, but Lila was gentle on the controls, holding the wheel lightly, eventually just sliding her hands softly, swaying gracefully as she turned to avoid the gullies that crisscrossed the primitive paths of the Sudanese—Chadian border.

At the fringes of the encampment, Lila told Sol that she was going to drive a new road to enter camp, a longer trip, but smoother, having seldom been used by vehicular traffic. They passed an area of particularly ragged people hunkered in front of ten-square-foot, bare shelters fashioned from twigs and leaves. There were no plastic tarps or grass mats. A few skeletal souls milled about aimlessly, others sat on the ground using their fingers to pull tiny globs of yellow mush from hollowed, dried gourds. With each nibble, they licked their fingers noisily, never taking their eyes off their microscopic portions. The men were wasted, but it was impossible to judge the well-being of the women, covered, as they were, from head to toe in dark robes with the most inadequate slits for their eyes,

When Sol shook his head, Lila mumbled, "The outcasts, the ultra-religious, absolute *Insha'Allah*, the if-God-wills-it faction. These are the ten percenters. They won't take food from us because we are infidels, impure. The very fact that we want to give them food is profane. To them, cleansing means only to submit to God's will."

Sol pressed her. "Well, if it isn't God's will that we showed up with food, whose is it?"

"That's the point. It is not God's will that we are here, it's the devil's will. That's their reasoning. One of the more religious checkers told me we, we whites, are destined to rot in hell because we have laid eyes on Jews, and once you've seen the devil, there can be no salvation, no matter what you do."

"A checker looked you in the eye?"

"When they think they can get something out of you, they will. Not so religious when it's useful. *These* people won't look at you, though. Extreme fundamentalists. Shame, really."

Fifty yards further along the road, they rolled up to an area of six-foot-diameter, grass-mat huts with woven roofs covered in plastic. A group of thin woman fed the morning fires with strands of thistle plant that blew into camp with the wind. Others ground coffee beans with primitive stone mortars and pestles. Two women cut paper-thin slices of wilted ginger root, the ladies eventually tossing their precious contributions into pintsized clay pots of boiling water. Finally, to the shrieks of laughter from the women, a squad of nude children tossed in heaping cups of sugar.

Lila stopped the jeep, forgetting to use the clutch. As the engine jerked to a stop, she explained. "That's *jabana*, desert coffee. I think it's been here for five hundred years. Very thick and sweet. Spiced as well. Desert dessert. Really good stuff. This is my favorite spot in Umm Balla. These people are quasi-refugees, you might say. They came with the rest of the miserable, but they staked out land under trees, built proper huts, are growing a few crops, and somehow manage to get food on their own, even coffee. That's why the women are only terribly thin, not simply skin and bone like their mates back there. I guess there are always the rare souls who refuse to suffer. Bloody amazing. So how did I do?"

"Bloody amazing. Why am I not surprised? One more lesson and you're on autopilot."

"Fine. So why don't you drive the rest of the way into camp? I'm exhausted." She pulled at the sweat-soaked material of her blouse near her underarms. "Perhaps you believe me. Yes?"

Sol had to sit for a moment to calm himself before nodding and walking to the driver's side. Lila gave directions, and he let the

194

clutch out too quickly—the jeep lurched to a stop, and the engine stalled. She giggled but put a hand in front of her mouth before laughing aloud. He glared at her then chuckled. As they approached main camp, a stench wafted toward the jeep, and Sol scrunched his nose. He turned to Lila. "Is that you?"

"No, you monkey. That's the defecation zone. Remember?"

Before Sol could answer, he noticed an old woman squatting in the fields, her *tob* pulled up to cover her face while her privacy was exposed to the world. She remained hunkered but shuffled around and placed her back toward the foreigners as the vehicle passed. Looking through a slit in the material, she saw Sol's head turned toward her and drew a second patch of the *tob* across her face. Lila shook her head. "We'd dig latrines, but they won't use them."

"I heard. They want to know why we want to collect poop in one place. They think we have ulterior motives."

Sol soon recognized the hospital and feeding centers from the new direction they had entered the camp. The children raced toward the Rover as it pulled up. Sol yelled, "*A Salaam Aleikum*," setting off waves of laughter as the youngsters rushed to surround the jeep.

"*Aleikum A Salaam*," a few kids called back, but most screamed "Hellooooo Meeester!" And as on his first day, the children fought gently with each other to shake his hand. A little boy stepped up, wiped his dripping nose on his palm, and extended it to Sol, who grabbed it and laughed. Several teams of older children pushed through to stroke Sol's arms, marveling at the white skin and hair.

Sol was mesmerized by the dazzling eyes and the openness of the children. He reveled in the simplicity of their affection, the accepting innocence, but it took only seconds before the plague of flies and beetles clustered about their runny noses and crusted eyes abruptly flew from the children to engulf Sol. He thought back to the surge of insects that had assaulted him on his first morning in camp and realized this was an exponential plague. The children squealed as Sol bellowed, "Jeese, get the hell off'a me." They laughed louder he when pounded at the flies, dispatching several dozen with each blow. The kids joined, smacking at him, though avoided stepping in the heap of carcasses that accumulated at his feet.

With a smile in her eyes, Lila breathed heavily, "Ah, yes, the cologne."

"Okay. I get the point," he mumbled, but the children were hooting so raucously, Lila did not hear.

Sol told Lila he felt comfortable going up the hill to the ramshackle clinic and starting on his own. She looked at him askance but tapped him on the arm and smiled. The regiment of children followed, several jockeying to hold his hand. Halfway along the path, it dawned on him that he had not yet gone near one of the refugee huts, so he left the path and walked slowly and obsequiously toward a grouping of eight-foot-diameter lean-tos.

Most of the refugees, young mothers and ancient grandparents, looked up and smiled. The few who didn't greet Sol scattered and dove into huts as the white apparition approached slapping at flies.

He moved deeper into the neighborhoods, small patches of arid sand claimed by individual clans. He spotted some women coming in from the desert hauling firewood teetering on their heads, the stock little more than twigs, though piled four or five feet high. Other women hefted five-gallon plastic gasoline cans of water, also balanced on their heads, cornrows safeguarded by small towels rolled into toruses. The younger girls sat on the earth grinding kernels of *durra* between flat rocks, searching doggedly for every single nub that slipped off the grinding stone.

As Sol moved through the zone, the entourage of children grew until more than three hundred diminutive boys and girls tramped along, forming a ring of dusty, barely clothed, miniature troops. He stopped and asked a woman who was boiling water in a battered pot if he could look into her hut. He used hand signals, and her face froze, for minutes it seemed, but she eventually turned away. Though Sol took that as tacit permission to examine the shelter, he didn't actually enter. He knelt and scrutinized the door, a few twigs she latched closed at sunset with a wisp of reed. He peered inside: a couple of donated blankets lay rumpled on the bare sand; hung from the walls by a twig were a few fragments of faded clothing. A small, rotting cardboard box held a plastic, liter soda bottle half-filled with cooking oil. An assortment of small packages wrapped in newspaper were strewn across the floor. It was the weekly allotment of soap, one bar;

milk powder; and a few teaspoons each of sugar, tea, and dried okra. Dug into a small hole was a plastic bag of *durra,* perhaps five pounds, a corner of the single blanket partially covering it as if to hide the grain from marauders. At the back was the nubbin of a single candle wedged into the grass mats. As Sol withdrew his head, he noticed, stuffed behind one of the quarter-sticks supporting the *tuchel,* a schoolboy's book bag embossed with colorful Chinese characters.

Sol crawled away from the opening and thanked the woman. She barely looked up. For a moment, he played with her eighteen-month-old daughter who sat in front of the hut, the child's eyes never leaving Sol's. Finally, he bent down and gave the baby a kissing monster smooch on the top of her head, fearing he had gone too far and a burst of terrified screeching would draw Lila and the checkers. He imagined he would be reported for assaulting the life-blood of Chad's future and sent home summarily, if he was lucky, or imprisoned for life in a Sudanese penitentiary. But the child giggled, reached up, and grasped his nose. The kids, now assembled in circle after circle as spectators, exploded in laughter. When the mother gave in and smiled, Sol sang to the baby in a falsetto that brought an uneasy hush to the neighborhood.

At the top of the hill, a mass of children rushed to line the path into the clinic. Their eyes opened as wide as moon pies when he stepped across the threshold to do whatever it was white specters did behind *their* walls. The tiny girl in the pink princess dress who had succeeded in working Sol for a few teaspoons of water on his first day crossed the line in the sand and thrust her red cup up into the doctor's face. She waited silently.

Sol laughed, and the girl smiled. "Hey, wait just a minute. I know you, young lady. You got me in trouble a while back. I'm not allowed to give you water. It's the rules." He laughed, and she laughed. In an instant, though, the cup was back an inch from his eyes. When he didn't pour her a drink, she grasped one of his canteens and pulled at the neck, struggling to free it from the canvas case. He lifted her up gently and placed her back in the mob. When she started forward again, the boys tugged at her, and soon the mass of children retreated down the hill, the little girl laughing, moving easily with the flow.

Sol gazed into the camp below. Slowly, the women emerged from their huts, pulled grass mats over the openings, and locked the front doors with tufts of thread. They gathered their children and walked dolefully toward the line that was forming in front of the clinic.

Achmed swaggered up the hill and stomped past Sol as if he had never before laid eyes on him. Sol shook his head, sneered at the man's back, and considered bellowing, "Weren't you the one who was going to get me laid? So, today, what, you don't recognize me? Must be so many of us white doctors buzzing around Umm Balla. And we all look the same, huh?" Sol shook his head and dropped into his crumbling folding chair.

As the first mom waddled forward, she extracted a twenty-pound four-year-old from her *tob*. She struggled to lift the wriggling body to show Sol that the baby was sufficiently alive to screech and raise his stick-like arms a few degrees. Sol smiled, nodded to the woman, slid forward in his chair a few inches, and smiled again when the baby disappeared under her gown. He reached into the box for two packets of rehydration salts, waved them at Achmed, and then toward the woman.

Instead of launching into the standard rehydration algorithm, Achmed snapped at the woman, "Fool, let *Doctori* see your kid. What the *hell* is the matter with you?"

Sol took a breath to upbraid Achmed, but Sol was so shrouded in flies, he ignored the checker and slapped madly at the pests. Lila slid into the clinic and stopped behind him. She bent forward and whispered in his ear, "You might give some thought to washing off the cologne." She called to a checker and ordered a basin of water, a patch of death shroud, and a bar of soap.

When it arrived, Sol retreated to a dark corner and soaped the scrap of death shroud. He was about to open his scrub pants but saw Lila watching. "I don't need you peeking."

She answered without emotion, "At what?"

When Sol retook his seat, he examined his patient's ears to discover, through the detritus of sand and bugs, an eardrum as inflamed as the setting African sun. He rubbed his chin in deep, therapeutic thought and prescribed Amoxicillin, their only pediatric antibiotic. He spoke to the checker, instructing him to advise the mother that the child needed a capful of medication when the sun first rose, another when the sun was directly above, and a final dose when the light of day began to fade into the distant horizon over Chad. The checker stood, took a bottle of the pink-powdered antibiotic from a cardboard box, poured in a few ounces of water, shook it uncaringly, and handed it to her with a sullen smirk. She remained squatted, unmoving, until he motioned with the back of his hand to dismiss her. Three paces outside the clinic, she opened the plastic bottle and sucked down the ten-day prescription in one long swallow.

Sol's jaw dropped. He was nearly out of his seat to challenge the woman, but Lila charged over and halted inches from the woman's face. She spoke in English, hiding a smile. "What in the bloody hell are you doing? Is your understanding of Western allopathic medicine so fragile that you would challenge a *doctor's* order?" She winked at Sol. "That medicine is for your kid, not you."

Lila ducked into the hut to summon Achmed, who strode forward, wagged a finger in the woman's face, and repeated Lila's declaration.

The young mom, eyes pointed toward her bare feet, mumbled, "My kid's fine. Healthiest one in the neighborhood. I only came to get the medicine bottle for a place to keep a little extra water."

Achmed's open palm moved toward the woman's face as he screeched in English, "I slap you into this year, *abed*, stupid *ewe*." But Sol lunged for the man and shoved him away before he could make contact. Achmed lost his balance and landed at the woman's feet, a small cloud of dust lifting from the earth.

Lila howled, "Stop it, the both of you!"

Sol wheeled around and started down the hill, ignoring Lila's calls for him to return. At the hospital, he found Muhammad and asked him to suggest another checker for the clinic. He chose Suleiman, a tall, light-skinned man with a kind face and gentle manner. They climbed the hill and passed Achmed, who spit on the ground in front of Sol. Suleiman whispered, "*Doctori*, ignore him. He is not one of us. He is from Khartoum. He is Muslim, yes, but not righteous like we are. It is the way they act, the faithless."

Sol saw four dozen patients over the next hour, though Lila commented relentlessly from the back of the hut that they were falling behind. Sol smiled and called over his shoulder, "Yes, Roxanne."

"Who?"

"That was my nurse in Whitaker, at my last clinic. She used to slip threatening notes under my door if I spent too much time jawing with cops or pilots. Whatever. Okay, let's shift into overdrive."

"What *are* you babbling about?"

At eleven, he took a short break. He'd seen a couple of hundred children since nine. The great majority were named Muhammad Hamed Idriss. He wondered how many would live to become aerodrome laborers, primed to change the course of human events by refusing to stop digging a hole in a third world runway. He stretched out on the sand at the back of the hut and fell into an uneasy nap until a commotion at the doorway roused him. An older woman stood smugly erect, a pair of rusted, hand-forged, Eighteenth Century scissors held tightly in her right hand. The fingers of her left hand snapped inches from Lila's eyes. What had awakened Sol actually came from Lila, who repeatedly pushed the lady's hand away.

Suleiman translated, though he grew redder in the face with each volley. Sol stood and listened for a moment in the shadows until Lila sensed his presence and turned to him.

"I don't believe this. She wants us to come to her hut and use our medicine to help her daughter before they cut off her clitoris with those rusty scissors."

Sol stood bolt upright. "What are you *talking* about?"

"Are you unaware of female circumcision?"

"Never heard of it. And it sounds like you're flirting with a couple 'a dozen lashes yourself."

Lila shook her head sadly. "Bloody hell. You're not serious. You said you did your reading. Infundibulation? Female genital mutilation?"

"Nope. Sorry. I don't know what you mean."

"It is not one of your jokes, is it?"

"Nope."

"Are you unaware that girls are circumcised around here? I can't stop it, but I'll be damned if I'm going to facilitate it."

"Lila, as usual, I admit, I'm an ignoramus. Tell me what the hell's going on, please."

She heaved a disappointed sigh. "*Doctor*, the culture here, actually in many places in the Middle East, prescribes that little girls have their clitorises cut out before age twelve. And just to make sure, they cut off the labia as well. Then they sew the whole bloody thing together. It's to ensure they don't mess around on their husbands, an insurance policy, if you will. No arousal, no sex for love.

"The women believe, or at least they tell the kids, that if they don't snip off the clitoris, it will grow and hang down to their knees by the time they're old enough to have babies. And that would make them impure in Allah's eyes because everything down there is corrupt and unclean. So, they have to excise the evil, every millimeter of it, before the child matures. If they don't, the girl will never find a husband, and the family will be ostracized and suffer a loss of honor. Then they'll be turned out alone into the desert, and that means certain death. You can't live on your own here. Very powerful incentive."

"Who does the surgery? Special doctor like a *mohel*?"

"Some places, yes. I've heard that's the custom in Somalia, where you hire a man, but here, it's the older women themselves who make sure the custom continues. They administer and do the whole process themselves. In Darfur, the men have nothing to do with it, at least not directly, but if a mother refused to let her daughter be mutilated, she'd be stoned to death—by order of a man, your friend the *quadis*, the good judge next tent over."

"That sucker ain't my friend. So, what happens when the girl starts menstruating?"

"Precisely. What happens? They leave a twig in between the bleeding lips. They take it out for a few minutes so she can pee, then back in until the incision heals. So, in the end, there's a permanent little gap. She can have her monthly, but the hole's tiny, and it's near the anus. How's she supposed to keep it clean? They've never heard of loo roll."

"I'm not getting this. If there's back pressure on the urethra, especially with all that bacteria, there's going to be constant urinary tract infections, then kidney infections and renal failure. You can't live like that."

"Want to wager? Many of the girls die of nephritis or fallopian tube infections. We see it all the time."

"I still don't understand the anatomy."

"Must I draw you a picture? Have you no experience? When they cut off the labia, they sew the bleeding stumps together with whatever string is lying around, or a vine if that's all there is. I saw the needle. It's blunt and rusted, like a Phillips-head screwdriver. They pull what's left of the lips together, sort of, hoping they'll heal and seal off the vagina."

"Sort of like the tools I used on André."

"This isn't funny!" But she had to force herself not to betray a smile. "Most of the time, the string doesn't hold, so the girls have to lie on their backs in the huts for two weeks. Their legs are lashed together with strips of rag to keep the skin joined until it all scars down, except for the small hole. Mama feeds them and puts more rags under them so they can pee. Half of them get septic from wound infections, and the other half from urinary tract infections. Some of them die within a few days of the mutilation."

"Okay, what happens when she gets married?"

"Husband doesn't care if his wife likes it or not. She's there for his pleasure, not the other way 'round."

Sol was wide-eyed. "No, I mean if they sew the vagina shut, how is there penetration?"

"They don't sew the vagina shut. Just the lips around it. He pokes until he gets through the manmade barrier then rams through the hymen, which I understand is a lot easier than the scars. It's a double whammy. Girl still has to show blood for the tribe the next day, or same problem—the girl's a whore, and honor is lost, and it's off into the desert, or just get stoned to death, if you're lucky."

"Lila, don't be mad if I ask if it's every woman."

"I told you, it's play along or die. When I was in Khartoum, I had dinner at the Hilton with a Sudanese woman; over six feet tall, gorgeous, a PhD student at the University of Khartoum, in sociology of all things. I screwed up my courage and finally asked her about the practice, if she had undergone mutilation. She smiled and calmly told me, 'It's much more sanitary, don't you think?' This was a graduate student! Then she bragged to me that her crotch was as flat and smooth as the palm of her hand. She smiled and said, 'What man could want more?'"

"Whoa. Okay, so what's *this* lady want?"

"She wants us to come and numb up her daughter so it doesn't hurt so much. For her own daughter, well, it's fine to protect her, but to hell with the rest of the kids. They're going to be doing three girls today. One's seven years old. And she also wants us to give her new scissors. She thinks the ragged edge on hers is cruel. And you wonder why I've become jaded."

"I didn't say you were jaded."

"No, but it's in your eyes."

"What are you going to do?"

"Kick her arse out of here, of course. What would you recommend?"

"When in Rome, you know."

Lila shook her head bitterly. "Sol, you've helped us very much in the past few days. I am grateful, but there is a limit. You need to take sides on this one, and if you're on the wrong side, I will personally not work with you for one more moment. Now, make a decision, or I leave!"

"Lila, please. I haven't had time to think about this."

"There is nothing to think about."

Sol walked out of the clinic, around back, and sat on the sand. He gazed into the scrub and followed the tiny patches of thistle brush that extended into the valley as far as he could see, over the border into Chad. It was the first time he realized he was not far from the very center of Africa. He wondered how he, or any other human soul, could have landed there.

Suleiman came around and sat with him and offered a primitive cigarette. Sol took it without hesitation. He let the thick, blue smoke veil his face, then drew a deep breath, stood suddenly, patted Suleiman on the shoulder kindly, and walked to the front of the clinic. Inside, Lila was sitting in one of the folding chairs staring out at the meandering lines of women waiting in the half-mile queue. Sol came up to her. "I will support whatever *you* believe is right. You've thought it out; I have not. At this moment in my life, I respect your opinion above all others."

She leaned forward and touched his hand softly. "That shouldn't be good enough, but I guess it has to be."

She left the clinic and hunkered outside the door, a couple of feet from the woman. The scissors were thrust back into Lila's face, and the fingers snapped even closer to her eyes. Lila nodded for Suleiman to translate. "Madam, I would like to help you, but you are harming your daughter. Do you understand that?"

"No," the woman answered softly, "we must do what we are told to do in the Koran."

"Madam," Lila demanded, "please show me where in the Koran it says that you must mutilate your children. Show me."

"White woman devil *jinn* Jew, I cannot show you. I cannot read. But I have been told by the mullah. So…"

Lila waited for the woman to finish, though there was only a shrug followed by silence. Soon the scissors were up again waving, poking millimeters from Lila's mouth, but she pushed the woman's hand away so sternly, the scissors dropped to the ground. Lila came to her feet and walked silently into the clinic. Suleiman picked up the scissors, dusted them off on his *jellabiya*, handed them to the woman, and helped her up. He nudged her away from the tent, but she worked herself around the checker, feinting left, then right, to poke the scissors back into Lila's face. The checker took the woman gently by the shoulders and pointed her down the hill.

Sol ripped through the next fifty patients, stopping every few seconds to slap a palm against his thigh, dispatching scores of flies with each blow. As he brushed the corpses from his scrub pants, a hundred more took their place, and soon both his hand and leg hurt, so he turned his attention exclusively to examining patients, albeit from afar. This new examination technique sped the delivery of medical care so dramatically, he decided he'd write a paper for the Journal of the American Medical Association on how to see several hundred patients per hour, and perhaps merit a study grant from Blue Cross.

But his musings were disturbed when the thuds of a new uproar poured into his little clinic. He peered through the door to what had been a well-ordered line of waiting patients quickly degenerating into a sea of stooped teens scattering toward the far corners of the camp. He caught a glimpse of a white jeep speeding up the hill, nearly whacking a few dozen of the slower women.

Lila, who had been quietly separating medications, looked up abruptly and muttered, "Oh, bloody hell. What next?"

The vehicle skidded to a stop in the front of the clinic and blocked the entryway. A dozen more women darted off. Before the dust settled, a short, pudgy African man in a safari suit rolled out of the rear seat and waddled toward the tent. Lila bristled from the doorway, but a soldier in pressed green fatigues on the passenger's side of the jeep threw his door open and trained an AK-47 at her. Several dozen more women tore away.

Lila stopped short in her tracks, though her expression did not shift. She stared at the little man. He offered his hand, leaving her no choice but to grasp it. He held it for many seconds, leering at her face, sweeping her body with his eyes. He finally locked his stare on her breasts and covered her right hand with his left. When he finally let go, she brought her hand behind her back and wiped both sides on her scrub pants.

"Mademoiselle Lila. It is a pleasure to see you," he grunted in a heavy smoker's tone, his accent overly British. "I hope that we may drink tea later and chat." She smiled weakly, and he went on. "But pleasure must wait, I fear. It has come to our attention that you have an undocumented doctor in camp. A *man*. Am I correct?"

Sol rose from his folding chair, crunching through the debris of insect bodies. The man eyed Sol vigilantly as the doctor emerged from the darkness. The guard's AK-47 swiveled toward him. Lila half-turned. "This is Mr. Aswad. He is *very* important. He is *the* Provincial Commissioner of Refugees for Darfur Province. Without Mr. Aswad, we could not exist. We are very lucky he supports us so generously."

Sol proffered his hand, though Aswad just stared at it and shook his head. Finally, he scowled. "Ah hah, so you are the new doctor. I know about you. I am afraid you do not have a permit to practice medicine in my province."

Sol cocked his head. "Oh, sir, excuse me, but I do. I went through the Ministry of Health in Khartoum."

"But you have not received the stamp from *me*. It is my duty to decide who may, or may not, work in Darfur Province, for I must protect these poor people. Do you have *my* stamp on your documents?"

"I do not, sir. But I would be happy to do whatever you want to satisfy your requirements."

"Very well. I must tell you that the permit is five hundred US dollars."

"Sir," Sol sighed, "I paid that in Khartoum."

"Do you have proof?"

"It's in my *tuchel*."

"How long will it take to bring it to me? I have no time to waste. I must visit several other camps this afternoon. There are many so-called doctors operating here, lining their pockets at the expense of these sad refugees."

"We can send the runners. Maybe an hour, maybe less."

Aswad huffed, "There is no time for that. We will settle with you in a moment. Now, to the conditions here in Umm Balla. Doctor, do you see the filth in this camp?" Sol sucked in a breath to answer, but Aswad went on. "These poor people are barely living. What kind of service are you providing? I want…"

Sol interrupted, "Excuse me, sir, but I just…" He stopped and thought about the credo his father had taught him, the one that demanded he not live by the excuse. "I just…I just want you to know that we spent tens of thousands of dollars on food shipments. We will feed these people first, get their strength up so that they have the energy to clean up the camp. And, actually, I'm glad you're here, sir. We could use your help making sure the trucks get through. I spent a week…"

Aswad's eyes burned into Sol's as he interrupted, "Doctor, I am not in the transportation business. I am here to ensure these suffering people are properly cared for. We have warned Please Help the Children in the past. If you do not improve these conditions, I will have to shut this camp down." His nose lifted, and he spat, "Look at you. Even the doctor is covered in flies around his…"

Out of the corner of his eye, Sol saw Lila stifle a laugh before she stepped between him and Aswad. "Okay, Mr. Aswad," Lila smiled coyly, "you are, of course, completely correct. The doctor is new. He doesn't have any idea what's going on. We *have* been lax. We will work harder in the future. In fact, we have requested an insect fogger and an engineer from our office in Khartoum. That should help, don't you think?"

Aswad was about to answer, but Sol interrupted. "We want the best for these people, too. You are the Commissioner. Maybe you can get your colleagues in Khartoum to fly the engineer and his stuff out here. That would be us working together. Newspapers in Europe and the US would love it."

Aswad thought for a moment, shook his head, and mumbled, "Newspapers do not come here, Doctor. As I have said, we cannot be your shippers or couriers. That is why *you* are here. You brought this upon yourselves with your foreign policy. This famine is the fault of the Jews and the Americans." He paused. "Perhaps it is time for me to speak with Mademoiselle Lila, if you do not mind."

Lila nodded for Sol to step away while she and Aswad went inside the clinic. They emerged less than a minute later, and Lila called Sol into the shelter. She placed her hand softly on his arm and sighed, "Just behave for a moment. Listen to me. He will go away if we give him American dollars. Do you have any cash on you?"

"I do, but I was warned by your office in London not to pay bribes under any circumstances. We can get kicked out of Sudan if the government finds out."

"Doctor, listen to me. He is the government. The bloody bastard will close the camp in five minutes if we make him lose face in front of his driver, his guard, and these people. You just paid tens of thousands of dollars to keep the camp open. Another few hundred…Soli, it's just the cost of doing business here. Please."

Sol undid the string of his scrub pants and fished around. Aswad gulped; Lila hid her smile. He handed her several bills. She counted and groaned, "You heard him, five hundred."

Sol cursed under his breath, but dug his hand into the bag, and drew out two more bills. "May he get crotch rot of the fingers from touching these."

Lila sneered, "Yuk," as she pinched the bills in her nails, holding them far to her front.

Outside, Aswad took Lila's hand again in both of his. She slipped the bills into his fist as he ogled her chest one last time, craning his neck to look down the front of her blouse. He stuffed himself back into his vehicle and snapped his fingers for the driver to move on. Sol waved goodbye, the back of his hand facing the jeep, his middle finger just a bit more extended than the others.

"*Mademoiselle Lila*, what the hell was that about? He seems quite fond of you."

She snipped, "Jealous? In his defense, though, you must understand that he is paid a salary not much greater than a street sweeper. It's all 'tips.' And, he is required to make payments to his superiors all the way up to the top. If I understand correctly, Aswad gets half, the next bloke keeps half of that, and eventually, Bashir pockets a small percentage, but it's a thousand times a day. Aswad's job is to control these people. If he can make money along the way, like by squeezing us, the people stay. As soon as the government's bled us dry, that's when the Janjaweed are dispatched to kill or capture the refugees for the slave trade. It is a very well thought out and complex equation. We are so far from civilization, they can, and have been, getting away with this for decades. Just like he said, no one cares."

"You care."

"And so do you. But no one cares about us. Tell the world when you get home. See what difference it makes. A five quid check from a housewife in London? That's all the difference it will make."

"And how does he speak such good English?"

"I'm embarrassed to tell you."

"You taught him?"

"No! Cambridge. British government scholarship for six years. Bloody English conscience. And you washed the perfume from your arms and face. Did you forget to wash elsewhere?" she asked, wrinkling her nose teasingly.

They finished the day at camp later than planned. It was after six when they left the camp to check on André. He was tottering about camp, though his gait lengthened to a goosestep when he heard the

Rover approaching. Lila paid the runners a few cents and a round of pita each then sent them off. Before they left, Daud laughed, "Madame, hellooooo." He stumbled for words, but gave up, pointed at the sun in the western sky, and allowed his finger to trace a great circle arc across the sky to the east. He touched the shoulder of each of his compatriots and turned to Lila.

She laughed and pronounced carefully. "Too-mah-row. Yes. Yes." She pointed at each of the boys, making them say the word five times.

The boys improved with each try, but Zahra appeared from the kitchen hut wielding her wooden spoon. The boys darted off, though Daud ran twenty-five yards, stopped, turned, and squealed, "Madame, hellooooo. Too-mah-row. Yes!" Zahra shook the spoon at him, and he joined his comrades.

When the screams of "too-mah-row" faded into the savannah, Zahra shook her head, wiggled the spoon at them again, and turned smugly to Lila. "Madame, make good eat mister. Sun go…eat."

Lila thanked her and walked to André's side. His entire face was swollen, the tissue around his eyes black. The seeping blood from his nostrils had dried on his upper lip, a few withered trickles crusting the corners of his mouth as if he had grown a purple Fu Man Chu mustache.

Lila winced as he turned toward her, but she took him by the arm and sat him on the picnic bench outside the common hut to recount the latest headlines from the camp. He listened without expression, and Lila's lips pursed, her eyes welded to his. When André did not reply, Lila burbled, "Well, whatever, the good news is that all is not lost: Zahra is planning a special meal for you at sunset."

"*Merde*, sheet," he hissed and hobbled away into his hut.

Lila turned to Sol. "We need to chat."

They sat in the common hut. Zahra brought tea. Lila sighed, "He's not all there. Getting worse, actually."

"Are you sure he's taking his meds?"

"I don't know. I've watched him swallow a few times, but he's a sly devil, you know. Could also be a subdural from the fall."

"Well, he's not dying any more, at least. He's probably too young for a subdural. And I don't think he hit his head that hard. I'm going out on a limb and betting on malaria. Anyway, they can't drain a hematoma in his brain, or in the maxillary sinus, in El Fasher, or at least, I wouldn't let them try, even if that turns out to be the problem, which I don't think it is. We can't get him back to Khartoum tonight, or even to Nyala until late tomorrow, and all they'd do there is put him back on real anti-malarial meds, which they don't have, and we still do, so for right now, we can do just as well as they can. We've got enough Artensuate left for a few days, but that'll be the end of my pretty lady's endowment, and it'll cost us one more bag of IV fluid." Sol shook his head sadly, "Each one of his doses would cover ten kids. I guess we've decided André's life is worth about a dozen Africans. Sound about right to you?"

Lila added quietly, touching his arm again, "So, we treat a sick man, a patient, as hard as we can. Maybe today we won't save the world, just one person. Not bad for a day's work, eh what?"

"Touché. Let's go talk to him. May have to tie him down. And I'll do it if I have to."

André was on his back, staring up into the thatch. He barely moved when Lila sat on the edge of his cot, or when she revealed they planned to treat him that night and evacuate him the next day. Lila turned to Sol, who had drawn up a syringe with a few ccs of Artensuate. She nodded. He found a vein on André's arm and slowly pushed the plunger. "*Mon ami*, this is the second time today I've had to hurt you. I am really sorry." André did not twitch until Lila and Sol rose to leave.

That brought a shriek. "Do not bring me ze food of zat woman. Zis is already ze worst day of my life."

Sol laughed. "Okay, I'll eat it."

"Zen zer will be ze two generations of ze doctor die."

Lila pared some of the fruit Zahra had found on her trip to the market in the next town and added a few tablespoons of fresh camel yogurt and sugar, from which she carefully picked out the gnats. She brewed a cup of coffee, exhausting the few beans remaining at the bottom of André's bottle. She brought it to him on a wooden board, but as she set it by his bed, he groaned, "I am so weak…"

"Do I have to feed you like a baby?"

André eyed the fodder and whispered feebly, *"Oui, s'il vous plait."* As Lila touched his lips with the first bits of sweetened yogurt, André opened his mouth with a tremor. After a few bites, his eyes rolled up into his head and his breathing became agonal. When Lila gasped, all movement ceased for fifteen seconds, but he sat up abruptly, snatched the spoon with a laugh, and finished the fruit compote. "So, you see, I am ze fine one...better suddenly."

Lila's eyes narrowed to slits, and she knocked the coffee into his lap. "Very humorous. You can clean yourself."

She stormed out and sat alone in the common hut until Sol came in, freshly showered, in a clean pair of scrub bottoms and a tee shirt with an FBI logo given to him by a patient halfway across the globe. When she didn't look up or even blink, he bent down near her ear and whispered, "Excuse me. Are you catatonic?"

"It's not funny. Don't you start. We already have one wise arse in our midst."

Sol laughed, "You want to take back the Artensuate we just wasted on him?" He thought for a minute. "We don't choose our patients, do we? We treat all comers, even the despicable." Lila's lips curled up a millimeter, and Sol went on. "And it's the worst day of his life, after all, malaria and a broken nose operated on by someone who's never fixed one before. Well, I take that back, sort of. I saw one done on a drunk old lady in an ER in the South Bronx. This second-year resident is tugging and pulling, doesn't know what the hell he's doing, and she's vomiting up purple T-bird all over him. I had to run out."

Lila shook her head, interrupting. "Are you daft? Do you ever stop jabbering?"

"What I mean is, let's let him slide on this one."

"You can, but I know him well enough to guarantee he's been planning this all day."

Zahra appeared in the doorway with a bowl of what smelled like meat and another of steaming grain topped with slivers of green onions. She smiled warmly, pointed to the plate, and asked, "Mister eat?"

"No," Lila smiled blankly, "he's not strong enough to eat that. He took some fruit and yogurt. But thank you."

Zahra left shaking her head, and Sol grabbed from the bowl what appeared to be a very small chicken leg. "I don't believe it. Roast chicken? It may be the worst day of André's life, but it's about to be the best of mine." He brought the tiny drumstick to his mouth and clamped down on the meaty knob. He waited for the juices to run, for the meat to come away from the bone and fill his mouth. He would chew and chew and forget what had become of him, if just for three minutes. But his teeth sprang back, for the meat was as tender as the spare tire on the Rover. He tried again, and on the third bite, he wrenched so hard to separate the meat from the bone, the drumstick flew across the room, caromed off the wall, and skidded to a stop on the floor. A cloud of dust juddered around it.

* * *

The evening was particularly chilly, and he said good night to Lila early. He brushed his teeth and trudged to his hut, so exhausted he tripped on a small rock just outside the door. As he fell to a knee, he saw the cloth of his scrub pants discolor with blood. He hissed, "Shit, what next?" The answer came with a whoosh just over his head. The thatch above the doorway split, a dark rod coming to rest in front of his face. He jumped back, imagining a branch holding the roof in place had cracked, but as he inched cautiously to the door, he saw in the moonlight that the stick was tipped with a triangular blade as wide as his palm. He pulled and freed it from the roof. It was an African spear, the razor-sharp front blade counterbalanced at the tail with a coiled steel band. It had been aimed at him, and would have poked a silver-dollar-sized hole in his head or his chest had he not tripped on the stone.

He ran to the common hut where Lila still sat staring numbly at the wall. She looked up, first into Sol's eyes, then at the weapon in his hand. "Where did you get that?"

"Someone threw it into my hut. Came through the roof. Just missed me. If I hadn't tripped..."

"What are you talking about?" she interjected sharply.

"This spear, Lila. Someone threw it into my hut. Let me try and guess who it could be."

Lila muttered, "You're probably right." She hit her fist on the arm of the chair and hissed, "Bloody bastard. Okay, we're going into camp right now and get this sorted out."

As the Rover bumped along the moonlit road, they saw two men walking away from the compound, so Sol sped up, but with the sound of the approaching jeep, one man dashed right, the other left, both disappearing into a clutch of huts. Sol gunned the accelerator. "Hang on. We're going to be in camp before whoever did this gets back. We'll call a meeting and see who's missing."

As they pulled up to the checkers' compound, several of the men jumped from their large tent to block Sol's entry. Lila, a step or two behind him, slid to the side and barked, "Meeting, now. Here. Anyone who doesn't attend is sacked. No pay, no ticket back to their home town."

Suleiman came out and stopped in front of Lila. "Madame, checkers very angry."

"Angry? About what?"

"Oh, yes, very angry. You see, we have no moving water, no 'lectric. All things you have in you compound."

Lila heaved a deep breath and spoke sharply. "Suleiman, I don't like your tone. You know very well we don't have running water, and very little electricity. And you knew quite clearly when you came here what the conditions would be. This is your country, not ours. We are trying to help so that you will learn enough to build a new society here."

Muhammad walked up next to Suleiman. "And people thank you very much, but you must treat equal, not *abed*. We not to work until have run water 'lectric."

Sol took a pace to stand inches from the man. "You listen closely, both of you, all of you," he roared toward the tent, "I came from halfway around the world, left everything I had. I'm spending all my savings in this place, and I'm doing it for you. One of your pals, and I'm sure it was Achmed, tried to kill me tonight. He wants to *murder* me because I stopped him from hitting a *woman*? So, you know what, all of you can kiss my ass. I'm leaving in the morning. I'll be back in London in two days and tell them, and there will be no more money to pay your sorry asses. And then all of you can rot in hell with the *jinn, al hum de le la*. Lila, let's go." He paused for several seconds before proclaiming very slowly and succinctly, "Lila, we drive to Nyala tonight. Tomorrow, El Fasher. Report all checkers to police." He waved an index finger at them. "You know how much money I have in El Fasher? One hundred *thousand* US. I pay police to kill off every bad checker man, *al hum de le la*. We go back to Khartoum in two days. By time police come here, we *khawajii* at home in London. Then police make refugees dig hole in shit field to bury all sorry fucker checkers." Sol swept his hand toward the array of motionless, staring young men. "I am done. I go home."

Though Sol expected Lila to protest, almost hoping she would, and force the checkers to concede, she nodded and muttered, "Let's go. I'm done here as well."

On the trip back to the compound, the Cruiser illuminated the same two men walking on the road. They looked up as if deer in headlights. One dropped a bottle onto the road as they crossed in front of each other and fell into the dust, but as Sol sped forward, the two crawled madly into the brush. Sol turned off his headlights, retrieved the bottle, drove a hundred yards toward the refugee camp, and backed into a slip between two trees. He convinced Lila that they should wait, hidden, until the men reappeared. When the two tottered onto the road, Sol delayed a few seconds, started the jeep, and darted out of his warren, right foot pressed to the floorboard.

Lila screamed, "Don't! Are you mad?"

"You're damn straight I'm mad, pissed off, crazy; those assholes tried to kill me. Not you, *me*. But calm down, young lady, I'm just going to scare the shit out of 'em." The two men tore for the sides of the road, once again crossing paths and stumbling. Sol skidded to a halt less than two feet from the quivering bodies. He sprang from the jeep and yanked one of them to his feet. The other he left passed out on the dirt. Sol turned away from the odor of alcohol and screamed into the night sky, "Hey, cocksucker Achmed, you want to kill me, prick? Here I am, coward. Take the first shot."

Sol pushed the man away, taunting him to take a swing, but Achmed collapsed to his knees, a stream of urine soaking his pants. Sol barked down at the cowering man. "Get on your feet. I'm taking you to the police in Nyala." He snatched a rope from the tool compartment and tied Achmed's hands, wrestled the whimpering man into the jeep, and bound his feet behind him.

Lila put her hand on Sol's arm. "Let him go. He's just going to slow us down. And the bloody coppers don't give a damn. They may even arrest us."

The ride back to camp was silent. Lila jumped from the jeep and ran to André's hut. The Frenchman was reading by candlelight. He looked up, shocked. "My Lila, I did not sink I would ever see you again. You can please forgive me. My head, 'ee is not right."

"Heeee has never been right. But..." Her eyes dropped, and she began to shake, and soon her sobs filled the *tuchel*. André stood uneasily from his cot and took her hand, pressing her gently down onto the corner of his bed. He poured a glass of murky water and handed it to her. She whimpered, "This has become a nightmare. When did it all go sour?"

"Long before we arrived, my Lila."

Chokingly, she related the evening's events and drew a deep breath. "It isn't safe here anymore. I'm leaving. Sol's leaving, and you are going with us."

André nodded. "It is time. Zer is ze food for ze long period now. Ze checkers can be in charge, or if we want to kill ze people, we put Zahra into ze refugee kitchen." Lila gasped, chuckled, but soon broke into a fit of laughter. André's shoulders lifted a bit. "Zat is ze first time you have laughed in ze whole life, I sink." André helped her up, hugged her tightly, and walked her to the door. "Now we must pack ze sings. I will miss you."

Sol was loading his duffle bag when André stuck his head into the doctor's hut. "Soli, I am so sorry zis 'as all 'appen. I know zat you 'ave give up so much to come 'ere."

"André, and you too. But the madness. We can't even trust our own side. Let's go back to Khartoum. Maybe there's another refugee camp we can go to together."

"No, my friend, I sink I am done. I am going 'ome. Become ze real doctor, come to ze States, and make ze million dollar. And I sink Lila is tired. It is dangerous if she stay in ze Sudan. She is ze most beautiful woman, maybe in ze world. She was different when she first come to 'ere."

They collected their bags at the Cruiser. Sol removed the tires from the Rover, pulled the distributer from the engine, tossed it angrily into the back of the escape vehicle, then pulled the drain plug on the gas tank. Lila ran to the kitchen and shook Zahra, who was asleep on the dirt floor. She clutched a club in her right fist, one she'd wielded when gangs of local Umm Ballans infiltrated her kitchen hut to pilfer the larder. Lila handed her a hundred US dollars, whispered good-by through tears, hugged her, and ran out. The older woman's eyes clouded as she watched the foreigners packing.

Sol asked, "Do you think we should make one more sweep of the camp to see if we've forgotten anything?"

Lila snarled, "Who cares? It's over. Please, let's go."

Sol took his place in the driver's seat but turned to Lila and asked, "Sure you don't wanna drive? Good chance to get some night experience."

She hit him with a bag of stale pita and laughed but soon began sobbing softly. André turned from the front seat and put his hand on her leg. She grasped his hand, squeezing it so hard he winced.

To get to the road that led through the desert to Nyala, they had to drive out of camp for a mile along the same path that led to the refugee area. At the crossroad, they could turn east where they would be safer dealing with the *jinn* and the Janjaweed than with their own minions. They had gone half-a-mile when they saw bright orange oil torches, a dozen at least, moving down the road toward them. Sol stopped the jeep a hundred yards from the fires, and the three Westerners stared as the fires approached.

André brayed, "And now zey come to burn us to des."

But Sol muttered, "I don't know. I'm not sure. They wouldn't announce themselves like this if they meant to hurt us." He opened his door and shouted heatedly, "Who goes there? Who are you, and what the hell do you want? We have two guns, and we will use them."

A voice called in English, "*Doctori*, I am Suleiman. Maybe you remember Suleiman. Please do not kill checker with gun."

Sol stuck his head in the jeep and asked if his companions had heard the response. André nodded but whispered, "Do you sink we must trust zem?"

Lila sighed, "André, we don't have any choice, do we? We can't run them down. Let's see what they want."

Sol grabbed under the front seat and pulled out a rusted pipe wrench. He pointed the handle with both hands toward the men and growled, "Move forward slowly. I will fire my gun if there is any trouble." When they were thirty feet away, Sol bellowed, "That's far enough. State your business."

There was silence, and Lila whispered, "Sol, I do not think they understand what that means. Tell them to send one person to talk to us."

Suleiman answered that he would like to speak to the foreigners, and that he would come alone, but pleaded again, "Please do not kill checker with gun. We do not have even knife."

Sol beckoned the man forward but waited until he was twenty yards away before pointing the wrench halfway toward the ground. When he was sure Suleiman had seen it, Sol slipped it into his belt, keeping his left hand on the handle, a landlocked pirate captain. Suleiman approached with his right hand extended, and Sol took it hesitantly at first, but with the warmth of the Sudanese man's grasp, Sol tightened his hand.

The American began, "Suleiman, this has been a very bad night. We don't know what you want, but if you try to hurt us again, I will have to use my gun."

"No, *Doctori*, checker not to hurt you. Checker Achmed and Checker Ramadan to hurt you. But we punish." Suleiman turned and waved his arms. Several men broke from the rear of the mob and came forward dragging two Western-clad objects, both of which were flung at Sol's feet. He could barely tell the lumps were human. Their faces were so bloodied and swollen, Sol did not recognize them until Suleiman said, "This Checker Achmed. This Checker Ramadan."

Lila jumped out of the car and screeched, "Was this really necessary? We were leaving. You could have had your running water that never ran, and the generator that doesn't work, and all the food that isn't there."

"Madame," Suleiman began, eyes cast down, "Achmed tell lie to checker. He speak you have all this thing. He speak *Doctori* have Moslem women in compound.," He turned his eyes away and whispered, "Make sex. He keep Moslem women as *abed*. He say *Doctori* make him come to compound to watch make sex to Moslem woman, watch eat, watch wash with move water, even hot in morning."

Sol barely looked up as he shook his head sadly. Finally, he yelled, "So this is what you get for protecting a woman? You die?"

Suleiman answered, "No, *Doctori*. Achmed lie, hurt checker, hurt poor people, so Achmed die. He live Khartoum. Arab government. He spy."

Sol growled, "What do you want from us?"

"We kill Achmed and Ramadan, you come back?"

Lila's voice cracked, "If you kill Achmed, we will have the army put you in prison. We came to Darfur to help people, not to kill them."

"Madame, if man try kill friend, must kill him. To *our* life, man do bad, must pay for all of life. You white say forgive, turn other cheek. Too hard for us to understand."

Lila grit her teeth. "Suleiman, you are a wonderful man. And I respect the law of the desert, and how you have tried to help us, but it is not our way, and the people who gave us their money to help Sudan do not want this. Achmed did wrong. You have punished him enough. Let him learn to be a better man. Please, as my friend, do not hurt these two anymore."

"Madame, I speak to checker. We do not want white leave. But not all us so stupid. We know this camp important to us for all our life, what we learn from you. I beg you stand here. I talk to many checker."

Both Sol and Lila got back in the jeep, and Sol slipped a disc of his music into the CD player. A piece of classical began slowly. The syncopation and tone were so poignant, the three friends leaned back, faces relaxing as if they had been transported to Paris and were sitting in a grand concert hall. André's eyes closed as he spoke softly, "Soli. Zis music. It is like ze medicine."

"*Rachmaninoff, Piano Concerto.* To me, the best piano concerto ever written. Maybe the best piece of classical music, ever."

Lila added so softly, it was hard to hear her whisper, "*In C Minor, Opus 18*. Poor man almost killed himself writing it to prove he was a great musician. He was in a terrible despair after Tolstoy told him to his face that his music was useless. Maybe there is life after depression."

Sol turned the volume up, and the three remained quiet until the checkers, who had been gesticulating animatedly, suddenly quieted and looked toward the jeep. A minute of silence passed in both camps before the checkers pushed Suleiman forward. He stopped near the jeep and nodded subtly. "Music is of power. You to stay we ask."

Sol beckoned the rest of the checkers, and the two worlds clasped hands and departed in opposite directions. The three Westerners sat in the jeep, wordless.

André spoke softly, "Maybe we listen again?" As they drove back to their compound, he murmured, "I sink, Doctor, we are ze real United Nation."

Outside the common hut, they stood silently in prayer, hands grasped, squeezing hard, until André whispered, "Amen."

Sol lay in bed reading *The Good Earth* for several hours until the lantern flickered, out of oil. He fell off and slept through to dawn, the first time since landing in the Sudan.

CHAPTER SIX

The morning brought a sky Sol had not yet seen in Africa. At first, he thought a *haboob* had blown in during the night to choke the heavens with dust and sand, but he sensed a peculiar stickiness in the air, a scent he did not recognize. He came out of his hut, and as his eyes accustomed to the diminished light, he realized it was not dust but billowing clouds, some very dark, some pure black, all masking the ferocious equatorial sun. Even the temperature was unusual. An unpleasant coolness clung to his bare arms. It felt as if there was going to be rain, but he knew better, for there had not been precipitation, even fog or dew, in Umm Balla for half a decade. When clouds had occasionally formed and thickened over the dry years, the moisture that fell from them was virga, rain that evaporated before it touched the ground.

When Lila stumbled out of her hut, Sol called to her and asked if it was possible the clouds meant rain. She shook her head. "Seen this a time or two. Never amounts to anything. Burns off by noon, and then it's hotter than usual and terribly sticky. Enjoy it while you can."

Sol drifted toward André's hut. He was still asleep, and Lila came up behind Sol. She whispered over his shoulder, "Let's let him rest. I think we should talk over breakfast."

Zahra had put several rounds of speckled pita on the table, along with a pot of boiled water. Lila brought out the marmalade and a box of mildewed tea. She called to Sol, "Are you dining on my fare, or are you still fixated on your chocolate oatmeal and roast chicken?"

"Nah, I'm with you." Sol handed Lila a warm pita, and she lifted the jar of marmalade toward him, but he shook his head and gushed, "After you, *Mademoiselle* Lila."

"Enough of that. Yesterday was a big payoff for that bastard. Let's hope we don't see him for a fortnight, at least." She spooned into a region of the jar where the green filaments of fungus were sparsest, fewer and fewer of those areas remaining, and spread the jelly carefully on the pita. She offered it back to Sol, though he pushed it toward and smiled, "Ladies first."

"No, the best people first."

Sol touched her hand. "That's you, Miss Lila. Don't know how you've made it this far."

They were silent for a moment but looked up curiously to what sounded like an engine in the distance. They both turned at the same moment to see if the Rover and Cruiser were still parked where they had been left. They were, and when Sol saw the open hood on the Rover, he groaned, "Now I'm gonna have to figure out how to get that distributer lined up and get the tires back on. Young lady, do you still have the timing light in your *tuchel*?"

She twisted her face but didn't have time to answer before the sound drew so close, it was unmistakable. Lila spat, "It's that bloody arsemonger again."

In seconds, though, a green Land Rover pulled slowly up to the gate of the compound. The two sat frozen and Sol shook his head to clear the mirage. When it did not disappear, he rose and went to the gate to open the lock with the key he carried around his neck on a lanyard.

A Caucasian man in his mid-forties emerged from the driver's side, marched up to Sol, and extended his hand stiffly, in a decidedly European fashion. "I am Johnny Tomich, chemist. I arrive from Burroughs Wellcome to rid the flies." When Sol didn't take his hand fast enough, Johnny snapped a crisp salute.

Sol laughed, "Chemist. Central Africa. Okayyyy."

"Yes, organic chemist. Master's degree. University of Zagreb, founded 1669."

"Well, glad you're here, and let me ask, what did you say about flies?"

"Oh, you do not know? Well, my company, that is Burroughs Wellcome Fund, received desperate request from Umm Balla medical team. They said a 'Lillian' writing. She was begging my company to bring pest control services to Chadian border. Burroughs Wellcome are very famous for control of insects in third world." Johnny pointed to the trailer behind the Rover, a two-wheel platform covered in meters of twisted copper pipe terminating in a two-foot- diameter metal cone on a swivel six feet off the ground.

Sol nodded. "Very impressive, your device there," then muttered barely audibly, "Looks like an African tuba." He smiled at Johnny and asked, "So, would you like to join us for breakfast?"

Lila stood to receive the visitor, her eyes expanding as Sol introduced the very tall, deeply handsome man. He mentioned their visitor had come all the way from Yugoslavia.

"Croatia is my country now. Thank you very much."

Sol took a breath to apologize, but at that moment, André emerged from his hut to stagger toward them. "My friends, I am feeling like ze *merde*. Ze malaria, it is ze work of ze devil. I am sorry. Please, now I am ze burden. I never believe it could like zis. *Mais*, you must go to ze camp and work. I take ze rest." His body straightened as he locked eyes with the white stranger. "*Mais*, am I see ze *fantôme*?"

Sol laughed. "Nope. This is Johnny Tomich. He's here to kill the flies."

André tried to speak. "*Oui, la mouche*," but that was all that came from his mouth before he began weaving. Johnny jumped forward to steady him.

"Well, first," Sol sighed, "let's take a look at the nose before we blame malaria. Sol jammed half the pita into his mouth, chewed a few times while breathing out, took a long gulp of tea, closed his eyes, and swallowed. He guided André into the common hut and peeled away the bandages. André barely winced as the plugs of cloth were pulled from inside his nose.

'Ah ha!" Sol laughed as a pool of yellow-green, foul-smelling liquid drained from André's nostrils. "What 'a you know? A good old bacterial infection. No sweat. Gimme an old-fashioned staph abscess any day over malaria. Two days and you'll be driving us into camp, God forbid."

222

Sol gathered a syringe, antibiotics, a foot-length of rope, and a roll of tape from his hut. He asked Lila to twist a rope around André's upper arm and tighten until a vein appeared. He injected the medicine. "We'll do another dose tonight. You're going to be fine, but here I am putting all this pain into you, and such a good man. You know what they say is the definition of hell?"

"Where you must eat ze food of Zahra?"

"No, Escoffier, that's where you're forced to torture the innocent."

"*Mais non*, Soli. You 'ave saved my life. Maybe someday I will to return ze favor. *Al hum de le la.*"

Over breakfast, Lila laughed about how Sol had stood up to Aswad, refusing to pay for the provincial stamp. "Soli told him he had already paid bloody enough in Khartoum, and had papers to prove it."

Sol interrupted. "Well, I do. I mean, I was supposed to pay, but I tricked 'em, bastards. Great story."

André asked, "Who you treek?"

Sol laughed, "I had to go to the Ministry of Health in Khartoum to get a license to practice medicine in the Sudan. I mean that's like an oxymoron. Anyway, I went through maybe ten offices before I got to the Minister of Health. Big fat guy in a green room, bare walls except for the dripping mold. He's sitting at this empty, beaten up, old desk. Had a phone and nothing else. He looked like a camel driver off the street.

"When I showed him my diplomas, he shoved them back at me and said they weren't in Arabic. I said, 'You speak English so well, sir, I bet you can read them.' But really, he couldn't because he couldn't speak English worth a damn, certainly couldn't read it, and anyway, they were in Latin. I think he was embarrassed, and I know he was pissed. So, he picks up the phone, listens, then slams it down. No service, as usual. He told me to take all my papers to some guy at the University of Khartoum, the medical college, some Doctor Mondour somebody, and have him translate all of it into Arabic. Told me to bring five hundred US for the guy. When I got it all done, I was supposed to come back to the Ministry of Health and begin the process all over again.

"So, I went out in the streets and found a man who had gentle eyes and looked like he could read and write. I told him I'd give him ten bucks to translate and write down on a paper what I told him, and then sign it with the name of the guy at the medical school. I also bought him tea and lunch, so he did an extra good job. Gave him twenty. Guy damn near had a coronary.

"I went back to the ministry late in the afternoon, waltzed into the anteroom, and smiled at the secretary. I walked over and picked up her phone. She didn't know what to do; must 'a thought it was a European custom or something to float in and take over an office. When I was sure there still wasn't a dial tone, I put it down, smiled at her again, and knocked on the man's door. He picked up his phone, slammed it down, and I paid the fifteen-dollar fee in cash. Dropped it on his desk, but he wouldn't take the ten because it had a tiny little tear in the corner. All I had was another hundred, so he told me to give him that and he would sign the papers. I said no way, so I had to go to a bank and exchange the bad bill. They took my passport and had me write my address in the Sudan. I sat for twenty minutes, and when the bank manager came over he demanded a seventy-five-dollar fee. I told him it was all the money I had, and that I wouldn't be able to buy dinner, and that I'd have to go to my embassy to beg for food, and they would ask why, and I would have to tell them, yada, yada, yada, so he charges me fifty dollars for the transaction, and I was still stuck with the bad ten. I won that day, sort of, but they bilked me five hundred for a three-dollar travel permit the next morning, so, who really won?"

During Sol's yarn, Johnny discovered Lila. He stared at her when she wasn't looking, and she looked back when he was laughing at Sol. She left and asked Zahra for more tea and an egg sandwich for the visitor. When she sat back down, she asked with a hardened façade, "So, Professor, how long will it take for you to kill these bloody, damn flies?"

"Just one day, Madame. I will fog today and be gone tomorrow morning. I go to Foro Boranga to do my work there. Then back to Khartoum and fly home in four days to Croatia and back to the classroom."

"Are you teaching at the University?" Sol asked.

"No, I am teacher at special secondary school."

Sol screwed up his face. "Organic chemistry in high school?"

"Of course. Now we are starting in the eleventh year for most of our students. When do you start in your country?"

"College, second year. But only people in chemistry, biology, and pre-med have to take it. Stuff's too hard for most people."

"No, not hard. Physical chemistry is hard. That is for the high school seniors. But I miss it very much, the students. I have taken three months from class and wife and children." There was silence for a moment, and he went on, though more slowly. "But I think I am very happy I come to Umm Balla."

"Well, we are as well," Lila added. "When will you start?"

"If you would like, I can make circuit through compound here."

The three brightened, and Johnny nodded with a grin, finished his tea, and mounted the trailer, pouring gallon jugs of variously colored liquids into the tank behind the tuba. He started a lawnmower engine under the funnel, and a green mist puffed out in gusts. He drove the jeep around the compound in concentric circles, directing an extra blast into the latrine and shower areas. Sol followed behind and walked to the shower, pulled the door quickly, and jumped back. Not a single creature had entered its death throes, and he called to Johnny, who turned back and yelled, "Not to worry. Just wait!"

* * *

They drove in a convoy of two vehicles into camp. Sol was frozen when villagers ran from their huts with empty baskets held forward, begging for *durra*. Lila laughed, "In the old days, when we were a couple of dozen strong, we had six rovers, and we'd stop here in the village and dump a cup of *durra* into each basket. Sort of like Santa Claus."

On that morning, with Sol and Lila in the lead, and Johnny a few yards behind, the three just stared straight ahead, never making eye contact, even with the four-year-olds holding out upside down, battered pots.

At camp, Johnny Tomich looked about, plotting the orbit he would ply in the few hours he had to change the lives of ten thousand of the planet's irrelevant. He gathered a dozen young boys and spoke to them in Sudanese Arabic so fluently, the early teens did not laugh. He hired them to walk ahead of the fogger trailer and move the indolent from their infinitesimal patches of earth before he drove by and blasted the camp with toxins. Johnny looked with a critical eye at the throng of boys who coalesced about his fogger. Daud was the first chosen to board the trailer and shift the tuba left and right at Johnny's command.

When the team passed the hospital, Checker Nasr sprang out and snapped his fingers in Tomich's eyes, braying that he could drive a Land Rover better than any *kafir, al hum de le la*. So Johnny gave Nasr the keys, and the jeep bucked off into camp. Johnny walked alongside in his bleached-white socks and tooled leather sandals, riding crop in hand, pointing it brusquely for the boys to train their gusts of venom.

When Sol set up his clinic that morning, Suleiman followed him in and approached with a package wrapped in yellowed newspaper. He proffered it in both hands without looking up, and Sol accepted it with both of his hands. He asked if he should open it right there. "Yes, *Doctori*, it is from checkers. We present of you."

Sol tore the paper gently to find a used *jellabiya*, faded by the years, yellowed in places, browned in others. But it had been washed, now fragrant with the scented Sudanese soap the checkers used to bathe themselves. Sol unfolded it, modeled it in front of himself, and walked to the door to look at it in the light. Suleiman mumbled, "It is biggest we could find."

Sol turned it front to back a few times, noting the identical pockets and neckline on both sides. Suleiman piped, "Oh, *Doctori*, you can tell which way by stain on front, right here." He pointed to a deeper, amorphous brown patch then looked up with a contented smile.

"Suleiman, it is beautiful. I will start wearing it tonight."

"*Doctori*, checkers no good listen bad man. Checker know Achmed bad man. He always say sex on Umm Balla woman. It against Allah say. And is he lie."

"Let me ask, is he okay? Achmed? I mean is he able to walk?"

"Yes. Madame tell checker no kill him. But must go today."

Sol nodded. "Yes, he must go away now. We will pay for his bus ticket. Please give him some food, and we will return it to you tomorrow. Is that okay?"

Suleiman was silent for a moment, deep in thought. He finally mumbled, "You white too kind. Achmed bad man."

"Yeah, very kind." Sol's voice tapered off, his attention drawn to the darkening western sky. "Suleiman, can you go get Miss Lila and ask her to come up here?"

As Suleiman headed down the hill, a young, very dark man appeared out of the savannah to approach the clinic. He waited until Suleiman was out of earshot then bowed slightly and took a position in front of Sol. His face only inches from the doctor's, he announced, "Meester, I am Joseph."

"Joseph. Okay. What can I do for you, Joseph?"

"Meester, you see, I work Foro Boronga Camp. Miss Norine. She give letter."

Joseph pulled a crumpled envelope from a pocket of his threadbare *jellabiya*, gently withdrawing a sheet of lifeless paper. He thrust it in Sol's face.

To Whom It May Concern:
Joseph Mugabi worked at the Foro Boranga Refugee Camp for three months.
Norine Abbott
Please Help the Children Foundation
Camp Director

"Joseph, if you are looking for a job, I am sorry, we have no work here."

"No work, Meester?"

"No work. I am sorry."

"Meester, you give money for bus?"

"And how much is that, Joseph?"

"Maybe seven pound, maybe ten, Meester."

Sol ducked back into the tent and pulled a few crumpled Sudanese pound notes from his backpack. He stopped for a moment, sighed, and unzipped the outer pouch. He pulled out his emergency supply of oatmeal and cocoa. "Joseph, are you hungry?"

"Meester, Joseph hungry every day."

"Well, here's a few pounds for the bus and some oatmeal and cocoa. Do you know what this stuff is?"

"No, Meester."

"Well, you boil water and put this in it and stir, and wait a few minutes, then stir it again and eat it. Okay?"

Joseph nodded and took the money and food without a word. He stared into Sol's eyes before turning and starting down the hill. He waited until he had gone ten yards then opened the packets of oatmeal. He poured the flakes into his mouth, chewed a few times, and tossed the paper wrappers away, scraps of life that caught the wind. As he looked up indifferently into the darkening sky, several women scurried across the sand for the blowing wastepaper, the chasers blocking and maneuvering until the fragments had been seized. By the time Sol looked down the hill, Joseph was gone.

Sol set up his table and chair and dragged the cardboard box of dry antibiotics to the sand by his left foot. The jerry can of water, he placed to his right. The women coalesced into a line meandering for what looked to Sol to be miles. With the clouds, the air was a few degrees cooler than the day before, and the refugees held their children in their arms, in the open, while they smiled and chattered with girlfriends. Sol looked for a checker to commence clinic, but he was alone.

Lila, who had been on her way up to the clinic, was intercepted by a checker who babbled that several dozen old Chadian men had staged a wildcat strike. They demanded a raise after one of their cohorts had fallen from his eight-foot-high platform and twisted an ankle. Lila detoured to the Distribution Center.

When she arrived, the checker stood in front of the strikers and told Lila the reason the man had fallen was because he had been guzzling sesame beer, a liter of it, before his shift. But one of the protestors stood from a hunker and huffed, "Old Muhammad, he can hold his liquor just fine. It is the terrible conditions the Jews have brought to us that threw him to the ground. The Jews, the *jinn*, the white, they come here to kill us."

When Lila asked where the Jews were hiding in the camp, the man barked, "You all have big red noses and white skin, so you must be Jews. You think you can trick us? *You* are the *jinn*, all of you, Jews. You, for one, carry money. A woman who carries money in her pocket and gives it to men! It is blasphemy." He had become so short of breath, he was unable to speak and glared at Lila, grinding his gums furiously. He finally gasped, "You talk back to men. You tell men what to do. You *live* with men. You sit in the front of a car. We can see your arms." He weaved about panting, until he steadied himself against a tree trunk "You must be a Jew; you are the devil."

His colleagues jumped from their squat to roar agreement.

Lila waited without expression until everyone rehunkered. She reached up to the breast pocket of her scrub suit, the men's stares locked on her hand. She pulled a notebook and pen from the pocket, eyed each man in turn, wrote a few scribbles, and ordered the checker to inform them that she was going to Nyala that very night, where she would pay the police to investigate the consumption of alcohol in Umm Balla. "Tell them again that I have written the names of the guilty. She waved the notebook at them and laughed, "The sin of *ithm*. They have a committed the taboo of consuming drink that is forbidden by God."

The checker paled and asked her if he could speak to her privately before he delivered the threat. They walked off a few feet, and the checker came close to her face. He whispered that perhaps the police might find things that were not altogether good for the camp.

She shook her head angrily, her expression hardening. "You tell them I am going." She turned and began to march stiffly toward the children's hospital, though called over her shoulder, "*ITHM*!" as she swung her butt ever so slightly.

The checker looked down his nose and hissed in Sudanese Arabic, "The *khawajii* woman *is* going to Nyala. You *abed* are as good as dead. Every one of you. The *khawajii* says she will pay money to make sure each of you fools gets one hundred lashes for the sin of *ithm*." The men's eyes widened as they chattered nervously, and with much grumbling, climbed to their platforms, grabbed scoops, and waited silently to drop an extra, illicit ounce or two of *durra* into the baskets of their kinfolk.

Sol called the first woman forward. She looked left and right, up and down, and when comfortable no checker was hiding under the table or in the cardboard box, she peeled the rags from her baby. Sol took a quick peek in the ears, glimpsed the fire-red eardrum, filled a plastic amoxicillin bottle with water, gave her the sun-here-and-there directions, touched her bare forearm, and asked the next patient to waddle forward. The first mom, though, did not move. She sat hunkered, frozen, looking at the spot on her arm Sol had touched, waiting for the skin to slough. The second woman pushed past her, and an encore performance ensued, and then the third and fourth, until hundreds of women had passed through the primal clinic.

When Sol saw the sun directly overhead, he walked to the opening, smiled at the women, pointed up, closed the grass mat doors, gulped a bag of raw oatmeal, drank a full canteen of muddy water, and stretched out in the rear of the hut, crushing down a corner of the cardboard box to fashion a pillow. Though the flies congregated over his prostrate form, he was so deeply asleep in minutes, even the monstrosities of the Sahel could not wake him. For a few minutes he dozed, dreaming of a horrible building fire at home in New York, in a very tall building next door to the apartment where he'd grown up. Sol was standing near the flames, unable to move until his father, long dead, floated into the scene and mumbled without emotion that Sol needed to do something. So, he ran into the inferno, pulled a woman to safety, then dove back for another soul. When he had amassed dozens of survivors, he looked to his father, but the old man stood behind the victims silently, unblinking, without expression. Sol wondered in the dream if the lack of communication on Jimmy's face meant he hadn't really helped a soul, but one of the women he'd dragged free, her face blackened by the fire, touched *his* arm gently. He felt a tender warmth, and his body relaxed. He was calm and tranquil—a sensation he had never before experienced.

Then, without warning, the broiling air stirred and light blasted into the hut. Sol woke staring into the eyes of a refugee woman hunkered next to him, her emaciated baby inches from his face. He rose and grumbled, barking at her to give him a few moments of peace, but she continued gaping at him, and he realized that if he kicked her out, he'd never be able to forget the act, so he took the baby to the table. There was dehydration though no infection, so he handed the mom several oral rehydration packets, but she snapped her fingers in his face and pointed to the little plastic bottles of antibiotics. He started to argue, to explain the need for the judicious use of antibiotics, for those medicines to be limited to prevent resistance, but stopped his hand signals, filled the bottle, and just as he began to tell her when to dose the child, she pointed to the sun, then to the eastern horizon, overhead, and to the west.

He laughed. She laughed. He smooched the baby's feathery-haired head; the young woman touched his arm, and he gave her a tiny tap in the shoulder. The next mom shuffled up, followed an inch or two behind by one more young woman, and another, until a hundred souls had passed through Sol's office before his lunch break was over.

By mid-afternoon, Johnny was on his second sweep of the camp, hundreds of barefooted boys trailing, taking turns to hop aboard and work the fogger. Several squads of young teens had scrounged tree branches and wielded them as swagger sticks, marching behind, mimicking the aristocratic Westerner as he pointed impatiently at swarms of vermin that had escaped the first volley.

When the troop neared the adult hospital, Johnny told one of the boys to close the flaps over the door so the full blast would not soak the patients. As the boy stretched the matting to draw it across the opening, Johnny saw a large, dark object just inside and ordered the jeep stopped so he could investigate.

As he walked in, his foot sank into a mush of mud, which he found curious, as there had been no rain in Umm Balla, he'd been told, for as long as anyone could remember. An instant later, he was hit with the odor of very fresh manure wafting from the puddle into which he had stepped. He looked up to see the rear end of a horse, not a great sized Arabian, but one large enough to carry the nomad who stood beside it holding the reins, two wisps of string tied through the creature's nose.

Johnny shook his head to dispel the mirage, but the odor convinced him, and he nipped at the man in Arabic, "Sir, you do not bring a horse into a hospital."

The man shook his head, trying to clear his own hallucination. He did not answer, but finally turned and went back to selling camel yogurt to the dead and dying.

"Sir, get that damn horse out of here. It is filthy. This is a hospital, not a barn. And clean up this mess."

The beaten mare passed a loud, long, rank blast of gas, followed by another bucket of scat, droplets of which sprayed on several of the nomad's emaciated clients. Johnny marched to the nomad, snatched the string from the dumbfounded wanderer's hand, and turned to yank the mount out of the tent. The man gasped, redid his *immah*, and struck Johnny in the back of the head with the tree branch he used as a riding crop. When Johnny spun around and slashed back with his own swagger stick, the horse spooked, jumped for the door, and broke into a sprint, knocking over children and huts, plowing through the shit fields as it galloped into the distance.

Several of the checkers, who had allowed the man entrance for a small percentage of the take from the sale, sauntered over. They spoke among themselves and agreed the foreign devil controlled much more in future income than did the nomad, so they dragged him out of the hospital, handed him his manure-stained *immah*, and barked at him to disappear.

When Johnny turned to leave, one of the checkers hollered at the nomad, "Get the hell out of here until the *khawajii* bastard leaves. Come back tomorrow."

Johnny growled, "I heard that."

The man left shaking his fist at the European, who ignored him and walked back toward his jeep. The platoon of kids retook position, though nothing moved—all eyes glued to the nomad in his obscene *jellabiya* crossing the defecation zone, head down, following hoof prints into the hills.

At three, Lila dragged herself to the clinic. She pulled the box of medicine wordlessly from under Sol's table to restock it. She nodded to him but said nothing, her eyes reddened and distant. Though Sol stared for a moment before turning back to the next patient, he couldn't ignore her and rose. He handed the baby down to the mother, winked, and told her he'd be right back.

Lila sat on the ground, her eyes closed. Sol hesitated for a moment. "Are you okay? Is there anything I can do?"

"Doctor Soli, there is nothing God can do. Thank you, though."

"What's wrong?"

"It's the final straw."

"What?"

Lila told him of Johnny's fight with the nomad and explained, "There was a lot of hub-bub around the place, and the checkers started pushing refugees around to impress Johnny. One refugee actually fought back, and Johnny heard the argument. Turns out, the so-called refugee was actually a local from just outside Umm Balla. The man was so mad at the checker for calling him an *abed* in front of his family, he told Johnny he was a farmer who had just sold his tobacco fields to some of the checkers for the right to live in the camp forever. Part of the deal was that he was not to be abused or extorted by anyone in the camp.

"He told Johnny that more than twenty percent of the people in the camp are locals who refused to sell their farms, but are living here until they harvest their crops. They have to pay a lot of their rations to keep the checkers quiet. Then he said he found out the real refugees are paying the checkers part of their rations so the checkers don't make up crimes against them and turn them over to Sadiq, the local lasher, who the checkers pay extra to be particularly mean to victims who talk back." She sighed. "It's all been a ruse, dear boy. Your life and mine. André, too. It's bloody awful to say, but he was right. We have been funding a cesspool. It's the last straw. Let's go."

Her eyes locked on his for longer than they had at any time since they'd met. Sol's chest tightened, and his legs felt wobbly. He stood above her for a minute, shoulders tensed, searching for words, thinking of touching her lightly, but went back to his station and finished the afternoon. He saw in that one day nearly as many patients as he had in the busiest month since he'd become a doctor, even during residency.

At 5 P.M., Johnny drove up to the clinic and sat next to Sol, erect and bright-eyed. "I am finished with the mission of Umm Balla." Sol could not help himself and peeked at the plague of insects still hovering about the half-mile of women waiting to see him. He recognized some of the women as having lined up for a third time that day.

Johnny smiled comfortably. "Doctor, you must be patient. You shall see."

The three, along with several of Johnny's helpers, drove back to the foreigners' camp at sunset. André was up, but trembling as he walked laps at a shrunken pace around the compound. The runners, their numbers now fully reconstituted, followed André, welding their attention to his every wavering. Zahra also followed, thumping the boys with her wooden spoon if they ventured too close to the incredibly pale man. When she whacked one boy, two more drew closer to keep André from falling.

Daud, however, was absent. He had remained in the refugee camp, having learned to drive that day when Johnny fired Nasr, who had been caught extorting a few pennies from the boys to sit next to him. Daud had wanted to come back with his compatriots to care for André, but his tribal family insisted he remain for a grand party to celebrate his exploits and the two dollars Johnny had slipped into his fist.

Lila paid the boys a few tenths of cent more that night, and they left for home. The hooting and squealing could still be heard when the runners pranced through the hamlet of Umm Balla, a mile away,

The four foreigners supped on Zahra's double-boiled okra, a scrap of double-boiled mutton, and stale pita. Johnny looked at his new friends and sighed, "I am sorry to have to tell Lila today of the farmer problem. Maybe it is not so bad to feed the farmers. If they are willing to give up their home to live here forever, their life must be very bad, and you are helping them. And maybe I am crazy to say that.

"I will miss you. In every other camp, the volunteers fight all the time. That is what they do even when they should be at work. And usually there are twenty or thirty of them, and no one does anything except plot against the next one. You are very different here."

Sol laughed gloomily, "Tomorrow is your last day? I mean in the field?"

"Yes. Foro Boranga. Fifty volunteers." He shook his head dejectedly.

Sol laughed, "You gauge your work by the number of Caucasians, not the number of flies?"

"Have you been to the larger camps?"

Sol shook his head. "This is my one and only."

"Well, you are very lucky. You have no idea what Africa does to good people. But I am done. After tomorrow, I will drive to El Fasher, give them back their Land Rover, and then fly to Khartoum. I cannot believe in two days I will be in Zagreb, clasping my wife and kissing my children. We will see one fly in the month of May, and my family will run after it for an hour with rolled newspaper. No more flies. I cannot imagine it."

Lila sighed then spoke in a whisper. "We are blessed to have met you. Thank you for coming. *You* will not be forgotten." She stood and asked the team to rise and hold hands. She sang *Amazing Grace*. The four nodded silently and went to their *tuchels*.

CHAPTER SEVEN

A n hour before dawn, Sol was awoken by grinding gears and the grumble of a tired engine as Johnny putted out of camp. When Sol left his *tuchel* to take a shower, he gazed into a sky darker even than the day before. The air was soaked with a humidity that had him dripping before he took five steps. At the oxidized shower cubicle, he jammed his nylon towel in front of his face and pulled the door open with a jerk, hurtling backward reflexively at the same instant. There was, however, no buzzing, whirring, or croaking. At his feet was a collection of deceased insects, frogs, and tiny mice. They were heaped in a mound that rose an inch off the muddy floor.

He went quietly to the fence around the compound, pried free a stick, and poked at the accrual until the water from the night before trickled into the drainage ditch. The monkeys screeched more vituperatively than usual as Sol showered in the freezing water. He laughed that if his bath in ice water was the worst moment of the next twelve hours, he'd have had the best day in a month.

When the three gathered for breakfast, a quiet sadness hovered until Sol finally broke the silence, shrugging, "What a good guy. Let's just thank him quietly."

André had gained strength overnight, announcing, "I am going to ze work today. You cannot stop me. I am ze *capitan* of my ship!"

Sol snorted, "Yeah, good, and I'm an admiral on the same boat, pal. You can go if you want, but I'm doing the driving, *al hum de le la.*"

When it came time to leave, Sol sat in the jeep, calling to André, "You don't get going, it'll be the next century before we get to camp." With no answer, Lila went to André's *tuchel*. He had fallen asleep, and Lila pulled down the mosquito net, tucked it in, told Zahra to keep an eye on him until the runners arrived, and climbed aboard the jeep with Sol.

At camp, Sol dragged up the hill to his workstation. Suleiman caught up to him and followed a few paces behind. The sky was darkening by the minute, and though Lila had assured him again the clouds would amount to nothing, that Sol would be long home before a single drop of water ever fell from the western Sudanese sky, he tensed, making out bolts of lightning in the distance as they tore from the desert floor skyward. At first, the thunder was twenty and thirty seconds after the flashes, more a rumble than clap, but the wind picked up, and soon there were crashes so deafening, the refugees grabbed their meager flotsam and jetsam, hurled it into their huts, and dove inside. A pack of six and seven-year-olds playing with twigs jumped up from their game, screamed, and sprinted to the nearest tiny shelter, lunging inside to bury their heads in rotted blankets and straw winnowing trays. It dawned on Sol that the children had never seen lightning, heard thunder, or ever felt a drop of rain.

His reverie dissolved when a marble-sized globule of water crashed from the sky, thumping his eye. It was more grit than fluid, the clouds of dust that had hung over Umm Balla for nearly half-a-decade soon to return to Earth as solute in the coming tempest.

Sol rubbed his eye and cursed. Suleiman jumped to his feet, and Sol spoke tremulously, "I don't know what's happening, but I have a feeling it isn't going to be good."

"*Doctori*, you must go. There to be flood. Many people *mat*, die."

Sol ducked a few more of the swelling drops and yelled to Suleiman, "Well, then let's get all the checkers together and make a plan to stop that."

"No, *Doctori* not understand. Water come now. All go way."

"Suleiman, these people can't go away. We need to help them."

Suleiman shook his head as he started toward the checkers' huts, but as water began to gush about them, he stopped and lunged back to seize the bewildered foreigner by the arm, forcefully pulling him through the paths that separated the refugees' frail huts.

"No, you go," the frantic checker shouted, trying to be heard over the chaos of screeching refugees and howling winds. "Soon all gone, all gone."

Sol wrenched his arm free, but at that instant, what had been a garden variety, third-world torrent gave way precipitously to unbroken sheets of muddy water, not just falling from the heavens, but thrust down so harshly, Sol felt as if he was being beaten by a cat o' nine tails. A sudden bolt of lightning bashed one of the huts just feet from Sol. The grass mats and plastic vaporized before his eyes. Sol dropped to his knees to search for the occupants, but another bolt exploded. The shocking roar heaved him to the ground, and the back of his head smashed against a *durra*-grinding rock.

As the flash of light in his brain faded, he anticipated a surge of pain but sensed only a blanket of calm and a dearth of emotion. Though his head continued in the muddle, he was aware that he did not hurt, anywhere. He felt satisfied to lie there and let Africa and Darfur and Umm Balla fade into a faraway dream. The thought of a subdural hematoma weaved its way through what was left of his consciousness, but he absolutely did not care. He let his mind darken until his only connection with reality was a bare sense of the deeply blackened sky.

It might have been a minute or ten or a day, but his eyes opened when he choked on water seeping into his mouth and nose. He heard the sound of violent coughing but was unaware it was coming from him. Next, he recognized a sensation of sliding and, finally, the obtuse vision of a black form dragging him through the mud.

Suleiman was nearly screaming, "*Doctori, Doctori,* what do you do, what do you do?"

Sol tried to speak, and though he could hear himself forming the words in his head, he could not make them flow to his mouth. While he knew he should be frustrated over the lesion that had disengaged the fragment of his brain that cared if he lived or died, for just an instant, he was at peace, the world outside his fading vision no longer of consequence. Somehow, he knew he would never again feel that serenity during the span of his life, so he let his head rest on the ground as the mud built around him.

He next remembered waking on an uncomfortable cot, lying directly on the prickly twigs and branches out of which the primitive bed had been fashioned. Suleiman and several other checkers hovered over him wide-eyed, blocking his view of their barracks.

"*Doctori* live! Checker so happy."

"What happened?"

"*Doctori* fall on head. Great rain. Suleiman tell *Doctori* all go."

"What?" Sol started to lift himself, but a wave of speckled gray descended over him, and he eased himself back onto the cot. When he tried to get up again, Suleiman pushed him back, though Sol spoke softly, "I'm okay now."

He rose, swung his legs over the side of the bed, and sat for moment to let the blood rise to his brain. As his mind sharpened, he wobbled toward the light, pulling aside the moth-eaten blanket over the doorway. The hut was abruptly flooded by an intense shaft of light. He jammed his wrist in front of his eyes and spun back into the barracks. He tripped and landed on his knees. The checkers were mute as Sol righted himself and took a step back toward the door to push through the blanket into a new world.

At first, the sun was so overwhelming, the empty hillocks and hollows in the distance were just a field of blurred, bare sand. As his eyes adjusted, he could make out a large shed or two, and then a few scattered refugee huts. He had never been in the checkers' area during the day, and realizing that, he nodded to himself that they must have chosen a remote patch of land for themselves, far enough away to remain out of sight of the squalor of their workstation. As his vision cleared, though, he realized the large buildings were not far away at all, and he started off toward them, picking his way through bits of blue plastic snagged on uprooted tree trunks. Occasionally, there was a cooking pot or a grinding stone that had been lifted by colossal forces and returned to earth, now useless hunks of refuse half-buried in the sand. He bent forward to pick up wisps of shredded tee shirts and torn feeding center wrist bands.

There was movement near the food warehouse, and he set out, walking at first, but he broke into a mindless, uncoordinated jog, his eyes fixed on the few souls milling about main camp. Fifty yards from the warehouse, he saw Lila sitting on a rock outside the medical supply hutch. He ran toward her but became light- headed and began to weave in the wet sand. Suleiman, who had been following at a respectful distance, ran forward and grasped one of Sol's shoulders to steady him.

Lila jumped from the rock. She dashed to Sol, clasped his arms. and looked up at Suleiman. "What's happened?"

The checker began vibrating as if seizing. He sputtered, "Ms. Lila, *Doctori* sleeping, sleeping. Checker take him on bed, say no go..."

"Suleiman, please be calm." He stopped shaking but went on babbling until she brought her index finger to his lips. "Please...talk slow my wonderful friend."

Suleiman took a step back, unable to form words, and Lila asked, "Sol, can you tell me what's happened?"

"I slipped and hit my head on a rock, I guess. I don't remember. I woke up on a cot in the checkers' barracks. I must 'a lit outta there too quick. But I'm okay now. Just a headache. Are you okay?"

"I'm not sure. I've been down here assessing the damage. Half the huts were washed away, along with dozens of babies and kids. The refugees scattered; some of them are off looking for their missing, but Muhammad said most are running to get away from the angry spirits."

"Angry spirits? Jesus." He paused and stared into the sky. "Then again, maybe they're right. I guess when they get hungry, they'll be back. Did they take any food with them?"

Lila answered, "No. The *durra* and oil were locked up. The key was in the pharmacy. It's gone, the pharmacy, that is."

They made their way toward the warehouse, pushing through gullies running with red water. The building was nearly floating; a sludge of *durra* seeping out to mix with the crimson mud of Central Africa.

Lila speculated, "Looks like the burlap didn't hold up."

Sol rose and boomed, "I'll murder that son of a bitch when I get my hands on him."

Lila took Sol's arm and steadied him, though he pulled loose and took a few uneasy steps toward the locked doorway. He yanked weakly at the rusted lock and lowered his head as if he was going to walk back to Lila and Suleiman but, after two steps, spun about and jammed his foot at the hasp so hard, the door splintered off its rusted hinges. He kicked a second time, and a third, to free a path through the debris. That, however, triggered a collapse of the fifty-foot-long straw walls. The grass mat roof crumpled halfway down. He turned to the checkers who had drifted over. "Get the flashlights."

When no one moved, Lila yelled to Suleiman, "Torches. Get the bloody torches."

The bottom bags of *durra* were soaked, the burlap shredded, but the upper layers were dry. Sol turned to Lila. "That's why Mr. Chun told me to put a layer of logs down first. And we didn't. Can we get a gang of men in here to unstack the good stuff?"

"We can. We'll pay them in wet *durra*, but we need to get it out of here in a hurry."

The checkers gathered a hundred dazed refugees and broke them into several platoons. The *durra* was restacked in two hours. As the sun set, a skirmish broke out amongst the workers over the spoils. The checkers waded into the melee with sticks, slapping at the antagonists. Sol quipped, "Looks like they're swatting flies."

At that instant, Lila and Sol turned to each other and their jaws dropped in concert. She gushed, "Crikey Moses, there are no more flies! He did it. The bloke's machine..." Sol watched her eyes for a moment before turning to the interpreter. "Have the men carry the bags to the distribution center. That is, the ones that haven't dissolved."

While the sacks had weighed a hundred pounds dry, soaking wet they were in the two-and-three-hundred-pound range, and the refugees stood, unmoving, arms crossed arms in front of their chests. Sol agreed to allow four workers to man each bag, and added an extra cup of *durra* in compensation.

With the sudden activity, throngs of women descended upon the distribution center, heads bedecked with cooking pots and baskets. They queued in four parallel cattle shoots leading into the remnants of the straw building. Once in place, the hungry refugees formed into family bands and hunkered, pots still balanced on their heads. They waited, jabbering excitedly, to claim their cups of serendipity. Soon, rumors began to circulate up and down the lines that because the spirits had not seen fit to wash these particular folks away, the *khawajii* were frightened of them. These were God's chosen, and the foreign devils would grant them an extra helping of the spoils of the storm, *if* they knew what was good for them. In Shoot Number One, the rumor was extra cooking oil was on tap; in Number Two, speculation had it the *khawajii* would supply dried okra; in Line Three, it was sugar; and in Four, salt and soap.

The checkers sauntered about smugly, ordering the food distribution workers still alive to the center. They snarled there might be a few scraps of leftovers for them if they presented to their stations without a squabble. A bevy of old men hobbled in from the four corners of what was left of the camp to climb rickety twig and branch ladders to their elevated, eight-foot-high, rickety, twig and branch workstations. There, the men reflexively dropped into hunkers next to grass-mat ducts poking vertically down through the floor. Next to each tube, a worn shovel was connected to a stout, wooden post by a five-foot, padlocked, heavy iron chain. The worker's task was to wait until a woman stopped under his grass-mat tube. When the basket on her head was in place, a worker below raised his hand, and the man above dumped a shovelful of *durra* into the tube. Another worker smacked the tube with a tree limb, to free the last of the grains, then hollered at the woman to move on, to the rear of the building. There, a checker examined the load to ensure no extra grain had found its way into her basket.

The gates were opened, and the first woman was directed to the furthest chute, though planted herself under the nearest tube. She braced for the load, but nothing dropped from the upper level. A checker howled up at the men. Silence. He cursed, climbed the eight feet, and shook his head at the platoon of workers, hunkered stiffly, arms locked across their chests. He moved down the line shoving and kicking at the elderly refugees, but they remained squatted, protesting that the grain was so wet and heavy, it was inhuman to expect them to work that hard for a payment of just an extra cup of *durra*. They demanded assurances they would be compensated for their yeomen's service. Lila was called to adjudicate, and when she agreed to an extra half-shovelful for the upstairs laborers, work resumed.

But it was not for long. The line halted as two dozen women stuffed themselves together just inside the distribution center. They refused to accept their ration until also guaranteed extra cooking oil, grain, *and* soap. The checkers shrieked that the only reason they were getting the bonus rations was because of the flood, and that they should be happy they were getting anything at all. The women, though, shook their heads in unison, refusing to proceed to the exit at the far end for the standard checker inspection. They stood frozen until a twenty-eight-year-old hunkered and crossed her arms in front of her bare, pancake breasts. She pooched her lips in defiance. The squatting spread in waves. Soon, a hundred stick-like figures poked out of the sandy ground, broad pots balanced on their heads, a patch of upside-down mushrooms in the failing light.

Lila was called back. She explained patiently that night's rations were different than the standard weekly allotment. There was not a flicker of movement, so she gathered the checkers and argued with them for five minutes, then returned to tell the women that if they stood, took the food, and made their way to the exit, the ordinary checker inspection would be suspended, but just for that night.

"So," one of the women queried with a smirk, "if we leave now, the checkers won't sift through our baskets and accidently spill out a cup or two for themselves? Is that what you're saying?"

"Yes, you will be allowed to go straight home. But only this time. Tomorrow, God willing, when you come to the distribution center, the checkers will be there to make sure no one gets extra just because your grandfather works upstairs. Can't you see that we do this to protect you?"

There was a bit of rustling. Several women came to their feet and yelled up to the scaffolding, prompting their grandfathers to wait until they got under the shoot. "Then you chuck me an extra shovel-full because the bastard checkers had their eggs squeezed by the *Khawaja* woman. So, don't forget."

They danced along the line, madly inflated portions of sodden grain shooting through the straw tubes. As pots tumbled and *durra* spattered, a wave of cursing rose, then a howl of plaintiff *al hum de le* *la*s. The wailing created a grand vacuum, sucking in gangs of ladies from the other clans, all dropping to their knees to skirmish for the scraps. Lila's head drooped, and she walked from the structure to sit alone in the darkened jeep.

Sol found her and leaned against the side of the Cruiser. He was silent for a bit before groaning through the window, "We should 'a left couple 'a days ago. There ain't a thing you or I or André or Johnny Tomich are going to do to get God to change his mind about Umm Balla. He's angry at Africa. And I think we may be enticing Him to strike us down 'cause we just don't get it. How many times do you think He's going to thump us in the head before the final swipe comes? I just don't know what the hell these folks did to piss him off. All I can think is, it must 'a been somethin' big, and He don't want us messin' with his plans."

Sol slapped the side of the jeep. "I say we go back to camp, get André, pack just what we need, drive down to Foro Borranga, find Johnny, and all of us head for El Fasher. My treat."

She looked at Sol for a moment, fingers entwined on her lap as she breathed slowly. When she let her eyes close, Sol risked staring at her. He enjoyed the zing in his chest and tried to imagine another face so stunning. He had never seen her in makeup and wondered if she had ever used even lipstick. It didn't matter, though, for she was gorgeous, perfect, the curve of her jaw, the camber of her cheekbones. At the same time, he withdrew, starkly aware he had not an inkling how one captured a heart so impossibly distant.

When her eyes opened, she smiled and whispered, "I know."

Sol started the jeep and inched slowly over the ruts carved by the torrent. As he turned onto the path to their compound, Lila muttered, "Now what?" In the distance, a blur of yellow flames juddered. She asked, "Didn't we just leave the checkers in Umm Balla?"

Sol drove forward at a crawl, the sallow flames breaking into separate oily torches. He and Lila were silent as they pulled up to half-a-dozen men. They pawed at the jeep and whined in a jumble of Sudanese Arabic and local tribal dialect. "Do you understand them?" Sol asked.

"Of course I do. No. Do you?"

Sol opened the door, stepped out, and searched for a familiar face. One of the men, an elder, smiled gently and reached forward to stroke Sol's arm. The man made a wiggling gesture with his hand and arm and a pinching motion with his digits, abruptly striking at Sol's butt. Sol smacked his hand away and pulled back, but the man howled, "*Doctori, Ta'ala, ta'ala*," then pointed into the darkness. Lila mumbled, "I think someone's been bitten by a snake. He's saying come with me. I know that much."

Sol shouted, "*Hwar, hwar?*"

The man pointed into the distance, "Inderabiro."

Sol's head dropped, his remaining spirit exhaled with a feeble sigh. "That's a long drive at night. It's north of here along Wadi Azum. How did these people get here? And with the rain? The *wadi* has to be flooded. It must 'a took hours, so whoever got bit has long since flown to their salvation. There's no point. And what about André? No, no, we can't do it. Can you tell him?"

But the man rubbed Sol's arm, his black eyes pleading, then snapped Sol's behind again. Sol stifled a laugh and asked Lila, "What the hey. You wanna go see another cadaver? Can't get too many corpses under your belt if you're going to be a real medical professional, can you?"

She, too, tightened her lips and nodded. "André will be fine. Not to worry, he's on the mend. We probably won't get back tonight." She looked into his eyes, letting her smile broaden. "Not a chance, dear boy."

They loaded the old man and six of his elderly companions into the jeep and drove away from camp along the rutted, sand paths, drifting north, paralleling the *wadi*. The spokesman provided directions by banging Sol on the arm with his fist at each turn then pointing wildly. When they rolled into the village an hour later, a cluster of cachectic souls ran to the jeep and grabbed at the two *khawajii*. Sol relaxed and let them guide him to a straw hut at the outskirts of the tiny village.

He was towed into a mud and grass enclosure, six by eight feet, smaller than a cell in the darkest African prison. On a wooden platform twelve inches off the sandy earth, in the greasy yellow beam of an Eighteenth Century oil lamp, lay a long-legged, extremely thin little girl, perhaps eleven years old. On the ground below the bed sat coiled the rear nine-tenths of a serpent, a green mamba, Sol was sure. But when he thought about the course he had force-fed himself in tropical medicine before coming to Sudan, he remembered the mamba was not supposed to live that far north in Africa, the scant number of trees in the Sahel robbing the serpent of its favorite haunt.

As Sol eyed the helix, the old man ran from the *tuchel* and returned holding the viper's head between the thumb and index finger of his left hand. He took the head and slashed at Sol's hand, hissing more loudly with each swipe. Sol pushed the hand back, carefully avoiding the fangs exposed by the crushing grip. "Okay, okay, I got it."

Sol called to Lila, who was outside the *tuchel* stroking the mother's arms. "Hey, could you bring my bag? I wonder if the antivenin's still any good."

Lila looked at the snake and shook her head. "Green mamba, but they aren't supposed to live this far north."

When Lila reentered the hut, the child was sweating madly, her head lolling about like André's two days before. She swung her arms combatively, moaning loudly. Lila looked again at the serpent and added, "But it clearly looks to be a mamba, eh what?"

"It is looks like a mamba, but like you said, maybe not. So maybe it's a variant, a cousin. I don't know anything anymore. And you know, this kid doesn't have a lot of symptoms of Dendroaspis envenomation. She should be paralyzed by now, and she's swinging around like a break dancer."

Sol turned to the old man and shrugged his shoulders, asking with the pinching motion where the girl had been bitten.

The man pulled the child's *tob* up, pointing to her right buttock. Sol took the lantern from its mud ledge and placed it next to the girl's skin, focusing immediately on a single, tiny puncture wound. He mumbled to Lila, "One fang mark? I thought mambas strike over and over. And, there's some swelling and maybe a little infected fluid right below the skin, but that's not what snakes do. There should be some necrosis, skin death, with a nasty snakebite, not fluctuance. I'm not even sure the puncture wound's a fang mark."

Lila answered, "What are you thinking?"

"You are the first person who ever accused me of thinking. I just don't understand why she's not paralyzed. That's what a mamba does, better than anything on Earth. Maybe she got bit, okay, but maybe it was a dry bite. Mambas carry a lot of venom, but if they strike and miss on the first swipe, most of it gets squirted away, and there's not much left. Say George, here, snapped once before he got purchase and blew his wad, then he tried a second time as they like to do, and only got her with one fang because it's hard to penetrate a tight, spherical butt when your mouth's only half-an-inch wide. Okay, say he did get one fang on the second strike, and there's almost no venom left, but the kid sees the snake, goes nuts, and let's face it, venom or not, it hurts like hell. So, the village goes nuts 'cause the kid's acting nuts, and *they* see the snake. And if everybody believes something's real, it *is* real whether it is or not. So here we are, no venomous snakebite, I don't think, but a little bacterial infection from the one dirty fang. But that's not going to make her this sick—no way. You know what, I think she's got malaria, or maybe it's psychogenic."

"So, this is the antithesis of André?"

"Lila, lovely lady, this is Africa. Cause and effect took a holiday here about a hundred thousand years ago. And by the way, we need to get back and check on your André and give him his antibiotics. I don't want him developing an osteo. If the nasal bone gets infected, he'll get a saddle nose. He'll look light a prize fighter for the rest of his life."

Lila smirked, "He may like that. They can call him André the Giant Nose."

"Very funny. We need to get back and follow-up on him."

Lila became serious. "Are you saying you don't want to spend the night here?"

Sol paused in thought. He stared deeply into Lila's eyes as he spoke evenly, "I'll give her a shot of the antivenin, and we'll load her up, and her father, too. Keep her in the hospital overnight. We'll get her stabilized and back here in the morning before she catches something really deadly."

As they put the child into the jeep, another crowd of villagers descended on the Westerners, men and women waving madly as they congregated in a circle around the Rover. Sol, already in the driver's seat, slapped his hands on the wheel, but when he looked out of the window more closely, he saw the petitioners place another little girl on the ground. As he and Lila pulled themselves from the jeep, Sol's jaw dropped when he focused on the girl's enormous belly.

He lifted his hands and eyes to the heavens, "That's a world record, Lord. Headlines. Your *Daily Mail*, isn't it?

GIRL AGE NINE CARRYING OCTUPLETS—EACH
FETUS WEIGHS MORE THAN MOM.

Lila grinned but turned serious when the father snapped his fingers in her eyes and told her to save his child. He pointed with his index finger to the crook of his elbow, making the sign of an injection. Lila mumbled to Sol, "Well, let's have a gander, shall we?" As she hunkered beside the child, the man's hands were in her face again, repeating the demand for intravenous intervention.

Eventually, they determined the girl had been fine until dinner that night but suddenly began crying hysterically, her tummy expanding by the minute, until she deteriorated into a semi-coma. Had the family ever seen this before? No. Was the girl well a day before? Yes. Did she eat anything different than the rest of the family? No. And what was it that they had eaten? A man ran toward a *tuchel* and emerged with a hollowed gourd and pushed it into Sol's face then into Lila's. It had a bit of yellow mush in the bottom, threads running through it of the same green mold that had invaded the marmalade.

Sol first inspected the girl's abdomen with his eyes. It was the size of a soccer ball, but it wasn't red or hot. He palpated, pushing his fingers slowly into her tummy. The child did not stir. "Not a surgical abdomen. Plenty of time before real trouble," he muttered. He percussed her gut, placing his right index and middle fingers flat over her belly button and striking them sharply with the tips of his left index and middle fingers. It sounded like a kettledrum.

Sol announced, "Gas!"

Lila's lips turned down. "That's what Mum used to say when she told us about being a little girl in the war. That meant on with your mask. Not happy times."

"Well, young lady, you are going to need a mask in a few seconds, just like your mama. Would you get me some soap from my Dob Kit?" Sol had the father put a grass mat on the ground, an operating table, then turned the child over on her belly. He called for a pot of water.

The man cracked his fingers in his wife's face and ordered her to fetch the family bucket. She did not move, so two of her neighbors ran off while the mom stayed behind to wail and wave her hands and a mutton chop over the child's head.

When Lila handed Sol his bag, he searched it superficially and patted his pockets. He looked up at Lila and asked, "You got gloves?" He turned to the audience. "Anyone here got rubber gloves?"

"Just get on with it, Doctor."

Sol soaped his right index finger and had the girl come up on her knees and present her rear end. As he inserted his finger in her butt, the crowd shrieked, and the father grabbed Sol's wrist. He wore a look of fury that scared Sol so, Sol pulled his hand away, rose to his feet, grabbed his things and Lila's arm, and strode for the jeep.

The cluster of peasants began to buzz. The volume amplified until the man seized Sol's left hand, pointed at that index finger, and gave the nod to continue.

A geyser of bowel gas escaped, and the girl's eyelids perked. With a second gush, Sol rooted around deeper and pushed her belly at the same time. When she was down to the size of softball, Sol stood and clapped the man on the shoulder, though the father pulled away before the index finger could touch his manure-caked *jellabiya*. Sol gave him a thumbs up, and the man grumbled to his daughter, who jumped to her feet and dashed off.

The father left without a word, following his daughter toward their hut. Sol turned to Lila. "And thank you so much, alien ogre, for sparing my precious daughter's life. Oh, and by the way, fuck you and the horse you rode in on."

Lila chortled softly. "And thank you very much, Doctor, for remembering why we came here."

Sol nodded, and they started toward the jeep but were slowed by a building commotion behind them. Sol tried not to turn and look, but it became so loud, he stopped and twisted angrily. The father was approaching at a trot, a six-foot spear raised above his head. Sol placed himself between the man and Lila, gnashed his jaw menacingly, and raised his Dob Kit as if a dagger. The man continued forward, stopping inches from the foreigners. Without a change in expression, he came to attention, took the spear in both hands, turned it sideways, and thrust it toward Sol.

Sol tightened his grip on the Dob Kit, but Lila whispered, "Soli, I think he's presenting it to you…Take it, Sol!"

Sol turned and handed the Dob Kit to Lila. He accepted the spear with a bow and pulled a dollar bill from the bag in his crotch, which the man snatched and shoved into a pocket. He spun around and was gone before Sol had zipped the plastic bag closed. A few loiterers followed him, though the majority of the peasants lunged forward, shoving daggers, spears, amulets, coffee pots, gourds, colorful baskets, wooden spoons—and one old man, his flip flops—into Sol's face. He pleaded in his meager Sudanese that his money was finally gone, but the men poked at his privates, their mouths twisted sarcastically in disbelief.

They eventually drifted off, the vacuum filled by a party of the senile who came to articulate a litany of infirmities that would have kept an orthopedic hospital occupied for decades. Sol escaped by walking backward, bowing with each step, nodding to the supplicants, each of whom was pointing to the veins in the crook of their elbows.

* * *

As they drove the dirt paths toward Umm Balla, the old man and his daughter dozed in the backseat, holding each other. Both Lila and Sol whispered, trying to allow them to sleep. Sol finally asked her, "Are you going to tell me now? Have I earned it?"

"Tell you what?"

"Come on, Lila. A promise is a promise."
"Why do you want to know about me?"
"I'll tell you if you tell me"
"What if I don't want to know about you?"
"Okay, but I want to know what happened to you. Don't you trust me after all this, Sweet Pea?"

"Oh, for Christ's sakes. You Yanks—so nosey. You have no respect for privacy, do you? A nation of busybodies." She was quiet for a minute, and Sol pushed no farther. As the jeep came to a flat road and the ride calmed, she murmured, "Very well, but not in front of our guests."

"When then, in front of André, who already knows?"

"Alright, alright. I was married to a Senegalese prince. Have you heard of Senegal?"

"West coast of Africa. Dakar. Kingdom of Takrur in the first millennium, then the Jolof Kingdom during the middle ages. Fifteenth Century, the Portuguese, then the French."

"Jolly good. Brilliant, actually. We met at Cambridge. He was extremely clever. Honors, first class, you know. But he was also gentle and kind, never arrogant. Handsome, too. Beautiful, really. We would talk about going back to Senegal and feeding children. But there were so many bloody obstacles." She shook her head irritably and stopped speaking, abruptly leaning back against the headrest.

Sol interjected, "But you're here, in Sudan. I'm sorry, Lila, you can't just stop there."

There was another long pause. "Finally, the president of Senegal, Abdou Diouf, that's another long story, gave my husband permission to work in his home province feeding kids. Then *I* met the president, and he signed my visa himself. I think he liked me."

"Well, duh."

Lila cuffed him on the arm and heaved a theatrical breath. "Sorry, sorry. I didn't mean to do that." She rubbed his arm. "I guess the story is fresher than I thought. It was my first time out of the U.K. It was shocking, but we were so happy, like a fairy tale." She stopped again. Sol bit his lip and kept quiet. "Then he got cancer and was gone in two months. He wasn't afraid. Not at all. Where he learned that is still a mystery. He believed he was going to join the kids who had died, and that he and I would be working from both sides. I'm sure he's toiling away on his part of the bargain. Sometimes I worry he knows what a poor job I've done."

"Wow, young lady, I didn't know we had so much in common. And I didn't mean to open such a fresh wound. I'm sorry."

"Not to worry. Actually, I wanted you to know. Now you tell me."

Sol hesitated. "If I do, you might think I'm trying to compete with you."

"Is it that bad?"

"Pretty much."

"Soli, go ahead. I want to know what's made you so driven."

"Okay. We'll be going our separate ways tomorrow, so I guess it doesn't matter. I was married to great woman. Her name was Dana. She was beautiful and smart, like you."

"Enough blathering," and she tapped his arm gently. "Come on, let's get on with it."

"We had been married for four months. Sound familiar? My sister Michaela was a nun, brand spanking new. She decided to go to Korea and work there to thank the Koreans for how well they treated my father during the Korean War. He almost died there. Shot."

"Oh, my goodness."

"Anyway, I was working full time at this awful clinic and couldn't take a minute off, and Michaela had to go to New York to the Korean Embassy to be interviewed for a work visa, so Dana decided to go along, get to know her and all that. Said it would strengthen our marriage. Her interview was on 9-11 in the World Trade Center. No DNA evidence. Nothing. Both gone in an instant, like they never existed.

"I didn't want to live—my entire family was gone. On the other hand, I had been given this precious skill, or so they beat into our heads in medical school. I still didn't really believe it, but my priest kept saying God was not done with me, and that Dana and Michaela would never have allowed me to quit. Bunch of other things, and he agreed there was no reason to stay back there. 'Go forward, Solomon, and serve God,' he said so many times, I started humming it in my sleep. So here I am."

Lila did not speak. Sol drove a few more miles before asking softly, "There's still one more piece of the Lila puzzle. When I first got here, I thought you said something about me not knowing what had just happened. That's not it, your husband passing?"

"Far from."

"I got the impression, at the time, it was between you and André."

"Far from." She sat back and closed her eyes.

He mumbled, "Leave it alone, Forte."

"No, you don't have to. I'll tell you. And maybe you will help me figure out what to do."

"I'll do anything on this Earth for you."

"No need to be melodramatic. But I have made the decision to do *something*." Another long pause. "At first, I just wanted to forget it, but that was because I was weak and afraid."

"That doesn't sound a lot like you."

"Well, it was, but now that I know you, I'm actually regaining a bit of trust. Even in Americans." Now Sol was completely silent, barely able to take in a breath. "Remember when we told you we used to have a few dozen bodies around here?"

"Yep. Hard to imagine."

"I can't remember what it was like, either. A dream. More like a nightmare, actually. Americans, and British, and a few Europeans. We Brits didn't get on all that well with the Yanks. They accused us of being unfeeling pommies; claimed we were all cold fish, happy to live our lives without affection. All they talked about was who they were going to sleep with that night. We British women got together, and we made a pact not to go to bed with the Americans.

"So, that very night, we sat around drinking sesame beer. The Yanks, especially this one doctor from Philadelphia, got really randy on the stuff. He broke into my *tuchel* in the middle of the night, the bastard. You see, one of the girls had just gotten a package that day chock jolly full of sex toys. He pinched one, and I woke up with it buzzing between my legs."

Sol looked away from her into the mottled moonlight, but she continued. "That wasn't the end of the world, but when I tried to push him away, he sneered at me with his ugly, perfect teeth. 'Ready for a little lesson in human reproductive behavior, you snotty, pommy bitch? You're gonna get it until you come.'

"I was half asleep. He stuffed the bed sheet in my mouth and managed to get my knickers off. End of story." Sol was speechless.

She went on. "Oh, I fear, though, there is a smidgen more." Sol still hadn't yet taken a full breath. "I bit his ear off.

"Never saw the bloke again. Gone in the morning, he was. But by evening, the Second Revolutionary War had broken out. The French and Americans versus us pommies. The so-called team blew apart at the seams, and over the next two days, there was a mass exodus. The Brits blamed the Yanks, the Americans blamed us. The Germans just sat back and drank more sesame beer. They were the smart ones.

"Our office in London wasn't interested, at first, and told us to stop acting like children and work it out. But when one of my mates said she was going to sue if they didn't take it seriously and report the bloke, all they did was say that there was trifling evidence, *trifling* mind you, that in the middle of some rough consensual sex, one of the girls had had her feelings brushed up. No names were given, well, just mine, and the British and New York offices settled the matter after the barrister in London called it, what was it, a 'he said, she said affair,' and warned that the American doctor could sue me and British Please Help the Children for defamation of character, *and* assault and battery.

"So, you see, there was nothing to be done. I became the lightening rod, not that bastard. Can't imagine what they're saying about me on both sides of the Atlantic now. And all over the rape of a very strange woman who couldn't have minded, could she? After all, she had been screwing a colored."

Sol remained perfectly still until they approached their camp, and Lila commented that there didn't seem to be much damage from the torrent. Sol groused under his breath so as not to offend their fellow travelers, "Just goes to show how much God hates this place. Screw the black man, save the white. Still want to know what these people did that's so bad. Every one of them couldn't have been an executioner in a Nazi death camp, a Stalin, or Mao Zedong. What the hell happened here?"

Lila carried the little girl to an empty hut and placed her on the bare cot. After Sol injected her with a few drops of the remaining Artensuate, he loaded a second syringe with antivenin. Lila returned with water, stale pita from breakfast, and blankets. "It's all we have," she told the father, touching his arm. He nodded without expression. She turned to Sol and asked, "Two doses?"

"No, Florence Nightingale, I'm covering my bets and pumping in a little antivenin also. Probably too late, but then again, she's not showing any signs of envenomation."

"Then why are you wasting it?"

"Okay, then we won't use it on her."

"You bloody well better."

André had been asleep as they'd pulled into camp, and after treating the little girl, both Sol and Lila went to his *tuchel*. The runners were also asleep on the ground surrounding the hut. Lila tiptoed past them and woke André, took a seat on the edge of the bed, and told him of their day and the flood. He laughed sardonically that he wished he'd seen the rain.

Sol screwed up his face and asked, "Wasn't there *any* rain here?"

"Not at all. Dry like ze bone. Clouds of ze black, *oui*, but I spoke to myself, 'God is teasing, again.'"

Lila shook her head and whispered to Sol, "The ground's wet. Must have been *some* rain. He slept through it. I'm not sure if that's good or bad."

Sol peeled away the bandage from André's nose. Yellow drainage gushed from the wound and dripped onto Sol's pants. He jumped back and tripped on his bag, dropping the syringe and medicine to the sandy floor. He rooted through the pile and selected a relatively clean needle and a bottle of antibiotics, both of which he wiped on his grimy scrub pants. He was disappointed and scared that the infection was still as active as it had been twelve hours before, but he hissed to himself, "Calm down, boy, you know better. We'll see after forty-eight hours."

They checked on their guests. Lila tucked the mosquito net around the girl's mattress. Sol laughed, "It's like shutting the barn door after the horse's run off. A day late and a Sudanese pound short, don't you think?"

Lila laughed, "You're sure it's malaria, are you?"

"No, I guess not. But I'm not the angel around here. You are."

"The answer's still no."

They retired to the common hut, and Lila boiled water for tea. With the lantern flickering, they dropped quietly on the beaten couch, Lila letting her shoulder touch Sol's. Both leaned their heads back, propped feet on the log that served as their coffee table. and in moments drifted off. Lila's head flopped to the side onto Sol's shoulder, waking him, but he didn't stir; a moment later, her back was pressed against him, and her head was resting on his chest. The scent of her hair staggered him, a gift on so awful a day. Though he had grown to believe that all women were essentially the same, that they were no more perfect or magical than a man, and that there was really little difference between the sexes, he was frightened that her touch seemed so distinct. He bent forward to draw in her breath, hoping that would break the spell, but even that was captivating, and it weakened him. He peered down and thought of kissing her hair and caressing her face with his hand, but he stiffened and shook her awake, whispering, "Lila, we need to get some sleep. Let me walk you to your *tuchel*. I'll check on the kid."

She nodded and straightened up, but more slowly than he expected, her hand holding his arm long after he'd stood and helped her to her feet.

She whispered, "What a day. I have a feeling this might be the one we'll remember for the rest of our lives."

They talked quietly as they walked, shoulders brushing a couple of times; and they laughed a little surveying the camp, the dozens of empty huts. She sighed, "I'm glad they're all gone."

Sol cleared his throat, "You mean except for Johnny and your Mr. Aswad."

Sol waited for the punch in the arm, but Lila turned to him. "Mr. Soli, if the rest of the world was like you, we wouldn't need to be here."

"I thought you were going to say, "And it's still no."

Her thump was playful. "I hope there'll be a day we can talk. There'll be light so we can look at each other. We'll chatter for days. No famine, no drought, no flood, no Africa, just hope."

Sol looked away. "There will never be such a thing as no Africa. Not for us."

Sol woke from an awful dream less than an hour later, and the harder he tried to get back to sleep, the more his brain churned. He gave up and made his way to the little girl's hut. Her father was standing outside, staring into the sky, and Sol followed his eyes heavenward to the miasma of sand and dust that had already lifted back into the stratosphere, blocking much of the moonlight. The air was frigid, and the old man was shivering as he grasped Sol's arm and drew him inside. Lila was asleep on the ground next to the child, both covered in tattered blankets. The father pulled up the girl's skirt, pointing at her butt.

One cheek, on the side of the bite mark, was now bloated and crimson, a tiny, off-white punctum having formed at the center. The other side remained its normal, steatopygous, muffin-like contour, the size of a hamburger bun. Sol patted the little girl's back before slowly moving his hand south, barely brushing the inflamed tissue. She whimpered, but her father coaxed her in Sudanese Arabic to be tough, and the child buried her face in the pillow. She did not stir again.

Lila woke. Sol sighed, "It's an abscess. The skin's so taut, it may rupture just pushing on it. How could this have happened so fast?"

"She's compromised. She's probably not had ten grams of protein in the past fortnight."

"Then how did she mount such a fierce immunologic response?"

Lila's head dropped. "Soli, I do not know."

"And I don't either, Miss Lila." He took a seat on the corner of the cot and stroked the child's ankle, ruminating, declaring finally to no one in particular, "I still think it's malaria, but she also got infected from the bite. It's not the venom. No way. She'd be dead if the snake had got it even half-right. The guy was a dud. It was a dry bite, but a dirty one. Pushed a slug of staph or strep from his tooth under the skin. That's the best he could do?" Sol raised his voice a bit, punching his palm. "Lila, it's an abscess. We need to open it right now. She'll be in septic shock by dawn if we don't."

Her gaze locked on him for a moment. She barely smiled, "Nothing's ever what it appears to be, is it?" She rose and walked to

Sol's hut to fetch the tools to drain the carbuncle before it burst of its own weight.

Sol signed to the father what was going to happen, and the man nodded without expression, though as soon as Sol injected the first cc of lidocaine to numb the area, the child shrieked. Sol accepted what he had feared, that local anesthesia was not nearly powerful enough to save the child from horrifying pain. "Lila, we need to go back to the refugee camp and get the nurses together and put her to sleep. It's time for a dash of ketamine."

"I detest the stuff," Lila hissed. "Every time we use it, the kids wake up insane, if they wake up at all. We've lost a couple just from the anesthesia."

"Well, it's got to be quiet when you're waking up or you get hallucinations. That's why we don't use it in the States, but a lot of people like it. I hear it's a big street drug. You and I could try it first."

"Please be professional, if it is possible."

"Not gonna happen, and it's fine for here. Fast down and fast back up. No respiratory problems. Don't need to intubate. We'll just make sure it's quiet."

"It's never quiet in camp."

"Will be right about now."

"Wanna bet?"

* * *

It took an hour to rouse an anesthesia team and find four lanterns and enough kerosene to last the thirty minutes Sol predicted the procedure would cost. The child lay silently upon a filthy grass mat on her tummy, staring at the sandy ground. Sol tapped her on the shoulder and showed her one of the Nike nylon gym bags he'd brought from the US to lug his supplies. He touched her cheek and smiled, "Little one, when this is over, I'm gonna give you this." He tousled her corn rows and pushed the bag toward her.

Muhammad spoke in Arabic, "Go ahead, it's yours, child. Take it. The *doctori* gave it to you." She grinned and gathered the bag, holding it close to her bare chest as if a doll.

The girl looked up at Muhammad and spoke almost stridently, "She say, '*My* father is a digger.'" The old man deflected the accolade with his hands, but she added, "*He* owns a *shovel*! It's the only one in Inderabiro!"

This time, her father shook his head no, but his neck straightened, and he suddenly had the courage to look Sol in the eye. He breathed heavily, imploring through the checker, "Please, foreign infidel man, *jinn* man, ghost with your skin inside out, help my daughter Kaltuma. That was my mother's name."

Sol nodded to Muhammad, who started an IV into which Sol injected a tiny amount of ketamine. When the child's eyes glazed over, and the tautness of her spindly muscles slowly softened, Sol gently brushed the swollen buttock with his fingers as a test. The whimper was joined by silent tears running across her dusty cheeks. Sol nodded to Muhammad, who had not taken his eyes off the girl. The solemn, coal-black man controlled the syringe so deftly, Sol believed perhaps only five or six additional molecules of ketamine had been injected.

Kaltuma's eyes closed as slowly and delicately as Muhammad had pushed the plunger, and now there was only stillness when Sol palpated the mass. He cleansed the area with gentian violet, speaking to Lila, his eyes locked on the child. "Young lady, this abscess is going to be so contaminated, I wonder why we're wasting medicine cleaning the skin."

"Ah, yes, Joseph Lister, let's get on with it. Do you want me to glove and assist?"

"Of course I want you here."

Sol made a tiny, superficial incision. He placed a piece of death shroud over the wound, in case he had cut too deeply, and opened the pressurized abscess. He watched the girl's eyes intently for the slightest tremor, and when the child did not stir, he lengthened the incision, snapping off bleeders with the prehistoric kit of surgical instruments that had likely bounced around Darfur Province since the British had been run out of the Sudan a century before.

"You ready?" he sighed. Sol plunged the scalpel deeper, automatically jamming the cloth into the wound, keeping it just a millimeter behind the knife blade. This time a putrid fluid oozed around the makeshift sponge, and he lifted the dam slowly to examine the effluent. The stench of fecal bacteria infecting the child billowed so fiercely into the mass of observers, several of the less medically passionate tore from the area, kicking up a miniature cyclone of sand and yesterday's dried feces, all of which settled into the open wound.

Sol shook his head and hissed, "Damn. So, our serpent pal didn't even get that right. It wasn't the staph or strep on his fangs. It was the fecal material on her skin, from never ever having bathed, that got shoved under the skin and took off like wild fire."

He scooped clots of reeking discharge until he was able to put his index finger into the cavity to break up compartments of pus that had walled themselves off to fool the unwary practitioner. His finger probed deeper, and then deeper, meeting only trivial resistance until his knuckles were blocked by the incision. "Man, I'm still not there. Gotta make it bigger. No choice."

"Do you think we should stop, Soli?"

"Yes, I do, and I wish I had never started, but what the hell, it's just dead tissue. If we don't get it all out, what we leave behind will keep festering, and there won't be anything left of her by sunrise."

He nodded to Muhammad, and the nurse pushed a bit more ketamine. Sol watched his patient's face closely as he moved the scalpel a quarter of an inch. Without a flicker of her facial muscles, he opened an additional patch of tissue and worked his whole hand into the wound, sopping up the rest of the infection. He ran a bit of the IV fluid into the cavity, sloshed it around with his fingers, and wicked it out with more cloth. He sighed again, closed his eyes, mumbled as if in prayer, then asked Lila to hold the flashlight over the wound. "Shit, that's what I was afraid of."

"What is it?"

"Bad news. We're down to the acetabulum, and there's our old friend the head of the femur. I thought that's what I was feeling. I just couldn't bring myself to believe it." He pointed into the gaping wound and nodded for Lila to look. "There's the hip joint. All the connective tissue around it's been devoured by the infection. She's screwed. Let's irrigate one more time, pack it, fill her up with antibiotics, and go home."

They waited in the hospital until the child woke. It was quiet in the camp, aside from the grunting of the horde of a new species of toad that had descended upon Darfur Province since the great flood hours before. But even they were beginning to die from the lingering glaze of Johnny's amalgam, and the croaking was slowly fading.

The release from anesthesia was so placid, Kaltuma was trying to sit up before Sol finished bandaging the wound. Lila took a couple of blankets donated by Brussels Airlines and covered the girl twice while Sol again proffered the nylon bag. He told Muhammad to let the girl know Please Help the Children was going to fill it with food for her and her papa. The nurse assured Sol he would find a blanket and a spot for the father in a corner of the hospital, and that he would make sure they had both *durra* and sweet tea.

Lila nodded with a gentle smile. "Thank you, Muhammad. Please make sure you give her as much as she wants. We are so happy the checkers are our friends again."

As Lila and Sol sat in the jeep ready to ride back to camp, he grumbled, "She'll be gone in a day, if that. I've never seen an infection move that quickly. Not from a superficial puncture wound, not in a compromised host who was barely able to mount an immunologic response. What is going on? Lila, I smell a rat. Somethin' ain't halal here."

He jumped from the jeep, jogged back to the hospital, found the father, and had Muhammad translate. "One more time. Ask him how long the kid's been sick."

Muhammad asked and answered, "Maybe three days, maybe five."

"Well, I thought the snake bit her only a few hours ago. When did the snake bite her, Muhammad? I want to know," Sol snapped.

"Just today."

"Then it wasn't the snake, was it?"

"The old man say of course it is snake. Snake kill people; doctor not kill people."

"But the time line? Tell him…" Sol stopped midsentence. He grumbled, "Thank you, Muhammad. But what does he mean a doctor doesn't kill people?"

"He say doctor give needle three day ago, so it is snake."

"What doctor?"

"Doctor come village Inderabiro with fat little man in white car. He make all children line up and doctor give every children needle in bottom. He say penicillin. Everyone father to pay fat man one pound. But how father know word penicillin?"

"He might if the kid was really given the shot. Muhammad, tell him it was the shot that gave his little girl the infection, not the snake. No, wait! On second thought, no, don't tell him. It really doesn't make any difference, does it?"

Lila was asleep in the jeep when he got back, and he moved off as smoothly as if he was driving a town car along I-19 through Whitaker. She didn't stir until they neared the camp, and Sol whispered. "We'll talk in the morning."

Sol could not fall sleep, so he rose, showered, brushed his teeth, and pulled on a fresh scrub suit—the one he had been wearing almost stood up on its own. He tacked a note to Lila's *tuchel* door, promising to be back after dawn, and checked on André, who was asleep. His skin was cool, the swelling and redness around his nose a bit less pronounced. As Sol shuffled, head down, toward the jeep to drive back to camp, Lila's door creaked open. She called, "Soli, wait, I want to go with you."

"You need to sleep. One of us has to remain sane."

"I want to go."

The jeep meandered the paths toward camp. Sol related his theory that the snake had had nothing to do with the little girl's impending death. "Like I said, everything here is a mirage. Maybe the world you and I come from is the only place where cause and effect is real. My father said nothing made sense during the war, either. Do you know about that insanity, I mean in Korea?"

"Sol, I know very well about the Korean conflict. I was a history major at university." xxxxx

"I had the impression you and your husband were both in medicine. When did you become a nurse?"

"I went down, I believe you call it graduating, from Selwyn College at Cambridge eight years ago. And I'm well aware of what that expression means to you Yanks. And I already told you that, that I was at Selwyn, didn't I? I'm getting senile from this place. There was no work for history majors; nothing meaningful, that is. So, I applied to nursing school. That's when I met Winston. Winston Fatouba. You and he would have become very close. Very much alike, the two of you. He'd do anything for another person, or even an animal in need, but it wasn't good to let him see you doing wrong, being greedy or callous. He simply couldn't tolerate bullying, when someone was picking on the weak. Your best friend, your worst enemy. I was so proud of him. He was reading international development at Pembroke College. They were very good to him there."

She was quiet for a moment, and Sol couldn't help himself. "Did you also know your pal Aswad when you were at Cambridge?"

"He is not my pal, at least not anymore, but we did date for a bit. I did it to make Winston jealous." Sol's jaw dropped, but Lila shook her head. "No, Solomon, he preceded me by a century, at least."

"Who, Winston or Aswad?" She did not answer, so he went on. "Why didn't you just turn around and go to the medical school at Cambridge?"

"In England, you don't just turn around and go to medical school. Especially as a mature student. Either you go to meds straightaway after secondary school, or you don't go at all. You have only one shot at the prize. We don't get second chances like in the U.S. In fact, I had to fight my way into the nursing program."

"Finish at the top of your class?"

"I did well."

Sol nodded. "I'm not surprised. And here you, we, are. Glad you took this path?"

"Well, I've not been very happy recently, but I'm feeling a bit more hopeful of late, the past few days." She was silent for a moment. "Okay, it's my turn. Why are *you* here? What are you running from?"

"You're perceptive, aren't you? And direct."

Her tone soothed a bit. "It's obvious. You lost your wife. It's a tragedy, the blow hitting so fast. I lost my husband. It was slow and agonizing. But you see, I'm fulfilling my end of a promise. You're out to prove something."

Sol grimaced. "Yeah, very direct. Okay, I've always wanted to tell you. I really screwed up. Maybe you'll say I'm a terrible doctor. You'll jump out of the Rover to get away from me."

"What did you *do*, Doctor?"

"Here goes. Couple 'a years ago, I had a patient, a real pain in the ass. State industrial patient, drug seeker. You have those in the UK?"

"That's mostly what we have."

"I was sure he was malingering. Always carrying on about the pain, the pain this, the pain that, howling in the waiting room and jumping around, and next minute, he's coming on to my nurse. Probably gave him more pain meds than I should have early on, but nothing to make the pencil necks at the medical board take notice." He was quiet for a moment, then smiled sheepishly, "Gotta admit, he did get a lot of Percocet from my office."

"Percocet?"

"Our oxycodone. I think you call it OxyNorm. Anyway, the way she, my nurse, explained it, it was such a hassle to deal with him, she was just trying to protect me, I guess.

"What was she *doing*?"

"I'll get to that. Suffice it to say he was the grand master pain in the ass. If you didn't give him what he wanted over the phone, he'd just show up without an appointment and harass the front desk and the patients in the waiting room until the receptionist had to park him in an exam room. Then he'd stand in the doorway of the exam room and badger the other patients as they walked by, 'Hey, did you know that Dr. Forte ain't treatin' my pain?' So, I had to stop what I was doing and go see him. This is like two or three times a week.

"Apparently, also, he was changing the number of pills on the prescriptions I did give him. And he always waited to get his scripts filled until after hours. So the pharmacy called just when my nurse was about to leave. You think they figured out he was altering the scripts? No, just wanted an okay or not to 'refill.'

"Roxi, my nurse, was tryin' pretty hard. She'd drag herself down to the record room to get his chart. But that day's chart note, or yesterday's, wasn't filed yet, so there was no way for her to know how many pills I'd written for—usually three or four. Took an hour, and she put in for overtime. Then the administration got on my case for not keeping my practice organized. 'No one else is charging overtime three days a week.' They threatened to take it out of my pay. So my nurse just started faxing in scripts over my name. I had no idea.

"Then one day, his girlfriend calls and says he's running around the house hitting himself in the head with a baseball bat because of the pain. And I had upped his meds to OxyContin. That was the final straw. I said, 'Sorry, lady, no more pain meds,' and she started to scream, so I told her to take him to the hospital. They admitted him for pain control."

Lila laughed thinly. "He was that good?"

"Well, they put him in a room and told him to stay in bed, but he got out and fell down. Broke his leg, right there on the floor next to his bed. X-ray showed a fracture in the proximal femur. It was around a weak point, a big hole in the bone, which turned out to be a met. So, all the time it wasn't back pain, but cancer in the leg. He was gone in a couple of weeks. Never found the primary tumor."

"They blamed you?"

"They blamed me for the meds. My argument was that I was treating cancer pain, but they said I didn't know it was cancer, so, therefore, it wasn't cancer pain as far as the authorities were concerned. So, I said whether I knew or not, I was sufficiently astute to recognize serious pain, and he really did have pain, but they dragged me before the State Medical Abuse Commission. They still haven't told me what they're going to do, but there's a new president of the board, some hanky-panky apparently with the last one, and they've been busy cleaning their own house. And who knows if they've even tried to contact me?"

Lila smiled warmly and looked into his eyes. She placed her hand on his forearm so gently, his chest clenched. "And who cares? They don't count. You will be fine. You're a great doctor, Solomon Forte."

Sol crept along as slowly as the jeep could go without burning out the clutch, wanting to make the time with her last, but they were upon the camp before he'd even gotten to the part where the State Commission had convened to end his career.

At the hospital shed, they found the night checker curled up on a fresh grass mat, snoring, so they wended quietly between the sleeping and deceased tiny bodies, barely able to tell one clutch from the other, both the living and the dead motionless on the ground. They came to Kaltuma, also lying stock-still, clutching the nylon bag. The airline blanket touching the bandages on her buttock was wet with drainage, though it was scant, and Sol chose not to wake her to repack the wound.

Lila took her pulse. "It's strong, a bit rapid, though nothing alarming. Not like hours ago, before you drained the abscess." The back of Lila's hand brushed the child's forehead. "She's tepid, but not sweating." Lila warmed her stethoscope, rubbing the bell against her palm before placing it delicately on Kaltuma's chest. Lila lifted her thumb and whispered, "Clear. You've done quite well."

Sol stood and lowered his hand to help Lila stand. She hesitated for a moment but grasped his fingers. He let his arm drop as soon as she was on her feet and turned to leave. At the entrance, he called over his shoulder, "Long time before camp gets going. Let's go back and check on André."

He waited in the jeep for her to ask him to restart the story, but her head sagged forward, and she was asleep. As the jeep crept through the village of Umm Balla, Sol noticed a light-colored cluster far out in the parched fields beyond the huts, one he was sure had not been there the day before. He slowed, tried to focus on the patch of relative white, then turned to drive into the fields to get a better look with his headlights. When Lila's head lifted, though, he said nothing and gently backed onto the road toward their compound.

At the gate, he fought with the Sudanese lock, noticing in the headlights that it had suddenly raised a patina of rust. He wondered how that could have happened to a hunk of metal that had never been exposed to rain or even one percent humidity until the past day. As he yanked and yanked, it finally gave way and broke into two sharp pieces which lacerated his palm. He wrapped his hand in an oily rag and drove forward without pulling the gate shut.

CHAPTER EIGHT

S ol slept until dawn, just as the cacophony of local roosters, sheep, camels, donkeys, monkeys, and the new plague of toads heralded the news that the Lord had granted Umm Balla another morning. André was sitting at the picnic table outside the communal hut wolfing down speckled pita and green-thread jam with one hand, a Duralex glass of black coffee in the other "*Mon ami*, you are well?"

"André," Sol laughed, "I don't know how I'm doing, but you look great. Did you get your dose of antibiotics this morning?"

"Of course. I injected to myself. So, you were right after all. I did not sink so, buy it *was* ze infection."

Sol snorted, "Well, I am very glad to see you're better, and that the malaria and the infection did not invade your brain and alter your personality. Is Lila up yet?"

"I 'ave not seen 'er, but ze door to 'er *tuchel* is closed. I sought she was at ze camp last night, so I do not want to wake 'er."

"Yeah, we should let her sleep. We had to go back there twice. She could hardly stay awake. I'm worried that she's getting near the end of her rope."

André thought for a moment then shook his head. "Let me knock and see if she wants ze tea. We can leave 'er 'ere today. An 'oliday."

Sol nodded and smiled weakly.

As André moved slowly toward Lila's *tuchel*, the little wooden door swung open in the wisps of the coming madness of whirling air. When André arrived at the hut, he knocked without peering in. When there was no answer, he looked back at Sol, his eyebrows arched. He called in, "Lila, you are well?" When nothing came, he ducked his head in the doorway. "*Mais*, Sol," he called over his shoulder, "she is not 'ere. And 'er sings are on ze floor."

Sol joined him. The mosquito net had been pulled loose from its attachments. The plastic bowl she'd used to wash herself before bed was lying on the floor, the spilled soapy water in a puddle next to the bed. Sol noticed the sand by the foot of her bed was ridged, and he followed the marks with his eyes outside the door and saw they crossed the compound, disappearing halfway to the gate. He grumbled, "Let's not get excited. We need to take a look around."

They banged on the shower hut, the loo, and the area behind the kitchen hut where Zahra and her children slept year-round in the open, on the ground.

André declared, "She is at ze camp. Come on, we go to see 'er and scold 'er for ze game she plays to get back at me. Very funny zis one."

They did not speak as André drove, Sol unwilling to waste his flagging energy arguing about who might be more proficient at the wheel. He tightened his seat belt, closed his eyes, and was actually beginning to doze when André gasped, "*Oh, mon Dieu*! Zer is ze fire!" He jammed the brakes at the first of the *tuchels* in the hamlet of Umm Balla, what was left of it, just tiny rivulets of smoke seeping from glowing straw filaments in the crushed mud walls. The two jumped from the jeep, stopping at several smoldering bodies behind the ruined huts, all women, their *tobs* pulled up beyond their waists, most with legs spread, tree branches protruding from their vaginas.

André screamed and pulled the tree branch from one of the women. Sol snapped, "Don't do that. We need to leave this exactly as we found it. Otherwise, there'll be no record."

"It is too 'orrible, Sol. I cannot leave zis."

"We gotta go."

As Sol turned toward the Rover, a glint near the ground caught his eye. There was another woman, nearer the huts, her unusually colorful skirt around her waist, though on the branch protruding from her vagina, an ornate crucifix was jammed into a cut in the wood. The thick gold necklace upon which it had hung was gone.

"Cocksuckers were sending a message," he hissed to himself. He thought about it for a moment and pulled the branch free, pried the cross from the branch, closed her legs, and neatened the skirt. He crossed himself and put the crucifix into his pocket.

André had watched and began weaving unsteadily. He collapsed into a pile of straw and vomited.. He tried to lift himself but fell back, barely breathing as he curled into a fetal ball. Sol grabbed him by the shoulders to yank him up from the heap of fodder. "You need to get strong, André. I am sorry. I know you are sick, we both are, but this is no time for weakness. You got me?" Sol dropped to his knees and lifted his hand to slap his friend but stopped and shrieked, "You got me?"

André looked up at Sol and straightened. "You are right. I must be strong. What we do?"

"And you are right. We cannot leave them like this. We need to check every one of these people to see if anybody's still alive. You are a doctor, my friend. Better than most. We can do that, yes?"

"Yes. I will do it."

They walked together amongst the bodies, seven by the huts, twelve more piled behind an empty animal pen, then eight in the fields, all women, all violated, all with throats cut or heads bashed. The two men did what they could.

Sol sighed, "*Mon ami*, all that matters now is that we find Lila."

"Zen we go to ze camp and find 'er."

"No way she's in camp. How could she have gotten there?"

"Maybe she took ze ride. She is not 'ere, so we do not know."

"Okay, we'll go and see. If she's not there, we need to get to Nyala and notify the UN. If we need to, we'll go up to El Fasher and contact the British Embassy."

Sol skirted the smoldering huts as he stumbled back toward the jeep. A tiny flicker of movement by a crushed mud wall caught his attention. He walked cautiously around the bodies, coming to a small scarlet mass covered in lumps of mud and ash, just a piece of cloth, he allowed, the shredded remnant of a *tob* rustling in the building wind. He shook his head and continued on, but a weak yelp stopped him, and as he twisted back, the cloth writhed. A muted screech tore Sol's breath away as a tiny, hairless head lifted out of the dirt. A chopstick of a hairless arm reached toward Sol. When the head dropped back to the earth, the sounds became a groaning, and Sol uncovered the rest of Might Joe Young's scorched body.

André had come up behind Sol and put his hand on his colleague's shoulder. "It is *terrible*. We must stop 'is misery." André took out his pocket knife, crossed himself, and cut Mighty Joe's neck. He pulled Sol to his feet and led him to the jeep.

* * *

Even before they came to the hill leading into camp, they could smell burning grass, though the scent from this distance was oddly calming, reminiscent of the fires lit to burn the autumn leaves at home in New York. Then wisps curled above the horizon, and as they crested the hill, André yelled angrily, "Foockers. I tell you many times. Foockers."

The hospital and administrative huts were charred, the larger poles having collapsed together, their remnants glowing and hissing, a dying, grand bonfire. The patch of ground that had been the pediatric hospital was now open to the world, no longer the dark, mysterious domain that had held within its grass walls so many tiny spirits during their interlude between this life and the nether world.

Sol walked to where he imagined Kaltuma's mat had been a few hours before. He picked up a chip of hard blue plastic, what was left of the nylon bag that had melted into the sand. Individual refugees, mostly very old men, wandered about aimlessly, picking at the earth for single kernels of *durra*.

Sol grabbed one and screamed in his ear, "Where are the checkers?" The ancient soul smiled sickly and put his hands together in prayer. Sol hugged him and stammered, "*Ana 'āsef, ana 'āsef,* I'm sorry, I'm sorry." The man stumbled away, headed nowhere.

They drove to the checkers' camp, but the tents were gone, even the pegs had been pulled from the ground, now just slits in the dirt where the wooden stakes had secured the shelters for that sad year. A man in ragged Western clothes came weaving toward them, an ancient AK-47 rifle held to his front, pointing first at Sol, then André, then back to Sol. There it remained, the barrel aimed toward the doctor's head. Sol raised his hands and shouted, "We do not have any weapons. Please point your gun to the ground."

The man stopped, staring beyond the two Westerners. He lowered the barrel a few degrees. "You take me ride El Geniena. I go home now. My mother is wait for me. I go home now."

Sol nodded. "Okay, we will give you a ride. We will take you to your mother. We will give her money. We will give you money. But tell us, please, what happened here."

When the man came closer, they could see his face had been beaten to the point that it was unrecognizable, the eyes swollen nearly shut, cheeks as bloated as if he and Aswad were the only obese men in the surrounding thousand miles.

Sol demanded, "What is your name?"

"You not know? I am Achmed. You make checker beat me."

"Oh, my God," Sol keened, "no, no, you threw a spear at me! Tell me you don't remember."

"You not shout me. I no throw spear."

As the barrel lifted again. André bargained softly, "Achmed, you want ze money? *Oui?*"

"You give money or Achmed shoot, *al hum de le la*. You give money take to El Geniena. You put up hand, *al hum de le la*."

Sol raised his hands again, though only in front of his chest. He cajoled, "Put the gun down, Achmed. I said we will give you money and a ride. Put it down or no money. We have so much money, but it is hidden. Put the gun down, or I will not tell you where it is."

The dazed man lowered the barrel again, but only an inch, and Sol took a small, slow step forward with his right arm outstretched, as if to shake hands and seal the deal. Sol offered gently, "I am going to go into my pocket and take out some money. But there is much, much more. Enough for you to never, ever have to work again. You can buy your mother a house with ten sheep, a hundred sheep. You and she will never be hungry again."

Sol pulled a few grubby bills from the front pocket of his scrub pants and started to unfold them with one hand. Achmed's attention was so riveted on the money, he let the weapon droop another several inches. When the front sights of the rifle sank below the beaten man's knees, Sol leapt toward him and yanked the weapon so hard, Achmed tripped headlong onto the sand. Sol gripped the barrel in both hands, raised the stock above his own head as if a sledge hammer, and screamed, "That's twice motherfucker. Now you *are* goin' to fuckin' die."

As the downward arc of the rifle gained velocity, André leapt forward and caught the butt in his hands. He screamed in pain, but held tight, spitting, "No, Sol, zat is murder. You stop now." He pulled the gun from Sol's hands and threw it wildly over the top of the jeep. "We need zis snake to 'elp us, *non*? Sink about it, Sol."

Sol cocked his leg to kick Achmed in the head, but his shoulders collapsed, and he walked to the weapon, lifted it, and retreated to the jeep. He jammed himself into the front seat and stared out at the featureless horizon. André hovered over Achmed, the fallen man having crawled into a fetal ball, mumbling in prayer. André hissed, "Where are ze uzer checker?"

"Janjaweed take, *al hum de le la*."

"'Ow you escape zem?"

"Achmed hide in sand, *al hum de le la*."

"What?"

"Dig hole in sand. Cover Achmed, *al hum de le la*."

"Where is Lila? Where is she?"

"Janjaweed take. Sell for Saudi man, *al hum de le la*."

André's teeth locked, and he kicked sand into Achmed's face. "Did not one of you *bâtards* 'elp 'er?"

Achmed answered tremulously, "Janjaweed have gun AK-47. Some man have AK-74. Why Achmed die for *kafir*? *Al hum de le la*."

When André's shoulders drooped, Achmed relaxed and raised his head a fraction, nodding, reaffirming the wisdom of his reasoning, the insanity of sacrificing for a *kafir*—a non-believer. André shrieked epithets in tear-soaked French, the anger of half-a-year honed to a laser point aimed at the lump groveling at his feet.

"*Cochon*, foocker, you die." André kicked Achmed's head with his sandaled foot then calmed for an instant and turned toward the jeep, besieging Sol to intervene. The American's eyes, though, were shut tight, his head pressed against the steering wheel, the air conditioning on high.

André swung around, dropped to his knees, and walloped Achmed in the head with his fists, a flurry of blows so violent, the Sudanese man's eyes closed, his taut muscles slackened, and the front of his western pants slowly stained with a dark, spreading circle. When André realized he had snuffed the checker's life, he slumped to the ground and rolled into a fetal ball next to his victim.

Sol still had not heard any of the beating, though after a few moments, with the swelter inside the sealed Rover a few degrees less than in the sun, he regained a modicum of consciousness and exploded from of the vehicle. He roared, "Son of a cocksucker," and sprinted back toward Achmed, to beat him until he agreed to serve as an interpreter for the days they would search for Lila. He would kill him when they found her. But when he saw both men motionless, he dove to the ground and searched the horizon for the sniper that had gunned them down. André finally twitched, and Sol crawled to his side. He looked for the pool of blood. When he saw no head wound, he became terrified that his colleague was shot in the abdomen and would live just long enough to speak a few last words, which Sol would someday have to deliver to André's parents in yet another foreign land.

But André sat up and shook his head. "I 'ave keeled zis man, Sol. I 'ate 'eem, *mais* 'ee did not deserve zis sing. What 'ave I done?"

Sol stood over Achmed, the Sudanese man's remains dusted with the red and yellow sands of Darfur, his arms and legs locked in the fetal position in which he had died. His eyes were tightly shut, the muscles of his lids locked in the same rigor mortis that balled his body. Sol thought back to the course in pathology in medical school, to the myriad corpses he had been ordered to scrutinize, bodies of the unnamed and unwanted hauled in from the streets of the South Bronx to further his education. He could not forget the Medical Examiner's van, the scent of recent death—not so different from that of life in those sad neighborhoods. The reek of stale alcohol and body odor hovered about the cadavers' uncleansed years of struggle on Bruckner Boulevard and White Plains Road. But Achmed's body was different—it was worse than the newly dead. It stunk of feces, more like the barely living patients in the hospital, late, late at night.

And while Sol had been solemnly advised by his octogenarian pathology professor, "Don't be fooled, Doctor, it is entirely possible for rigor mortis to occur just ten minutes after death," he had never once heard of the final gathering of locking calcium ions flowing into the deceased's muscles in forty-five seconds.

With a puff of wind off the desert, sand blew into the camp, and there was the feeblest quaver of Achmed's locked eyelids. Sol roared, "Wait a gotdamn minute. Bullshit. This asshole ain't dead." Sol grabbed Achmed by the faded Western shirt and dragged him to his feet.

Achmed screamed, "That *kafir*, he beat me to the death. Look what he do to face. Now I keeeeell him, *al hum de le la*" The man feinted toward André but did not fight back at all when Sol grabbed his arms and pinned them behind his back, or when Sol pushed him to the ground and held him there with his knees. The three froze, now the center of attention of a circle of refugees who had closed in on them. Sol lifted himself off Achmed when the man yelped, "You are keeeeell me," and spewed a string of rasping epithets in Arabic that brought the masses even closer.

Sol hollered, "André, get some rope from the Rover and help me tie this asshole in the backseat. We need to get the hell out of here."

André's eyes opened, and he jumped to his feet. As Achmed squirmed, André began to laugh and surged forward to resume the beating. Sol pushed him away, imploring, "André, get ahold of yourself," then spoke slowly, enunciating carefully. "We-will-not-kill-him-now.   We-will-cut-his-eggs-first-then-cut-his-throat-if-he-does-not-find-Miss-Lila-for-us."

They set out in the Rover, following the truck tire tracks in the mud that led toward the hills. Achmed was lashed to the backseat, his mouth covered with a gag fashioned from his underwear. They sped across the wasteland, the Rover moving so fast, the wheels spent little time on the sand. With a few miles behind them, the ground dried and the tracks grew fainter. Sol realized the rains had not deluged the entire region—it had surgically picked off only the truly vulnerable. They raced for an hour parallel to the *wadi*, shreds of man-made debris strewn on the banks. An object nearly masked in sand caught

Sol's eye. The jeep stopped, and as Sol climbed out, he was blanketed in the sensation he was being watched. He looked about guardedly and focused on a large mass leaning against the other side of a withered tree. He was sure it was a nomad. He reached back into the jeep for the AK-47 and chambered a round.

Sol yelled, "*Salam Aleikum.*" There was no response, not a twitch. He approached slowly, his finger slipping onto the trigger. Abruptly, a putrid odor blew into his face and stopped him. The wind shifted a few degrees, and it allowed him to take another two steps forward. He made out the face, a male, he guessed, for the hair was short, though the cadaver was so bloated and dark he could not tell if the figure was African or Caucasian. The body's western pants had been pulled down, though white socks remained visible. There were no sandals.

He held his breath and took a few more steps. Johnny's genitals had been amputated and jammed into his mouth. Sol vomited.

He and André tensely discussed what to do and agreed they had to transport the body back to Nyala. It was the only choice, yet as they bent over to move him, the odor made it was impossible. Gagging with each shovelful, they dug as deep a pit as they could and covered him with a few inches of sand. They rolled rocks over the grave in the form of a cross, and Sol took compass readings from several hillocks and noted the odometer reading. He recited the *Lord's Prayer* and drove on.

As they scrambled over the next hummock, Achmed began grunting madly, craning his neck. André cackled, "Sol, look zer, look, one of ze *camions*."

In a whirl of yellow dust, they caught site of a prehistoric, Russian troop truck less than a quarter of a mile in front of them. It had just begun a jounce up the foothills of a mountain whose peak was hidden in a veil of roiling sand. Sol could make out two figures standing in the back of the truck, faces wrapped in *immahs*, both training AK-47s into the cargo bed. Sol turned hard left, skidding the jeep away from the truck toward the hidden side of a dune. He could not know if his own churn of dust had alerted the Sudanese government's mercenaries, but he continued along the west side of the sandbank, coming to a revetment of reddened sandstone that flanked the mountain. He mumbled to André, "It's like being on Mars."

"I wish we are zere. It is safer zan Africa."

Sol backed into one of the fissures, turned off the ignition, placed his head against the steering wheel, and coaxed his breathing to slow. He turned to Achmed. "Hey motherfucker, I'm going to take off your gag. You shout, or you spit, and I'll have André slit your throat. Do you understand?"

Achmed nodded tremulously, and Sol pulled the obscene gag roughly from the man's head and hurled it against the window. The soiled material left an unctuous smudge on the dirty glass. Sol scowled, "Give him a drink of water." André poured a few tablespoons. Sol was silent until Achmed began whining and begging for more. "You listen to me. You are going to be quiet. One peep from you, and I'm going to cut your dick off and shove it down your throat. You got that?"

André laughed sardonically, "Not much of a meal. 'Ee will starve."

Sol turned away, not allowing Achmed see him grin. "First, Achmed, you are going to teach me how to use your fucking gun. No, first, you're going to clean it with pieces of your shirt, one part at a time. Then you are going to clean every bullet. When the gun's so clean you can eat your Wheaties off of it, shithead, *then* you will teach me to use it."

"What are you say eat? Achmed no eat *kafir* shit."

"Don't worry about it. I'll tell you what to eat and when. André, we will go up the *jebel* in the dark. I'll carry the gun. You follow. We'll put the rope on the dickhead's neck and keep his hands tied behind him, and for sure a gag. When we get up there, I will try to kill all but one or two of the Janjaweed, maybe wound a couple and have them lead us to Lila and Romey."

André thought for a moment and suggested, "*Mon ami*, do you sink it is better to wait until ze dark and zen head norse to El Fasher? If we fail zis night, zey will keeel us. *Pour moi, pas de problème*. I do not care for me, but zey will torture Lila. I cannot die knowing zis sing. *Non,* we must be smart, not ze cowboy."

Sol was quiet for a long time as he stared into the reddened dirt far beyond the edge of civilization. When he finally looked up, both André and Achmed had fallen into stupors. The temperature in the Rover neared one-hundred-thirty degrees. "Okay, you've got a point. But I'm going. At least I want to know what we're up against. You stay here. If I'm not back by dark, drive to Nyala and call the UN."

Sol snatched the AK, chambered a round, turned the weapon toward Achmed, found the safety with his fingers, looked at it quickly, and snapped it to off. Achmed's eyes burst open, and he dropped to the sand writhing like an eel out of water. Sol sprang forward and grabbed the man's shirt, ripped a few strips from it, tied the shreds together, and attached one end of the poor-man's sling to the barrel and the other to the stock. He suspended the weapon across his back and started up the blind side of the hill, trudging through loose sand and gravel, coming finally to a steep wall of shale. He pulled at outcroppings of volcanic rock until his fingers bled, though scraped a few meters higher until the wall was nearly vertical. He lifted himself onto a ledge but lay prone to avoid the sun on his face. He closed his eyes for a moment. When he opened them, he was looking straight down. He understood that he was trapped, unable to climb another step higher and incapable of descending, the footing so meager.

He lay there, sweat pouring with such ferocity, he could sense his dehydration building by the second, thirst charging from unpleasant to throbbing in minutes. He pulled at the skin on his arm as he had the dying children in the camp; his flesh tented critically. Soon, he had trouble remembering why he was climbing a mountain in the Sudan, then what continent he was on, and finally, he pondered what he had done so wrong in life to be condemned to suffer death by fire.

"Doctor, you will wake. I must take you down. Now, Doctor Sol! You will wake, NOW!"

Sol tried to peer at what was pulling him from the stillness of his swoon, but the dearth of water in his body had sucked away all trace of fluid from the surface of his eyes. They were cemented shut.

"*Maintenant*, now, Doctor. Take my 'and."

Sol rubbed his eyelids fiercely, grating at them with bleeding finger tips, until he pried one open. He was, though, unable to fix on André's gaunt face until his friend poured a tablespoon of water from his canteen into Sol's eyes, then one into his mouth. Sol grabbed at the canteen, but André pulled it away. "No, Sol. We must conserve. I 'ave ze rope. I convey you down."

He looped one end to a hook of rock poking just above the ledge. He tied the other end about Sol's chest, sat back, braced one of his own feet against a lip of sandstone, and pushed at Sol with the other until Sol rolled over the razor-sharp edge to disappear below the ledge. André growled, seizing the very last particle of strength left in him to lower Sol on belay, an inch at a time, until the rope slackened as the doctor came to rest on the shale below.

André pulled the rope from the knob of rock, wound the nylon into coils, and slung the mass over his shoulder. He lowered himself methodically over the sheer wall, until he was standing over Sol. Sol looked up at the face inches from his own. "*Mon ami*, how the hell did you do that?"

"I told you zat I am ze mountaineer in ze France. *Oui*? You must remember. But you do not believe me, *oui*?"

"You also said you were a race car driver."

"And I am, my friend. But only someday you will see. For now, we take zat pig and drive to Nyala. We cannot do zis sing alone. Please, Soli."

"Okay, okay. You're right. We'll get the helicopter. We'll hire mercenaries. We'll find her. I'll pay every penny that's left."

"You sink zey will let you, ze dogs in London? You must call and tell zem. Zey may say no, the money is for ze food, not for ze nurse."

"André, they gave me money to make this mission happen, so screw 'em."

"*Mais*, zey are ze administrator. Zey 'ave ze control. We must be careful. I 'ave seen zis in my own medical school. It 'appens even in ze France. Ze little man become ze big man. 'Ee go to ze board of ze director, and 'ee forget everysing but ze power of 'imself. Zey can call ze police on you. We must be careful, Soli."

"Sniveling, greedy little bastards. Same in every corner of the world."

André looked down at Sol. "It is funny what you remember so far from your 'ome."

Sol became unsteady again and let his head rest on the sand, but the anger inside him swelled, and he sat up. "You can't imagine what those asshole administrators said about Lila in London, the bastards. Don't worry. We'll find her, and then you can marry her and argue all day and night and be happy forever."

André's jaw drooped. "*Mais*, you do not understand, Soli. Zat is not what zis is. But we find 'er, and zen you will see."

Sol grasped André's hand and rose to his feet. "You got some water?" André handed him the canteen, but as Sol guzzled, André snatched it back.

"I tell you, conserve. Conserve."

Sol, though, had swallowed enough to clear his head, and the two scrambled down the last of the shale, coming to the empty jeep. Sol gathered a cc or two of molasses-like spit from his mouth and blew it into angrily into the wind. "Okay, so where is that jerkoff?"

André hissed, "*Merde*, I 'ad to take ze rope, *oui*? 'Ee say 'ee stay 'ere. I tell him we come back and save 'im from ze Janjaweed. Where is 'ee?"

"André, I think the cocksucker *is* Janjaweed. Why was he the only one they didn't take?"

"*Mais,* 'ee say 'ee 'ide in ze dirt. Zat is what 'ee say."

"And we should believe him? Why would he chance making it in the desert by himself? No, he left our little hideaway here to signal his pals up on the *jebel*. André, you were right. We can't do this by ourselves. We need to get to Nyala, at least. Call the UN. The guy who helped me get the supplies, Mr. Chun, he'll do something."

* * *

They raced west along a dried riverbed until André put his hand on Sol's arm. "Doctor, look ze compass. 'Ere. I sink we are in ze Chad. We 'ave crossed the border, I am sure. Zis is dangerous. We 'ave a vehicle. Zey will sink we are ze Janjaweed. Zey shoot first, zen zey ask ze question. Please, we must turn to ze east."

"We can't yet. There's no place to cross the *wadi*. Maybe it'll dry out soon. Let's keep on. Time is more important than our asses."

"*Mais,* let us take ze look at ze *wadi* 'ere. Maybe it is not so deep."

Sol nodded, stopped, and walked down into the water. It was a foot deep and five wide. He came back and gunned the engine, letting the tires drop over the embankment. Though the wheels spun, and the jeep nearly stopped, Sol pressed his foot to the gas pedal so hard, his leg cramped. The vehicle fishtailed and barely found purchase but slowly crept up the other side of the *wadi*. The sand on that side was not blanketed in thorn bushes as it was closer to Umm Balla, for here the wind had come from the south for centuries and cleansed the desert of the tire-shredding flora. Sol accelerated to about thirty, relaxing after several minutes as the jeep's bucking slackened. He watched closely for a change in the water temperature, but they were moving fast enough to allow the radiator to cool the engine, the needle going no higher than a millimeter or two into the red.

He nodded to André and was about to pat him on the arm to thank him for the good advice to put Chad behind them, but a flash of yellow exploded to the right, super-heated sand spewing into the vehicle, most of it into André's face. A second eruption burst in front of the jeep, and another hunk of shrapnel whacked through the windshield. With it came a blast of searing heat that saturated the cab.

André screamed, "*Merde, fils de putain*! *FILS DE PUTAIN*! Sol, stop, stop! *Mon yeux*!"

But Sol did not stop. Instead, he spun the wheel hard right, ramming the jeep into the sand behind a low hillock. When the rig rolled to a halt, Sol dragged André onto the sand and laid him down gently. "André, take your hands away from your eyes. Let me look. I won't hurt you."

As André slowly pulled his fingers away, Sol gasped. One cheek was gashed, and his left eye was cherry red. Sol could only see only a sliver of the globe through the swollen lid. A thready stream of blood-tinged fluid leaked through the nearly closed lids. Though he had not seen much in the way of ocular trauma since his residency, he knew the enormity of any high velocity wound to the eye, and that, if the globe had been pierced, there was no possibility that vision could be salvaged. The other globe, however, was intact, despite a lacerated lid, and Sol relaxed a single degree. He thought of a policeman in New York who only had one eye, a lieutenant, one of his mother's distant cousins. He grasped his friend's arm tightly, pleading, "André, André, can you see me?"

"*Oui*, I can see you, but it is so tangled, is zat ze word? What 'as happened, Doctor Soli? You will stay wis me, *oui*?"

"I will never leave you, *mon ami*." Sol grasped André's arms tighter and squeezed. "Never. But we need to get back to work. First, let's get that left eye protected, you know just like in the first year at medical school. You did pass the first year, yes?"

"In ze Congo."

"Let me take a better look at it." Sol calmed himself and growled under his breath, "No different, moron, from any patient you ever saw. Slow down, then slow down some more, *then* take a look, then look again, and when you're sure you know what's going on, stop and look again. Step by step."

He thought of the hematologist from whom he had taken the saddest course of his days as a medical student. "Oncology's not so bad," Dr. Shelly had half-smiled. "We're all headed to the same place in the end, some of us just a bit sooner than the next guy, but it'll be here in no time, Sol, no matter who you are. Kick and scream all you want. It's a year or two, plus or minus. No need to get crazy." Then he warned, "You're so New York. Slow down. If you want to make a difference, don't try to be a hero. All you need to do is ask, each time you come a crossroads, how you would want to be treated."

So, Sol took one of the plastic cups from which the kids forced down their toxic slurry, wiped it out with his tee shirt, placed the open end over his friend's eye, and fixed it in place with a couple strips of electrical tape he found in the Rover's door pouch. He helped André to his feet and smiled, "*Mon ami*, it's going to be fine. You will soon be the best doctor in France."

* * *

They rode east and came to *Wadi* Azum, where the desert was flat and smooth. As they sped toward Nyala, Sol played his American CDs. André remained silent, head back, eyes closed, facial muscles flaccid for several hours. Sol slowed every few minutes and checked André, fearful each time that his friend's luck had finally run out.

Unexpectedly, when Sol hit a pothole, André sat forward and spurted, "What is it, Doctor? Why do you love zis American music? In ze France, we cannot understand why you go on and on about your country. It is so young. You 'ave no culture; only ze 'amburger and ze violence. It is like being in ze 'ell to live zer. We see it every night on ze news."

Sol laughed. "André, you can't really believe that. Look, we'll be out of here soon. We will get Lila, and the two of you will come to the U.S. and be my guests for a year. She will be a visiting nurse, and I will arrange for you to attend medical school classes. You'll be an exchange student, anywhere you want—Penn, Harvard. I will make sure it's the best, for both of you."

"Doctor Soli, forgive me, if you please. Zer is murder on every boulevard."

Sol let the jeep roll to a stop. "Is this what you believe? André, I love my country. You will come there if I have to carry you." Sol paused and laughed again. "I love my country, André. Most of us do. And when you leave, you will cry. You'll see."

"*Mais*, I 'ave seen ze TV."

It was long after dark that the air conditioner began growling like a maddened bear, blowing tepid air that warmed more powerfully the higher Sol pushed the knob toward cold. It finally exploded a mile from the heap of loose sand that was the parking lot of the Hotel Finest Africa. André, who had been asleep, looked up and mumbled, "We are 'ere? Sanks Got."

Sol sat quietly with the engine idling for a moment. He leaned back, astonished they had arrived in a town sufficiently civilized to repair a tire. He told André to remain in the car while he went in to be sure there was room. On the cold tiles behind the counter slept the night man. He sensed Sol's presence and jumped to his bare feet. When his eyes cleared, he gasped at the white visage but gathered himself and offered Sol Suite Number 321, which had just been vacated by a VIP.

Sol collected his comrade, and the two men entered the lobby, the clerk almost losing consciousness as he gazed at the other pallid apparition, the one with a red plastic cup taped to his head. He pointed at the cup over André's eye, but Sol ignored him and took his companion by the shirt and led him up the stairs.

Their room was stripped of bedding, and the shower was clogged, but the ceiling fan was turning at ten or eleven revolutions every minute or so.

Sol settled André onto the bed and told him it was time to do an ophthalmic examination. He pulled the lamp from the desk, played the gloomy light onto his friend's eye, held his breath, and removed the plastic cup protector. The windshield glass had peppered the skin around the eye, and Sol picked at it with the tweezers from his Swiss Army knife before trying to move the lid. As he peeled away the crust of dried blood that sealed the lid shut, he desperately tried to remember the algorithm for treating ocular trauma. It was up to him. There was no one in Nyala or El Fasher, or perhaps even in Khartoum, to whom Sol would entrust André. He evaluated slowly and carefully, the most basic of medical laws.

He moistened the corner of a slip of death shroud and very gently softened the dried blood and crusted discharge. The lid relaxed slowly, and he was able to see the tiniest ribbon of the globe itself. It was red but did not appear to have collapsed. Sol forced himself to move his fingers more slowly than he had ever before on a patient. He picked at the blood, red cell by red cell, taking comfort in the lesson of a neurosurgeon he had been assigned to observe in medical school. At the time, Sol was astonished, and intimidated, by how the man sat for hours, silently, peering through a microscope, teasing one nerve fiber from the next, working his way down through the brain at a pace that might keep him there all night. Finally, he got to the tumor, and Sol was happy; for the operation would soon be over, and he could go home to eat and sleep. But that was when the neurosurgeon slowed even further, ensuring it was only cancer he was extracting, molecule by molecule, vigilant to fulfill the oath he had sworn the day of his graduation from medical school—"First, do no harm."

Now, fifteen years later, Sol forced himself to work more slowly, and eventually he freed another bit of the lid. A single, tiny splinter of shrapnel had wedged itself on the cornea. The metal was already rusting, a record of chemical deterioration, faster even than the corrosion of the lock on the gate at Umm Balla.

Sol held the lids open and dribbled a stream of water onto the globe, but as he expected, the sliver did not budge. He did not bother to ask André to remain perfectly still as he gently swiped at the sliver of metal with a corner of the death shroud. It caught on the cloth and pulled free easily.

Sol gasped, and André asked quietly, "Zer is ze problem?"

"No, André. No problem. Nothing's pierced the full thickness of the cornea. The globe is intact. The iris opens and closes normally." Sol picked away the few remaining shards of glass, laughing aloud as he worked. He blurted, "It's a miracle, André. I thought back at the mountain that you had lacerated the globe, the liquid and all, but it was just tears."

"I 'ave plenty of zose."

Sol went into the street to find something safe to eat. He returned in half-an-hour, passed the sleeping desk clerk, and left on the desk a round of stale pita, a handful of pigmy dried dates, and a hardboiled egg the size of a grape. After dinner in the room, Sol cleared a dead mouse from the shower drain and flung it out the window. It bounced off the head of a parked camel. The creature snorted loudly, which set the others growling and nipping at each other.

Sol led André to the bathroom for a shower. The water was freezing for the first few minutes then too hot to stand. Sol took his turn and swore in Italian as the water turned abruptly cold.

Long before dawn, André awoke and showered again, washing away the sheets of dust-contaminated sweat from the night. He fell asleep squatted over the toilet hole. Sol shook him and urged with a laugh, "*Mon ami*, it is ze time to go to ze El Fasher."

André smiled as broadly as Sol had ever seen. "Finally, you are learning to speak ze English."

They found a gas station in which a dim light bulb glowed behind the single pump. Sol banged on the door of the hovel and offered a fistful of dinars to fill the tank and the jerry cans, and patch two of the tires. In minutes, they were on the semi-paved highway, pushing the shaky Rover toward El Fasher as fast as the engine could burn the barely-80 octane fuel. Drugged by the heat, Sol did not notice the water temperature gauge creep into the mid-red or the oil pressure droop to the left.

André looked up as the stink of hot metal wafted into the jeep. He gasped, "Ze engine failure, 'ee is imminent. I know zis from ze days I am ze race driver. We cannot go on."

"André, my friend, we have no choice. It could be just a low oil level. There's two quarts in the back. I'll dump 'em in and see. If we have to, we'll leave the jeep here and flag down a truck or a bus."

Sol expected André to argue, correctly, that if it was just a matter of a low oil level, the temperature would not be climbing, but André nodded and whispered, "Maybe you are right. We try."

Sol stared at André, astonished, then checked the level. It was low. He walked to the back of the jeep and opened the rear hatch to fetch the two quarts of emergency oil, but noticed a tiny bead of blackened oil seeping into the sand. He dropped to his knees and followed the leak to the oil pan. A steady, delicate filament oozed from a half-centimeter, jagged hole. Sol scrubbed about on the desert, picking through the detritus, searching everywhere for a thorn to pack the fissure, but found nothing. When he told André, the Frenchman huffed and thundered, "*Mais*!" But his good eye spotted the slip of cigarette-pack aluminum foil Achmed had tossed uncaringly on the back floor of the jeep. "Put zat in ze 'ole. It is ze low pressure down zer; it will last forever…or until 'ee does not."

With the two quarts, the oil pressure rose, and the water temperature inched to the left, stopping at its customary place in the early red. They looked at each other, shrugged, and jounced into the parking area at the United Nations Quonset. It was a bit before dusk.

Sol snorted, "A hundred-and-twenty miles, ten hours. That's a Twenty-First Century Darfurian record."

When they could not find Mr. Chun at the warehouse, they motored to the UN living quarters at the north edge of El Fasher, an unpainted, cinderblock building facing north, the very distant deserts of Chad, Libya, and Egypt glowing saffron on the murky horizon. Chun was sitting in the common lounge reading a month-old *Seoul Times* and nursing a cup of tea.

"Doctor," he looked up, shaking his head as if seeing a ghost, "I am so surprised and happy to see you. We hear much trouble in Umm Balla."

"Yeah, floods and Janjaweed. We had to leave. This is Dr. André Anseau, from France. He is my colleague in Umm Balla. We came because…"

Mr. Chun's eyes hardened, and he barked, "Where is the Englishwoman?"

"We think she was taken by the Janjaweed. That's why we are here."

Chun snapped, "Why you no call me?"

Sol was startled by the timbre of the man's voice. "We tried from Nyala, but the lines were down."

"I am sorry, but we witness violence epidemic. There soon no other but Sudan soldier and Sudan refugee in this nation, one or other. All foreigner will be dead or running for life. There no food for population, only for army, feed them so they have energy murder all day."

"Mr. Chun, you have contact with the UN office in Khartoum. Is an official protest in order?"

Chun did not answer but slipped on his shoes and lifted the telephone. "Dead, very big shock." He slammed the receiver down and walked to the door. "Come with me."

They followed in the Rover as Chun drove into the UN office complex. He snipped to one of the secretaries, "I speak Mignini on phone."

She manipulated buttons on the satellite phone and lifted her nose as she handed it to Chun, who placed it on speaker phone. "This Chun in Fasher. Mr. Prosecutor Mignini, we have situation. Englishwoman with Please Help Children take by Janjaweed. This time UN must act."

In heavily broken English, the voice on the phone crackled, "Chun, I tell'a you so many time, but a still you not'a understand. This animal, Janjaweed. Do only as'a please insure power. Get sex every night, money in Swiss bank. Not'a poor agenda, eh? Only avenue military. UN'a no power. You know answer. But I inform supervisor sit in New York, but no hold'a breath."

"Mignini, you listen Chun. They meet in committee, discuss with Khartoum office, in month come back, talk to you. She pregnant in three hour, dead in three day. I respect Mr. Prosecutor, but for one time in diplomat life, you need to get off ass, do something."

Sol rose and grabbed the phone from Chun. He shrieked, "This is Doctor Solomon Forte. I am Italian-American. My papa and mama are *Sicilianu*. So, I am as well. What do you want to be thinking about on your deathbed, sir? Do you want this woman's blood on your conscious the moment you die?" There was no answer, and Sol assumed the officer had hung up, but he heard a breath on the other end, so he continued. "You don't. And, if you don't act now, I, personally, will track you down, and follow you, and never let you, your family, or your country forget what you didn't do here."

Sol slammed the phone closed and tossed it onto the desk as he stormed out to brood in the jeep. He listened to his music, eyes bolted shut, until a gentle knock on the window startled him. Chun beckoned Sol back inside with a nod and a smile. He poured tea and renewed the connection with Mignini. Chun spoke forcefully. "So, sir, I understand you come tomorrow in morning UN jet El Fasher. You bring Minister Defense Sudan investigate. Is correct?"

"*Si*, yes, but no crazy Siciglion doctor threaten Italian minister. This'a very *delicato. No problema, si*?"

"Mignini, you do good to UN. See in morning."

Chun had been glancing at André off and on, trying not to stare at the heavily bandaged eye and swollen face. When he saw André's head droop and his eyes close, he whispered to Sol, "French doctor is okay?"

"You can't imagine what he's been through. But I think this is the worst that's happened. He really cares for Lila, the English woman. They've been there together for over half-a-year."

"They are involve?"

"You know, Mr. Chun, I really don't know. I don't even know if they like each other. I can't tell. But they are always snipping, those two."

Chun laughed gently. "Oh, that mean they husband wife, for sure. Now you know why Chun stay Sudan for three year."

"So, it's the same everywhere."

"And for all time of human." Chun's eyes sank for a moment then looked up at Sol, "Never mind, I take my European friend to special room. We make good care friend."

He nodded at Sol to wake André, and the three walked to a battered shipping container. Chun pulled a ring of keys from his pocket and tried a dozen until one opened the padlock. As a narrow metal panel swung open, Chun reached in and pulled a string. A single light bulb barely glowed in the far corner, and he took André's arm to lead him into the eight-by-twelve box. Sol, who could not see past the two men into the primitive guest room, waited outside. Chun stuck his head out and nodded for Sol to join them. The container was a bare metal shell with two cots, a chair, and an air conditioner. He eased André onto one of the beds then took Sol by the arm and guided him to a cinderblock bathroom with several shower stalls and sinks. He held Sol's arm a moment before uttering, "You two men hero. We take care make you safe. We work hard find girl."

Sol's lips tightened. "What are the chances we'll find her? Do you have any feel for how they treat foreign women?"

"Only God know. Chun tell you, work very hard find girl. Good night Doctors."

Sol walked André to the loo and gave him a tiny bar of soap, a toothbrush, and one of the microscopic towels afforded guests who had dragged themselves off the Nubian desert. He set the shower water temperature for André, and when his friend staggered out minutes later, Sol took the thread of remaining soap and entered the mildewed stall. The water was, though, lukewarm, and as hard as he tried to pull himself away, he could not make his hand reach up to turn the spigot to off. He finally dried himself with his tee shirt, more content for a brief moment than he had been in the past year. He savored the touch of grace before the images of his lost wife and sister, his parents, and then of Lila, blurred the mirage of serenity.

In the morning, Chun took them to breakfast at the UN dining hall. André barely ate, scarcely able to hold himself upright. Sol waited for sweat to pour off his friend's brow, a sign, along with the malaise, that the stress of the eye trauma had lowered André's resistance and allowed the infection, and the malaria, to retrench themselves. He remained dry, though.

Sol wolfed the pita, wilted cabbage, spaghetti, mutton meatballs, and yogurt placed in front of him by a staff of delicate Sudanese women.

Chun's cell phone rang, and when he saw the number, he placed it on speaker. Mignini ground on about the heat at the fueling point at which they had had to land to attend to an engine malfunction. He grumbled that they were somewhere in the vast desert between the capitol and El Fasher, and that he was wasting battery power on the satellite phone by calling. "Chun, this'a better be *importante*." The phone went dead.

Forty-five minutes later, while they shared a third cup of coffee, and André began to perk up, the phone rang again, and Mignini's voice vibrated, "You'a meet us at *aeroporto*, fifteen'a meenutes, *si*?"

Several vans followed them, washed and shining, ready to transport the dignitaries back to UN headquarters. Mignini was first off the Russian Antonov-70 transport's airstairs. Following, came three high-ranking military officers. Sol recognized their uniforms as British, Pakistani, and Indian. He gulped at the UN's blend of nationalities selected to rescue a British woman, but put on his most obsequious smile, one perfected as a medical student and resident in front of attending physicians.

Chun walked to the delegation, bowed slightly, and made introductions. When the supporting staff of two dozen lesser military and civilian workers emerged from the An-70, Chun wagged his finger in the air, and the UN vans sped away. The entourage proceeded with its blue-bereted UN police escort to the dining hall, the only venue in the city sufficiently secure to accommodate a delegation of foreign dignitaries. As the men were seated, the Sudanese server women, nodding in greeting to Sol, stepped gracefully from the kitchen, their platters piled with pita, cabbage, withered spaghetti and meatballs, and yogurt.

The British soldier placed himself between the Pakistani and Indian officers and offered plates of food. When the Indian official snatched a pita round without using the tongs, a tip of his index finger grazed the platter. The Pakistani's eyes expanded, and his lips pursed. He turned his head and jabbed his nose into the air.

The Englishman pleaded, "Gentlemen, let us break bread together and approach our mission with open minds."

The Indian general spoke a sentence to his staff in Hindi. When several of the minor Indian delegates snickered, the Pakistani mocked in broken English, "You know, officer, *I* speak fluent Hindi." His complexion reddened, and he fumed, "You fingers touch pork. I never eat you touch."

The Indian stood and barked, "How dare Pakistan private speak in such tone to India general? Only untouchable in India eat pork. I never touch pork in my life." He turned to his delegation and pointed his finger in the air. "Ve go."

The contingent behind the Indian rose, came to relative attention, and left faced, though one, in civilian garb, revolved in the opposite direction, but only for an instant before joining the adagio swagger toward the door.

Sol suddenly remembered an older woman he had dated, a veteran of the 60s, a soul who had regaled him with tales of her good and bad LSD trips. This was, he wilted, the narration of the worst she had suffered. The room spun, Sol's heart rate escalated, his mouth parched, and his fingers trembled, though were numb. His emotions shifted like the sands of the Sahel. His life had gone from euphoria to terror in less than thirty seconds, from the hope that these men might fight to find Lila, to the fear that they would sacrifice her over a shred of bacon.

The British officer slammed his fist on the table. "Enough of this rot. If you two buggers want to spend the rest of your miserable, so-called careers as corporals, fine. I am here to right a wrong. You will act professionally, or I will put you both back on the aircraft straightaway, and you will have the forty-eight hours before I get back to Khartoum to gather your defenses. Had better craft them well." He pointed testily to the embroidered King Edward's Crown on his epaulette, then to the gold star on the Indian's shoulder. He glanced at the glowering Pakistani, not bothering to point at the colonel's epaulette.

The Indian delegation halted sloppily, and the superior officer nodded for them to retake their seats. The British general pondered the situation for a silent moment before looking up. "Gentlemen, and I hope against hope that I am using the term appropriately, we will act in concert to find this woman, not because she is British, or South Asian, Pakistani, or Sudanese. We will find her because she is an innocent, a woman who gave of herself to comfort these suffering people. May I remind you, that is why we are here. Doctor, please brief us, succinctly if you don't mind, regarding this woman and what you know of her whereabouts."

Sol spoke for five minutes. Chun added what he could about the Janjaweed of Western Darfur.

The general turned to Sol. "What do you need? A show of force, an attack, a delegation to negotiate? Tell me, and it will be yours straightaway."

Sol reeled with the gravity of his position. "General, thank you, sir, but I just came out of the desert. I've been there for a while. My mind is moving at Sudanese speed. All I know is that, given the capacity of the Janjaweed's dilapidated trucks on the desert, if they kidnapped Lila and the rest of the refugees, they couldn't have gotten any farther than Jebel Mara by now. I have heard that is where they have a local headquarters. The rebels who oppose the Janjaweed have no aircraft, so the Janjaweed are invulnerable on the mountain. From what I have learned, they regroup and resupply on the mountain, then set out for the coast, which one I'm not sure, but it's in trucks. They sell their hostages, and buyers put them on slave ships for the Middle East. That's weeks, if not months, of travel. Their tracks will still be clear if we get out there right away."

The room calmed, and the general nodded. "Gentlemen," he spoke respectfully to his counterparts, "please help me. I am an artillery officer. Colonel Ayub Kahn, here, is a Pakistani Air Force officer, a decorated jet fighter pilot, I might add. Colonel, can we track these bastards by air? What type of aircraft do we need?"

The man challenged, "Why you call dem bastards? Because dey are Muslim? Because dey represent Islamic government of Sudan, because…"

"No, Colonel, because they kill indiscriminately, because they mutilate women, and because they do it for money and for personal enjoyment. That, Colonel, is not in the great tradition of the Islamic faith, now is it? I am sure you do not condone that behavior."

"Of course I do not. But ve are sitting vit American in front of us. His people rape in Vietnam, and now Iraq, Afghanistan. He is so concern for vhite voman? He allow her to sleep among men vit out marriage. He is one who blaspheme name of Allah. He cohabit vit British voman. He vant woman back to go on blaspheme."

The British general brought the palm of his left hand to his mouth, as if contemplating an answer. His right hand, however, balled into a fist under the table. Sol watched the man's eyes harden. "Sir, let me handle this. It's my fight." The general nodded, and Sol went on. "Colonel Kahn, sir, let me assure you that I was not involved with Ms. Lila. My wife and my sister died together in the World Trade Center on 9-11. Perhaps you have you heard of that catastrophe?"

The Pakistani grumbled, "It is not clear vhere is responsibility for 9-11. Ve believe your President Bush plan entire massacre, not *jihadi. He* kill American infidel. Blood of your vife on his hand. And that is not matter for talk now. Ve must respect Sudan Islamic government. Vhen I am in New York UN office, I respect Christian law of U.S. Here, ve respect law of Sudan, *sharia.*

"So vhy Pakistan soldier die for voman who blasphemy law of Koran by live alone vit two men?" His voice raised. "You do this in face of Muslim refugee? Such disrespect." He stood and raged, "If I find dis voman, I send to Sudan government for lash, if lucky. Maybe stone and you next."

Sol nodded, loosened the muscles around his mouth, and smiled. "You, sir, are *suar.*"

The colonel, along with his staff, stared at Sol for a moment, unsure if they had heard him correctly. When the senior officer sprang to his feet, so did his contingent. The colonel glared at Sol, and from the depth of his soul, spit into Sol's face. The British brigadier stood, took a deep breath, and launched at the man, but Sol had already moved toward the colonel, blocking the Brit. Sol's body hit the Pakistani officer with such fury, the two of them fell backwards five feet. The colonel spit again, this time into Sol's mouth. Sol, on top, cocked his fist and drilled down so hard, the Pakistani's jaw dislocated. Sol could not tell if the man was facing left or right.

Sol jumped to his feet, grabbed André by the shoulder, and pulled him out of his chair. He steered him across the dining room, out the door, and into the blinding Sudanese afternoon. Left behind was a building shuddering so heatedly with shouts, it loosened the coating of grime on the metal roof, sending down a veil of filth that encircled the jeep. Sol threw the Rover into gear and peeled out of the UN parking lot, taking the first corner so abruptly, he nearly skidded into a pair of Darfur camels. One peered down at the jeep, roared his head back, and launched a wad of spit at the broken windshield. Sol rolled the window open, hurled his own hocker at the animal, jammed the Rover back into gear, and spattered the creatures with gravel.

The jeep peeled around the animals and sped onto several more roads until chancing upon a petrol station. Sol filled the tank to the brim, topped off the jerry cans, and dribbled gas into the water bottles. He paid for high test, the best gas to be found in the Sudan, barely eighty-five octane. He told André to clear the camel saliva from what was left of the windscreen, but the Frenchman folded his arms and did not move. "*Non*, Soli. Do you not know saliva of camel contain ze syphilis?"

"Don't give me that."

"*Mais*, it is true. It is a disease spread of ze bestiality by ze lonely camel boys in ze desert night."

At the first restaurant, Sol ran in and plead in his elementary Arabic, "Want food. Here money. You, honorable man, give bread, meat, *al hum de le la*." When the proprietor's eyes locked on the cash, he trotted to the primeval kitchen and filled bags with pita, chunks of steaming, braised mutton, and a salad of greens and reds. He looked at the money again and tossed in a plastic bag of watery feta cheese.

As the jeep rolled south, back toward the edge of town, Sol asked André to make a sandwich for himself. Though André had been nearly silent for the last hours, after a few bites his color returned, and he put his hand on Sol's forearm, asking, "*Mon ami*, do you sink we can do zis sing wis out ze 'elp?"

Sol did not answer, but when they came to the southern edge of El Fasher, about to reenter the desert, Sol grumbled, "André, you heard them. What choice do we have?"

They drove for an hour, neither bothering to waste the energy to shout above the grinding of the defunct air conditioner that could not be turned off. Over that clatter, though, came a sudden shuddering, which shook the vehicle, and then a loud, rhythmic, thumping. They glanced at each other uneasily, acknowledging the imminent death of the engine. Sol jammed his foot to the floor, spun the vehicle in the opposite direction, and headed back toward El Fasher. At that instant, an abrupt shadow engulfed them as if a solar eclipse was darkening the desert. Sol slammed the jeep to a halt. The windshield filled with olive drab. By the time Sol realized it was a helicopter, the ship had broken to the side of the road, setting down far enough from the Rover not to engulf it in a noxious mix of sand and camel dung. The plan did not work.

A figure in a Viet Nam War vintage flight helmet, the double dark visors down, bolted from the right door and sprinted toward them. André's face lost all color as he grabbed Achmed's rusted AK from the backseat and fumbled to chamber a round. He succeeded only in pushing a button that released the banana-shaped magazine. It clanked to the floor, and several rounds popped out to roll under the seat.

André roared, "*Merde!*" though thought quickly and aimed the rifle out the window, screaming, "'Alt, or I shoot."

Sol reached over and pushed the barrel of the AK-47 down. "André, that's Crisanto, Romeo Luzon's son. Put the gun away, man. And you call me a cowboy." The running figure stopped short in his tracks and raised his hands into the air. "I am Crisanto. You know me. I fly the food to your camp."

Sol yelled to Crisanto, jumped out of the Rover, and jogged to the Filipino pilot. He hugged him tightly. "My friend, so good to see you. What have you heard about your father?"

"That is why we chased after you. The Janjaweed have sent a demand for ransom. It is twenty-thousand dollars. They say we must give them the money before one more day, or they will kill him. They say they are holding him at Jebel Mara."

"They told you where they had him?"

"Yes, and they say we have to come in the helicopter to pick him up and give the money at same time."

"Do you have the money?"

"My family in the Philippines gave us some, and we only have to pay Singh for fuel and engine time. Maybe what is left will be enough."

"Crisanto, these are pigs. They will take your money and the helicopter. It's a valuable tool. They want it for sure, and your father is even more precious. They'll hold you for ransom and force him to fly missions. When they're done with you, they'll kill you both, even if Singh pays the ransom. So, you can't just fly down there and give it all away. Please."

"Doctor, what else can we do? They gave us three days. Almost two are gone before I got Singh to give us the ship."

Sol rubbed his forehead so hard it hurt. "Right now, the only game in town is the UN, and they are definitely not on our side. But I think I can get in contact with Mr. Chun. He might help. Tell you what. You go back to the airport, and we'll wait for dark and drive to the Hotel Obeid. They don't know me there…yet. Here's Chun's number. Ask him if he would meet us there at nineteen hundred. I got into a fistfight with the Pakistani military attaché. The Sudanese cops are looking for me, no doubt. I'm fucked in this town."

Crisanto's head dropped. When he looked up, the thinnest smile came to him. "Doctor, you sound like my father."

Sol and André made their way to a concealed corner of El Fasher and waited until just minutes before seven to creep toward the crumbling Hotel Obeid. They wormed the jeep through a back alley, stopping in a hidden crevice of the hotel. A man missing his right hand was squatted next to the hotel's stinking garbage baskets. Sol paid him a US dollar to guard the jeep. The stunned man saluted with his left hand, took Sol's arm, and squeezed hard, nodding exuberantly. Finally, he caught his breath and barked, "*Ana fahim, ana fahim, ana fahim!*" "I understand, I understand, I understand!"

Chun was waiting at a table in the far shadows at the rear of the dining room. When Sol and André dropped into their seats, Chun shook his head. "Dr. Forte, I think maybe idea good you not consider diplomat life." Sol tried to smile, but dread clutched his chest. By now, every expatriate in Sudan knew of the loose cannon American doctor sailing around the desert, punching out the lights of anyone who dared bicker with him. How, he froze, would he even get back to Khartoum, to say nothing of negotiating Sudanese passport control, to escape the country? And how would his fit of pique help save Lila?

"Mr. Chun, I overreacted. But I am not some kind of a rag doll. I don't know what iteration of the story is going around, but nobody says or does that to another man and gets to walk away, at least not where I come from. Do Koreans allow a man to spit in your face, in your *mouth*? I don't think so. You're the toughest people on Earth. So now, I have to pay. No sweat. I'm ready. What do I need to do?"

"You need do nothing, Doctor, except find colleague woman. I am assist you. But how you know word for pig in Urdu? Everyone think you language genius."

"Yeah, a real genius. You really want to hear?"

"You tell Chun. Chun know it good story. Wait one minute for tea, then tell."

Chun poured, and Sol cracked a smile. "Ready? In my office in Whitaker, I saw a lot of foreign folks. It was the best part of my practice. Word of mouth. Foreigners knew they'd be treated with respect in my practice. There was this family from Pakistan. I had a million patients from South Asia. Good people. Revere education. Anyway, this guy was an engineer; she was a housewife. They came to me because she was sick, real sick, coughing up blood, fever, chills, shaking so hard at night, the kids could feel it in the next room. So, when she got to my office, first thing I did was tell my nurse to get a chest x-ray. The husband went crazy. Jumped out of his chair like a bolt of lightning had bitten him in the ass. He's like screaming, 'Can the x-ray see through clothing?' Of course it could. Well, he had a fit, spit on the carpet near my shoes. Then he yelled, '*Suar!*' At least he didn't spit *in* my mouth. So, that's how I know. He dragged her out of the office. I wanted to call the cops, but the clinic CEO told me to mind my own business, that if I made a fuss, I'd be on the street looking for a job by sunset, and in jail by dawn for a hate crime."

"In America?" Chun asked, stunned.

"In America today."

Chun placed his lips against his templed fingers. "It help Chun understand. Anyway, Doctor, I must tell you we not have sufficient diplomat strength with Mr. al-Bashir government in Khartoum to intervene. Government deny relationship with Janjaweed, but Janjaweed arm of Sudan government. Of this, there no question. So, attack on Janjaweed is attack on al-Bashir himself. But that not important now. What I do is contact brother. He general in Korean Marine. He station Pentagon for two year. I ask him get high altitude photo Jebel Mara. We maybe not see one person, but we see many of people, and we see topography."

Sol's eyes lifted. "If we get enough intelligence, will the British brigadier do a rescue mission?"

"Never. He would be force leave country. I tell you, Janjaweed is Khartoum government. But first thing first. We gather intelligence. Then we go to British brigadier. I tell you, *he* not so angry about you strike Pakistani colonel. But I can say no more."

"So, what do André and I do, and for how long?"

"You follow me in Rover. Chun take you to safe house, but you must not go from safe house until Chun say word. Doctor not worry. They not kill woman. If dead, no good for sale. She worth more than one million to Saudi oil man."

André appealed to Chun, "Do you sink, *Monsieur*, zey will 'arm 'er?" He paused and went on. "You know what I mean?"

"Chun not know. Man here like cut clitoris. Maybe not so much in Saudi. But sometime. Chun guess she not virgin. So, Janjaweed sew up vagina hide she not virgin. Saudi man want white virgin. If sew up, maybe also cut clitoris."

Sol was about to grab Chun, to press him to divulge if he had seen this before, to demand how he could know such a thing. While he was silent, his lips tightened so, Chun nodded. His face hardened. "She worth much money. I know you not like hear, but she come here, and you come here, and no man force you to come. You come to hell on own. This not Time Square anymore." Chun reached forward and grasped Sol's shoulder, squeezing very hard. "You never be same after Sudan. This bad years for you, and you never forget, but someday Chun tell you his life. My father life in Korea War. You be happy for sure only you lose wife and woman." Chun hesitated, shook his head, and continued, "I remember American movie *Top Gun*. You remember? Colonel say he not blow smoke up Maverick ass. And Chun no blow smoke up doctor ass. Maybe you lose colleague. No way to tell future now. Very hard to hear my word, but you listen Chun. You listen *to* Chun," he corrected himself. "We work hard to make better world, but great cost."

Sol and André followed in the Rover as Chun drove the dirt paths of El Fasher, coming upon a single-story hostel of good size. It was neatly built and surrounded by shrubbery and colorful plants. Chun skidded to a stop in his UN jeep, ran inside, but sprinted back in an instant, and sped off. He acknowledged neither André nor Sol.

A man in a *jellabiya* darted out from behind the building and motioned for Sol to follow through an alley behind the building, pointing for the foreigners to pull into a straw and mud shelter. The Sudanese man grunted and waved his hands roughly, demanding André and Sol snatch their belongings and run behind him through an open parking area. A few dozen kneeling camels bellowed madly at the sudden disturbance. The men were led into the wooden building and through an anteroom, where several women were washing clothes in tubs. They did not look up. At a third hallway, a pair of Sudanese women in Western nun's garb met them and gently guided them into a spare room with two cots, a bare table, and three primitive chairs. They motioned for both men to sit and brought plates, bowls, spoons, and, finally, a platter of spaghetti. André's eyes rolled as he jeered, "Why do zese people sink I am ze Italian. Zat is you."

Sol laughed, but the women remained so serious, both men calmed and bowed their heads to eat.

"Where are we André?"

"*Mon ami*, did you not see ze cross in ze 'allway? I 'ave 'eard of zis place. It is ze Greek church of El Fasher."

"Greek Orthodox? Here?"

"*Oui*. Ze Greeks come 'ere many millennia ago. Amazing people, even more zan ze French, I 'ate to say. Zen in eighteen 'undreds zey come wis ze Syrian, trading ze goods, zen ze church come. I 'ave 'eard of zis. I sink we are very fortunate."

They ate, showered, and slept until dawn, when one of the sisters knocked gently on their door. She whispered in delicate English, "I have for you breakfast. You must not leave room."

As Sol cracked the door, the young Sudanese nun looked away abruptly and slid a tray of food along the floor into the room. "Spaghetti, André, hot, and a lot of it!"

André smiled, "You know, Soli, ze French man is ze connoisseur of ze world, but I must tell you, zis is not so bad as I sought. When I return to Paris, zis recipe will come wis me. Maybe I quit ze medical. Open ze Sudanese Spaghetti Emporium on ze Champs-Élysées."

They ate and drank *jabana* in a miasma of hopelessness, until a loud thud on the door startled them into consciousness. A young Sudanese man handed Sol a letter and tore away. Chun had written that he was working on the problem and would contact them the next morning. He reminded them not to leave the room. At noon, there was a gentle tap on the door, and another platter of spaghetti was slipped in. André quipped, "Very nice."

The men, with nothing to read, and nothing to do but wipe themselves free of unrelenting sweat, spent the day restlessly supine on their beds. At dusk, there was another sharp knock and the next dispatch from Chun. Plans had changed. His brother was unable to convince the Americans to do as he had hoped, but they were still not to budge, for he was working on a new plan.

Minutes later came the gentle knock. They picked at the spaghetti until about nine. Sol growled, "I need to make sure the Rover's okay. It's our lifeline. I'm going to sneak out and check it. I'll be back in a few."

But Sol got only as far as back door before the mother superior jumped from the shadows and placed herself between Sol and the exit. "*Doctori*, you know you must not leave this sanctuary. There is nothing you can do alone in the desert."

"Sister," he spoke with reverence, "I am a Catholic. We are the same. We are one. I have the mission of saving one of God's spirits from a hell she does not deserve. I do not care if I die. André does not care. We have our duty."

"And, *Doctori*, so do we have a mission. We cannot make you do anything, but we ask you to stay here until dawn. A man will come to see you. Perhaps he can help. You must trust us for this night."

Sol nodded and returned to his room. André listened, sighing, "Soli, she know more zan we. We are alone against ze world movement, you and me. It is more zan we can do. We wait, *oui*?"

CHAPTER NINE

At dawn, there was a sharp knock, and Sol cracked the door, stretching out his hand for a letter from Chun, but a Sudanese man in a filthy *jellabiya* pushed his way through and slammed the door behind him. "I Bra'heem. You die Janjaweed, yes?" Without waiting for an answer, he growled, "They devil. You die. Now go. Come fast."

He stood, hands on hips, glaring at them, as if his command had been so clearly sufficient to draw the two Westerners through the door to follow him to the farthest reaches of hell. But Sol raised both of his palms in the man's face. "Wait a minute. Who the hell are you?"

"Bra'heem. SLF."

"Okay, Bra'heem, so what is SLF?"

"Sudan Liberation Force." He took his left hand, fingers viciously extended as if an axe blade, and smashed it into his right palm. "No time. Go now. Die Janjaweed."

Sol snapped, "And where are we going?"

"You come."

Sol, nearly seventy-five pounds heavier than the young rebel, rounded his shoulders, flexed his chest, and sucked in his neck. Ibrahim backed a step as Sol took one forward. "You don't tell me what to do, Ibrahim. If you want to help us, we will help you with more money than you ever dreamed of. But you tell me what you can do for us."

"Go *khawajii* woman. You come now."

"How do you know about that? Where is she?"

"Every man know *khawajii* woman where. Go now. Patrol come die Bra'heem. You come."

Sol looked at André, who shrugged.

The man yelped, "You obey SLF!"

"And you need our money, because we have more money than you ever saw in your life." Sol pulled out two US tens from his pocket, flashed them quickly in front of the man's eyes, threw them on the table, but covered them with his hands. "American dollars. There's two hundred. I have thousands and thousands more." He spoke slowly and succinctly. "A million dollars." Sol jammed the bills back into his pocket. "If you help us find the British woman, it will mean a million dollars to you and your SLF."

"You come now. You go before come police. Police die Bra'heem."

The two Western men grabbed water bottles, a few stale loaves of pita, a can each of powdered milk and cocoa, and stacks of oatmeal packets. They went down the backstairs and past the kitchen, where a nun, busy draining an enormous vat of spaghetti, eyed them without expression. In the alley, they brushed away the camouflage of thistle weed from the Rover's hood. Sol waited for Ibrahim to go to his own car and lead them to his commanders, but the man jumped into the driver's seat and snapped his fingers for the keys.

Sol grunted, pointing his thumb over his shoulder, "Are you out of your mind? Get into the back. You don't know how to drive."

"You give…" Ibrahim hesitated and made the sign of a key turning in the ignition. "Bra'heem know to go car."

Sol called André to the rear of the jeep, where they whispered back and forth until Sol straightened and smiled at Ibrahim. "Okay, Ibrahim, you drive, and we'll sit in back. No problem." The two men took seats in the rear and leaned back peacefully. The Sudanese man looked over his shoulder and relaxed for an instant, until Sol lunged forward, knocked off the rebel's *immah*, and grabbed his hair. He placed his Swiss Army knife to the man's throat. "I am right behind you. You see my knife?" Ibrahim glanced sideways and down at the blade just millimeters from his right carotid. "One problem, and I cut your throat. Do you understand?"

He barely nodded and added quietly, "Bra'heem know. We go now."

He popped the clutch with so little skill, Sol was thrown back and nearly stabbed André. But the rebel soon gained control, pulled out of the alley, and moved slowly into the flow of foreign-labeled jeeps, motor scooters, taxis, and bicycles riding on bare rims. At the first traffic light, Ibrahim looked left and right violently, and Sol braced for the jolt forward, but this time Ibrahim came off the clutch far more gently. He drove a few blocks, and the Westerners relaxed, until the jeep turned with a savage swing of the wheel. Sol recognized that they were headed south down a dirt road toward the edge of El Fasher. As they approached the next intersection, Ibrahim ordered Sol and André to duck, swung the vehicle hard right into an alley, into another, and a third. He jammed both feet on the brake, threw the door open, and ran into one of a clutch of cinderblock and mud huts.

Two men toting dusty AK-47s, their *jellabiyas* caked with filth, ran to the Rover. They jammed muzzles through the driver's door into the faces of their foreign guests. Ibrahim took a place on the other side of the jeep and ripped open the rear door. He ordered Sol and André to lie flat on the seat. He jumped in, tied their hands behind them with rough hemp, and wrapped their heads in vile-smelling cloth. They were pulled from the Rover and tugged into one of the huts. Ibrahim commanded, "Now, you money. Take Jebel Mara. Die Janjaweed. *Khawajii* woman give you."

"Bra'heem, you take off the cloth. We talk."

"*La, la, la*. You money."

"Bra'heem, the money is in the safe at the UN house here in El Fasher. Did you think I carry all that money in my pocket?"

There was a choppy, guttural exchange in the background, and Sol took the opportunity to whisper to André, "*Mon ami, ça va bien?*"

"*Oui, ça va bien*, ze best day of all ze life."

Ibrahim snapped, "No speak. Captain speak go money now."

"Well, Bra'heem, it's going to look very funny, me with a rag around my head trying to get the money from the safe at the UN. Did you think about that?"

"Friend here. You run, no money. Captain die friend. He knife to neck. You know?"

Sol spoke to André quietly, "Not to worry, *mon ami*. They won't harm us. It's just talk. It was Chun and Mother Superior who arranged this whole thing. Anything happens to us..." He turned to the men and spoke loudly. "I understand. I will get the money. Do I have your word on Allah that you will not hurt my friend?"

"Money yes, no die friend. Money no, captain knife neck die." Ibrahim made the chopping motion with his hand, though this time with so much less violence, they could barely hear it.

Sol was guided, still hooded, to the Rover and pushed face down into the rear seat. Ibrahim jerked the vehicle onto the blazing streets of El Fasher. Sol worked a hand free and lifted the blindfold. He watched surreptitiously as the jeep twisted through neighborhoods, in and around droves of kneeling camels that littered the streets and sand sidewalks. They wound up back at the hostel where Sol and André had spent the last two nights. Ibrahim skidded into the alley and jammed the brakes. Sol slipped his hand back into the ropes. Ibrahim pulled him out gently. "You go now. Money. You go here. You no go here friend captain die him. Cut neck die. You know?"

"I told you, I understand." He pushed past Ibrahim, carefully though, barely brushing him. "You remember this, Ibrahim, if you hurt my friend, I will pay to have your family die by the knife." Sol drew his index finger across his neck, jumped into the driver's seat, and popped the clutch. Gravel and dirt hurtled down the alley, blanketing Ibrahim.

He went straight to the UN compound, but this time he was met by a wooden barrier crossing the usually open driveway, and by the palm-frond-like open hand of an exceptionally tall, cadaverous Sudanese watchman. The official was garbed in a desert-stained *jellabiya* and *immah*, the latter wrapped so high above his scalp, he had to bow far forward to exit his guard shack. With that, the *immah* toppled and unwound, snaking along the ground as it flapped in the grimy wind like a tattered kite. The man caught up to the blowing cloth and, without bothering to shake off the latest iteration of soil, lazily rewound it on his head, adjusted it carefully, then lurched back toward Sol in the ungainly gait of a seven-foot tall man.

"Sir, this is an emergency. I must see Mr. Chun. Please open the fence."

"You name." He handed Sol a nubbin of pencil and sheet of worn paper, pushing both through the driver's window. His hand came to rest an inch from Sol's eyes.

Sol pushed the man's hand back out of the window. "My name is *Doctori* Forte. Now, please open the gate. This is *emergency*. Do you understand emergency?"

"The man pushed the paper back into the jeep. "You name."

Sol scratched "Forte" angrily and waited for the log to be raised. The man bent forward to enter the shack, the *immah* fell, he gathered it from the ground, rewound it, adjusted the cloth twice, lifted a telephone receiver, and shouted, "*Slam, slam!*" He followed that with an angry "A*l hum de ley la*," as he dipped through the door and the *immah* slipped from his head. He caught it in his hands, redid it, and heaved his way toward the compound. When Sol saw him enter a Quonset, he jumped from the jeep, lifted the log, and sped toward Chun's office.

The Korean man looked up, surprised, but only for an instant, the slight shake of his head melting into a nod toward a seat. "You are persona non grata in UN, you know."

"I know, but there is an emergency. I need my money right away."

"Why?"

Sol related the story. Chun listened, stone-faced, then asked, "How much you promise to give?"

"A million."

"You have million?"

"No."

"So, what you do?"

"I'll give them what I have."

"No. Now they want million." Chun paused in thought. "But not all bad. You give some thousand now, more when you have girl. They never see money like one US thousand. You tell rebel your money in Sudan dinar now. Worthless to buy gun. Take time to change money to dollar. Government watching all money changing. Rebel know that. Come, we get some money, but after, you leave UN compound very fast."

The gorgeous Norwegian woman sat stiffly in front of the safe. She recognized him instantly, grimaced, and asked in clipped tones, "How may I help you?"

Sol spoke softly, his eyes cast down. "I would like to get some money from the safe."

"May I see your passport?"

Sol sucked in a deep breath, but kept his eyes planted on the floor and his voice tranquil. "Madame, my passport is in the safe with the money. This is an emergency. A woman's life is at stake."

Chun jumped forward in front of Sol and interrupted, "Sigrid, please, open safe give money. No woman life. He just say that. He need buy food for Umm Balla children. Much fire flood Umm Balla."

She rose suspiciously and placed herself between the men and the safe, to assure they could not scrutinize her fingers as she spun the dial, though neither Chun nor Sol were watching her hands. Sol took fifteen thousand in tens from the stash, placing five thousand in each of three separate plastic bags. He laughed, "Maybe they'll think it's fifties, the zero being five and reading backwards in Arabic. I'll tell them I'm giving them seventy-five-thousand."

"And they cut off head and keep money. Every fool in world know US dollar. You must go now. And you no talk about save woman. You are not army. Government have woman. They catch you, cut off head for sure."

Chun sent Sol out the back gate of the compound, using his key to open the fence. He mumbled to Sol, "Maybe next time you see Chun, it in Korea. I be poor man on street. Sack by UN for help American fighter doctor. No job, no money. Maybe you give fifteen thousand dollar Chun in ten dollar bill."

* * *

Sol raced through the streets of El Fasher to the airport, skidding to a stop in front of Calcutta Helicopter. Crisanto sat behind the building at a table in a grass mat lean-to, the maintenance hangar, working on an aircraft generator, a dozen pieces of the ancient device spread before him. He looked up at Sol, smiled broadly, and came to his feet. Sol asked, "Now you're the Calcutta Helicopter chief mechanic?"

Crisanto laughed and whispered, "You want Singh to service the helicopter?"

"You got a point there, Crisanto. I know I told you that you shouldn't try to rescue your father on your own, but I've gotten involved with locals who say they can get Lila back. We will make sure they find your father, too. But if we fail, here's some money. These people do negotiate. Here."

Crisanto shook his head in disbelief, weighing the bag with both hands. Sol added, "It's only five thousand US, but I hope it helps." Sol tapped him on the shoulder and rushed out.

A half-kilometer from the hostel, he went around a block twice, and when he was sure he wasn't being followed, sped toward the building, pulling into the alleys, past a herd of hobbled camels tied to stakes. The animals were nipping at each other, waves of spit arching like mortar rounds.

Ibrahim burst from behind a mound of trash piled nearly as high as the first- story windows. Sol imagined it to be the personal debris of the hotel's guests over the past two decades, the 80s the last time the garbage had been collected in Western Sudan. The wildly gesturing man demanded Sol approach, but the doctor pulled off the alley, stopping next to the largest of the camels, one nearly as tall as the refuse heap and with a stench more ghastly than the debris.

Sol climbed into the backseat, where he took another five thousand from the bag, reached under the cushion, and cut a slit with his knife. He shoved the bills inside the gash. He crawled back over the driver's seat and placed the remaining bag of money halfway under his thigh. He left the corner open to show the green.

Ibrahim ran toward the Rover, flip flops slapping through the camel dung, until he skidded to a stop in front of the jeep. He stood, hands on hips, "You money? No money man neck cut die."

"I have the money. A lot of it. Now, let's get your friends. We go now to Jebel Mara." Sol pointed at the bag under his thigh. Ibrahim's eyes swelled to the size of pitas. He cocked his arm and jammed it through the passenger window, but Sol clasped it with his hand and growled, "You will get the cash when I tell you you can have it!"

Ibrahim froze. He eventually whispered in disbelief, "You speak Allah name curse!" He started to cap his incredulity with an "A*l hum de…*" but became wordless and stood with his jaw hanging, arm still protruding through the window.

Sol drummed the back of Ibrahim's hand as if disciplining a naughty child, and the young man backed off. When Sol grabbed the bag and waved the money in Ibrahim's face, the proto-rebel gathered himself and snapped, "Bra'heem do car."

"Bra'heem. I drive or no money."

"No. Bra'heem dry."

"*Maht salem,* goodbye." Sol put the bag of money between his legs, jammed the jeep into reverse, and started to back out of the driveway, but Ibrahim threw himself behind the vehicle.

"No go, no go! Bra'heem speak."

Sol replaced his smirk with a deep scowl. "Speak what?"

"*Doctori* want neck friend cut die? You want?"

"Fuck you. You know what that means? That means '*kes en neck eighty*'."

When Sol popped the clutch, Ibrahim's eyes became even bigger than when he had seen the cash. He bellowed, "No go, no go! Why you speak '*kes en neck eighty*'? Bra'heem friend. *Khawajii* girl come back. We go."

Sol waited for Ibrahim to relent, revving the engine, playing the clutch. "Stand behind the car! Come on, keep standin' there!"

When Ibrahim ran to the passenger door, Sol grabbed him by the *jellabiya* and shouted, "Get in, sit down, put your hands under your ass, don't move them, and shut up." He pulled out of the driveway, demanding over his shoulder, "You will tell me the roads."

The young insurgent obeyed until they got a block from the safe house and then, no longer able to contain himself, screeched, "Now Bra'heem do car," and put his hands up as if steering.

Sol acquiesced. He accepted the blindfold and moved to the rear seat, but when Ibrahim started to tie Sol's hands, Forte snapped, "No ropes. Start driving, Bra'heem, or no money."

At the safe house, Sol sat up from the backseat, removed the blindfold, clutched the sack of money close to his chest, and marched into the ramshackle structure ahead of Ibrahim.

Inside, there were two, rusted metal cots with thin blankets covering the bare springs. André sat on one; the blindfold had come undone, and only one wrist was loosely tied with a piece of tattered hemp. He was sipping tea with the other hand. At the rickety wooden table in the center of the room sat three men also drinking tea, their AK-47s lying haphazardly on the ground in the thick dust near the door. One of the men, a squat fellow, five-three, if that, jumped up and sputtered in Arabic at Ibrahim, who pointed at André and muttered back a few angry words. Though the man was stubby, Sol was amazed at the size of his head and feet—it was as if all his growth had gone into the far reaches of his body. A second conspirator looked up, a man as tall and thin as the guard at the UN, and Sol's gut clenched. The man jumped from his seat so quickly, his *immah* toppled, and as he rewound it, Sol could see this was an ancient soul, one perhaps born in the 1930s. The man roared, "Bra'heem, Ra'as al Ghul, *suker khaljic!*"

Sol smirked. He turned André. "He just told the one with the huge gourd and Ibrahim to shut up. He called the head *Ra'as al Ghul*—Demon Head. Is that good or bad? Whata you think?"

André began to answer but stopped when the tall one barked an order to the third coconspirator, who could not have reached his fifteenth birthday. The youngster rose from his chair sullenly and grumbled, "Yes, DokDok."

André asked, "What are they saying, Sol?"

"Well, I think the tall one told the kid to go and get two more teacups. And the kid said, 'Yes, DokDok.'"

"What is ze meaning, DokDok?"

"You remember when one of the checkers was teaching the kids to read? One of the books was *DokDok*, He told me it was an old children's story about a DokDok, but I forget what that is."

"So, Soli, we look at ze playbill. We 'ave Ra'as al Ghul, ze Monster Head; Bra'heem, who is really Ibrahim, who is really Abraham, and ze stick figure who is DokDok." Why are we 'ere, *mon ami?*"

Sol considered an answer, but the kid returned with two glasses of steaming tea and placed them on the table for Ibrahim and Sol.

Sol studied André for a moment. He reached over to remove the remnants of the blindfold, using it to wipe the grit and sweat from his friend's face. Sol chose the least filth-caked corner, dipped it in his own tea, blew a few breaths to cool the liquid, then dabbed at the remaining dried blood from André's eye. Through the internecine howling of increasingly guttural and strident Arabic, Sol asked André, "*Mon ami, ça va bien?*"

"*Oui.* As I say many time before, 'I am ze 'appy one.'"

"I see we've been captured by the Apple Dumpling Gang."

"*Que?* What?"

"Nothin'. I'll tell you later. I got the money. But I'm not taking crap from these jerks. This is who's gonna save us? *Oy vey*, as they used to say at medical school."

Sol turned to Ibrahim. "Everybody needs to sit down and talk. I want to hear your plan." Ibrahim's eyes squinted, and his head turned like a dog trying hard to understand his master. "You do have a plan?"

Ibrahim cocked his head. "Plan? Plan."

"Look, Bra'heem, we need to get going very soon. Where are your soldiers?"

"Soldiers? Soldiers. Yes, many soldiers money give."

"I have enough money to pay you and an army, but you will get a lot, lot more when we have the girl." Ibrahim sputtered, and Sol shook his finger at him sternly. "This is many, many thousand American dollars." He pulled a wad from the bag and tossed it on the bed. The bills fluttered in the hot gusts, soon roiling through the hovel. This time, Ibrahim's eyes expanded to the diameter of jeep tires. With the sudden silence, Sol waited until all faces shifted from the money to him, then lifted his nose arrogantly and took a gulp of tea. It was so hot, though, he spit it out and moaned, "Jesus, is everything in this place deadly?"

Ra'as al Ghul laughed heartily and downed his own steaming tea in a single gulp. He sat taller and rolled his shoulders, pressed his lips together, and turned away from the foreigners. Sol laughed and undid the hemp around his friend's left hand. Sol muttered barely audibly, "I guess we're on our own." He wagged his index finger left and right as he bellowed, "Let's go. No money for SLF."

Ibrahim jumped forward. "No go. Money here, *al hum de ley la.*"

Sol laughed and hissed, "That's nothing. Now you *not* have million dollar. André, let's go."

Sol sprang to his feet and walked from the room with military bearing, adding a bit of a swagger as he passed DokDok. André followed, though slouched until he focused his good eye on Sol, and straightened into a robotic gait. The two Westerners marched from the building, but Ibrahim and Ra'as sprang out the other door and Ibrahim gushed pleadingly, "Now go die Janjaweed, *Insha'Allah, al hum de ley la.*"

He yelled inside, and the kid, followed by a limping DokDok, joined the two at the front and the rear of the jeep. There was strident quarreling until the teenager ran back into the room for the blindfolds.

Sol shook his head roughly. "No way. I'm driving." He put a few bills in the hands of each man, forty or fifty dollars, and maybe seventy in DokDok's scrawny fingers. It was more than all four, together, had ever seen or imagined could be in one place at one time. Sol smiled, nodded confidently, and hopped in the driver's seat. André took the passenger side. The four insurgents squashed into the backseat and another round of squabbling filled the jeep. Sol turned the key, slammed the Rover into first, and played out the clutch slowly. Ibrahim hollered, "No! No! Bra'heem two minute car. Two minute *khawajii* car."

Sol yelled, "Bullshit!"

André whispered, "I sink he wants to drive away from 'ere and zen you can drive ze car."

Sol sighed, André hugged him, and Sol tied the plastic bag of money into his scrub pants. The blindfolds were placed loosely, the car lurched, a few vicious turns were slashed, a series of *al hum de ley la*s importuned, and the jeep jerked to a halt against a curb a mile later. The blindfolds were removed and the two foreigners nudged into the front seats while the four Sudanese scrunched onto the floor in the back and the cargo bay. They kept themselves below the level of the windows. Sol drove, following Ibrahim's screeched instructions for turns to the left and abruptly back to the right. They traipsed back along the same roads until Ibrahim yelped a final command, sending the jeep shuddering out of town. They did not join the highway, but paralleled it southwest into the desert.

* * *

There were lefts and rights at various landmarks, a rock, a dead tree, or the skeletal remains of a long-deceased camel. After an hour, they bounced into a primitive settlement where Sol was ordered to stop. DokDok creaked from the backseat like a rusty gate opening for the first time in decades. He limped into a twelve-by-twelve grass hutch, "Ze 'ilton," André laughed. In seconds, two women flew out, tongues trilling piercingly drawing the ladies of the village of Lub from their huts to gather in a messy circle. The mass vibrated sideways, then forward and backward, the din of *al hum de ley la*s so piercing, André had to cover his ears. But every few steps, the women stopped to redo their *tobs*, and in all, very little progress was made in regard to where the battalion was eventually to settle, which in the end, was just a few feet from where it had started.

DokDok hobbled back to the jeep and spoke with Ibrahim, who translated to Sol, "Now money for soldier. Army SLF."

Sol argued, "We just handed you a fortune. Use what we gave you."

André shook his head and spoke forcefully, "Zey are ze women army? We pay for zis?"

Ibrahim, however, laughed hollowly, answering, "SLF no woman army." He sliced his open hand against the other palm, barely making contact, grunting, "Woman call man SLF Army, *Insha'Allah*."

And indeed, a few men drifted in from the fields. DokDok barked at them until they shuffled into a proto-military formation, the troops smiling expectantly at the two foreigners. Ibrahim stepped back to the jeep again to demand money. Sol jumped from the driver's seat, ran to DokDok, stuffed his hand in the man's *jellabiya*, and pulled out two tens. He handed one back to DokDok, and took the other to the largest man amongst the recruits, waved it in front of the man's eyes, and then toward his pals. As Sol's hand moved, the men's eyes followed the bill's every flutter. He handed it to the big man for a moment, snapped it back, and placed it in the next man's fist.

DokDok yelled, and one of the men jumped forward, saluted with his left hand, redid his *immah*, and rushed into a hut. There was a ruckus of pots and pans and boxes being tossed about until he backed out waving a key triumphantly above his head. He stood at attention, dipped his head at the accolades of his tribesmen, and jogged to the far end of the village. A moment later, with a rumble and a screech, a twenty-passenger school bus bumped to a stop in front of the troops. The engine continued bucking and coughing after the driver had removed the key and taken his place back in ranks. The exhaust, a far deeper yellow than what was left of the vehicle's paint, set off widespread coughing.

DokDok scuttled around to the gas cap, opened it, pointed to Sol, then took a ten and pretended to stuff it into the tank. André mumbled, "It is a waste of ze money. Ze bus does not go two kilometers. Zis is ze 'uman and ze bus graveyard of ze Earse." He slashed his hand left and right. "I do not ride in 'im."

"Not to worry, my friend, we'll take the Rover. I promise not to get you within a kilometer of this thing." They stared into each other's eyes, and Sol nodded. "I know what you're thinking, and you're right. How the hell do they figure they're going to sneak up on the Janjaweed in a truck bomb? It's a lost cause. Let's cut our losses. We'll go back to El Fasher, and I'll do whatever I need to do to get things back on track. Anything is better than this."

Sol started the jeep and began a crawl through the sand toward the hard pack that had brought them there, but DokDok yelled at Ibrahim, who sprinted toward the barely-moving Rover. He slowed twice to redo his toppling *immah* but caught up with the jeep when the tires became mired in the sand. "*Doctori*, Money gas. Little money gas."

"How much?"

Ibrahim held up five fingers, lifted his own ten-dollar bill five times, ran to a 55 gallon oil drum next to the first grass hut, and tapped it on the rusted lid five times. André mumbled, "Maybe it is only fifty, Soli. Nosing really to lose."

When Sol dug the bag out of his scrub pants, the women chortled, and the men whooped as they ran to their *tuchels*, dragging from them armfuls of matériel: rifles, some with tremendously long barrels, essentially muskets; some AK-47s; and one man, a crossbow and quiver of arrows with moth-eaten feathers. Each citizen-soldier also hugged a hobo's bundle the size of a basketball and a plastic supermarket bag with rations, water, packs of LIFE cigarettes, and a few toothbrush sticks.

The bus grunted out of Lub into the *wadi*. Sol and André crept along in the jeep a hundred yards behind, negotiating turns around the thorn branches, barely able to clear the minefield of tire-consuming spikes. After the first blowout, Sol cursed so loud Ibrahim heard him and leaned out of a window to stare at the Westerners. When Sol pulled out of the *wadi* onto the desert proper, the bus stopped and Ibrahim waved wildly for them to get back into the riverbed, but Sol grabbed bills from his pocket, waved them in the air, and then at the flat tire. A dozen men flew from the bus and descended upon the Rover, the tire replaced before *Thunderstruck* on Sol's CD was over. He gave a ten to the largest man, and they pushed off again.

At the next town, the same recruiting dance took place—food and water were loaded, most on top of the bus, but several men hung their bags on the hood, some behind the bumpers. The women produced a hodgepodge of rusty fuel cans, glass bottles corked with bits of cloth, and beaten pots filled with gasoline. DokDok examined each aliquot of fuel, sniffed it, touched it, and rejected a few bottles, those filled with lamp oil, and one cut with water. Sol pulled twenty more dollars from his crotch.

A half mile deeper into the desert, six additional troops boarded the bus with their armaments and hobos' bags. At one of the towns, DokDok petitioned for a hundred dollars to buy fuel, but Sol refused, placing five more tens in the man's *jellabiya* pocket. DokDok frowned and sent the recruits to a hut from which they hauled, on a litter fashioned from tree branches, a 55 gallon barrel of gasoline. They struggled to get it aboard the bus, where they collapsed, exhausted, on the cushionless seats. Several of them lit cigarettes.

The army trundled further into the Nubian desert. Hours passed, the temperature soared, and when Sol and André were nearly comatose, there appeared through the blowing sand an outline in the sky.

Ibrahim ran to the jeep. "Jebel Mara!"

The bus stopped, and the men poured out to gawk at the ten-thousand-foot mountain, one they had heard about since childhood, but never been the several dozen miles from their home villages to have actually witnessed. They were incredulous and stood in reverence, though a few turned and ran back to the troop transport and hid under seats. There they stammered about the *jinn* waiting to strike them dead for having let their eyes gaze upon so lofty a proclamation of Allah's power.

André announced to Sol he had counted forty men stuffed into the wobbly bus. "And zer is ze gasoline bomb wis zem. It incinerate 'alf of ze Darfur if our soldier not stop lighting zer cigarette next to 'im."

The army had come from seven desolate villages, the men having already travelled further that night than most had ever gone in their lives, perhaps all of them put together.

André shook his head and asked, "'Ow did zey find zese villages? Zer are no roads, nosing for many mile."

Sol mumbled, "Amazing. And how do they fit all these guys into a clown car?"

Sol wondered how much longer the recruiting was to go on, but Ibrahim came to the Westerners, head high. He halted with a flourish. An index finger poked the air above his head as he declared in a command voice, "Now have Army SLF. Now die Janjaweed." The chop to the palm had regained a bit of its vigor.

They stopped a little past dusk. Though the moon was magnificently full and one could see for miles in every direction, DokDok ordered armed scouts out to remote listening posts, but the men stopped just fifty yards into the desert. A fire was started, tea and *jabana* brewed, cigarettes passed around, and after the break, the men dropped to prayer mats.

DokDok finished his tea, squared his shoulders, and lowered his voice into a deeply grave timbre. He directed several of the men to smooth the earth for a sand table. Other men formed boundaries with branches from thistle trees. A few soldiers poured water into a hole to make mud that they used to create the features of Jebel Mara. DokDok clucked his tongue impatiently when an aspect of the model was not to his liking but did not touch the mockup himself, instead pointing with a twig and barking corrections.

André and Sol were excluded, and as they inched closer to watch, Ra'as shook his head and waved his index finger, dismissing them. Ibrahim tightened his face. "You no look. Secret for SLF."

DokDok continued to growl orders, his eyes fixed on the heavens as if drawing from a conduit of divine knowledge. His final command sent the men scurrying aboard the bus to vault back out in seconds, rifles clasped to their chests. They fell into formation at semi-attention, jaws locked, to stand inspection.

The next phase of the battle plan was delivered by DokDok, who lectured his platoon for but three minutes. He guided them through a verbal dress rehearsal of the mission, using his twig to point at salient features of the battle zone while Ra'as shouted out that element of the mockup. The troops jumped to their feet and moved in slow motion, feigning grunting and suffering. The final act was to pretend they were climbing over or working their way around imaginary obstacles.

DokDok became silent but continued his stare into the evening sky. He finally lowered his head and spoke in hisses to Ra'as, who barked that the troops would do it again, and then again, and once again, until they got it right. When several of the men griped and asked for another tea break, DokDok had them fall into formation. He walked the rows silently and glowered, shaking his head in disgust at every second troop. When he returned to his position at the front of the formation, he growled at Ra'as to order the men to run through the mission several more times.

André winked at Sol, who nodded knowingly and pulled a wad of cash out of the jeep, enough for one bill per man. When DokDok finally dismissed the troops for a smoke break, Sol asked Ibrahim obsequiously if he could meet with DokDok. They sat quietly around the fire as Sol handed the stack of bills to the commanding officer. Sol asked Ibrahim to inform the troops that there was ten dollars for each man, and much more for the officers, if they returned the girl unharmed. "These are excellent soldiers, sir," Sol nodded, "Thank you. You are a very good man."

DokDok nodded almost imperceptibly and went over the tactical mission another time. When he was done, the men sat in a circle speaking quietly, an occasional hollow laugh or two wafting into the desert night, until DokDok ordered them back into formation. He inspected the weapons carefully and found several men had forgotten to load their magazines. With a shake of his head, he dismissed the troops to sleep on the sand. André and Sol sat in the Rover, their seats reclined as they tried to rest.

At 10 P.M., Ra'as woke the men. Without a word, they climbed aboard the bus and ground off south. Sol followed at a distance, lights off, moving so smoothly and carefully he barely raised a puff of dust. With the full moon in the western sky, they were able to keep the bare outline of Jebel Mara in sight through the sandy haze, though as the moon passed behind the two-mile high peak, the craggy outline burst into razor-sharp detail.

The bus stopped when a portion of the setting moon, a sliver of gold, became visible to the flank of the grand mountain. The sphere soon filled the horizon. André muttered, "I once read ze paper on why ze moon is so big rising and setting. Do you know?"

"No. Bent rays, I guess."

"Zey could not figure 'im out. I sink it *is* ze bent rays of ze atmosphere, but zey say no. No answer. *Etrange, non?*" He sighed, "Soli, I 'ope we will see ze moon once again. One more night. But ze truth, I do not really care anymore, only zat she is okay, wis or wisout you and me 'ere."

Sol put his hand on his friend's thigh, "We will make it, and Miss Lila will, too. Trust me, I'm a doctor. I know about these things."

André smiled. "Ah, zey know it all, ze doctor. But sank you. I will never forget you."

As the moon disappeared, the sky blackened and the bus moved very slowly forward toward the mountain, creeping for several more hours, stopping every half hour to fill the gas tank with the sloshing pots first, the glass bottles next, and finally, the gas cans.

Sol worried the eastern sky might be lightening. At two miles from the base of Jebel Mara, the driver cut the ignition and allowed the bus to roll to a stop behind a copse of trees, well hidden from the mountain.

The men spilled from the coach. They were dressed in desert fatigues, their faces wrapped in dark brown *immah*s, all but their eyes hidden. Ibrahim told Sol not to move the jeep, not to speak, and for sure, not to follow the troops into battle. "Bring *khawajii* woman," he nodded, pointing to the ground in front of them.

The men broke into three squads, lining up separately behind a mark in the sand drawn by Ra'as. DokDok milled about mumbling to himself. Abruptly, he stopped stock-still to stare into the eastern horizon. After a minute, he nodded to Ra'as, who ordered the first group to depart. Watching a windup clock, he sent the next teams into battle exactly five minutes apart. DokDok and Ra'as stayed behind until they had established communications with their lead squad over a kid's walkie-talkie, gently tapping the mouthpiece in code rather than speaking into it.

Soon the pre-dawn light brightened the sky, and in minutes, the first rim of yellow appeared. The men had already reached the base of the mountain and taken concealed positions behind the loose boulders DokDok had simulated on his sand table. In minutes, the entire fiery orange disc of the sun spewed escalating light and heat. The bus had been parked east of the enemy position exactly along the path of the rising sun. Sol could see Janjaweed soldiers three hundred feet up the mountain sitting on outcroppings of rocks, smoking cigarettes and drinking tea. The light, however, blared into the eyes of the defenders on the *jebel* so intensely, they had no idea the bus was parked in the middle of the desert, barely hidden by a stand of pathetic trees, and that the rebel force was in position at the base of their stronghold.

As the air currents built, the desert became obscured in eddies of dust, and Sol could no longer make out the position of the army he had commissioned. The building wind covered the noise of the rebels, and he took a small kerosene burner from the bus to heat water for chocolate oatmeal.

He badgered his friend to finally try the porridge, but André groused, "I would razer die of ze starvation and 'ave ze pain of ze toose zan eat zis sing." But he tried the gruel, liked it, and finished the bowl. He was about to ask for another portion when the report of rifle fire from the mountain startled them. Sol dropped the empty bowl, climbed to the top of the school bus, and peered through the web of tree branches. As the battle intensified, clouds of smoke lifted from two positions: one high in the shale, one at ground level.

"André, come up here." They watched as the billows of cordite closed in on each other. When a series of larger explosions rose from the lower reaches of the hill, Sol hissed, "Shit, grenades. Our guys don't have grenades, do they?" André shrugged. A period of silence followed, and Sol cursed, "The battle's already over. We need to be gettin' out of here in a hurry."

André nodded in agreement but hesitated. "I do not want to leave wisout our friends...*mais*, zere is nosing we can do." His head sank and rocked left and right. "Yet again ze tragedy. You are right. Come on, Soli, we go." They loaded the jeep, but as they pulled out of the thicket, there was a beating sound, one that grew deeper and louder very quickly. Sol turned. "What the...it's Crisanto. I told him..."

With the Rover in the open, Crisanto recognized it, but the helicopter was at full throttle, sprinting at a hundred knots, thrashing the air not five hundred feet off the desert. As the ship flew over, Crisanto decided to turn and circle to determine what was happening on the ground. But by the time he passed the Rover, he was so close to Jebel Mara, and the aircraft was so fast, there was no room to make a turn. The best he could do was pull the nose up to bleed off energy and, he prayed, slow down enough to roll to the left before running into the mountain. As the ship rose, though, bursts of small arms tracers passed the cockpit. There was no choice—he had to try a turn. He rolled left violently. It was more stress than he had ever placed on a helicopter, and, as feared, the maneuver threw the ship into a hard skid to the right, a truck turning viciously on a slick highway. He watched breathlessly as the tip of the main rotor closed in sideways on a shelf of volcanic rock. His body tightened and, by instinct, his hand yanked the stick as far back and as far left as it would go. The G stresses became so large, he greyed out. When Crisanto regained full consciousness, the first thing he saw was that the sideward drift had stopped, the blade now just feet from the rocks, but getting no closer.

He regained control of the ship and dipped down to maneuver into a natural revetment shielded from the line of fire. Though both airmen were trembling, they broke out in fits of laughter.

They hoped that, while they had announced themselves to both the Janjaweed and DokDok's men, all sides would deduce the helicopter was coming with money to reclaim Romey, and all sides would cease their fire. They lifted off again and headed toward the open area behind the Janjaweed's position that had been described in the ransom demand. They would expose themselves and demonstrate their non-belligerent intent, then follow hand-signal instructions on where to land.

As they flew around the edge of Jebel Mara, however, tracers flew past the helicopter's plexiglass cockpit, all of it coming from the base of the mountain. He could see the Janjaweed's weapons on the *jebel* were not aimed at him, but at the base of the mountain.

Crisanto could not know that DokDok's men, in their wildest imaginations, would never have expected an airborne weapon to be sent in *their* support. The only aircraft they had ever laid eyes on were the ones deployed by the Khartoum government to murder Darfurian peasants, planes that flew above their rifle fire but easily rained down napalm and antipersonnel bombs on their families. The rebels screamed in defiance and stood in the clear, willing to die to bring the specter down.

Crisanto dove the ship back to the revetment and told his co-pilot to jump into the back and man the M-79 grenade launcher. Jati snatched a canvas bag of ammunition, dropped to the floor, and when Crisanto picked up again, he poked the grenade launcher through the open door and fired several rounds into the rebel SLF's position.

"André, we are witnessing the end of the world. We have just paid for our allies to kill each other while the fuckin' Janjaweed sit back and let it end. Then they'll go down, take the guns and the helicopter radios, and the fuel, and the bus, and us. Bullshit. Let's go and fix it."

"*Mon ami*, you are ze insane one. You know zis." But Sol wasn't listening. He was hurling gear into the jeep."

"Coming?"

When they reached a point a quarter-of-a-mile from the mountain, Crisanto spotted them and landed on a flat area behind the jeep. He jumped out, yelled something in Tagalog, swore in tainted English, counted the bullet holes in the fuselage, and spit on the sand with each puncture he tallied. Sol explained, and the young pilot smacked his head and howled, "Oh Jesus, we hit them with M-79 grenades. I saw some go down. Oh, my Jesus."

Sol pulled André out of the jeep on the pretext they were going to have a meeting, but without a word, jumped back in, gunned the engine, and disappeared up the stone road into the mountain. Small arms fire came from above, a thousand tiny puffs of smoke drawn together by the updraft through the cavern in which the one road wound. The spent gunpowder shot skyward as a dense cloud. When it got to a thousand feet, it spread into the shape of a mushroom. Sol mumbled, "World War fuckin' Three."

He should have been an easy target, but the road snaked through a corridor of craggy boulders, each the size of a house, and he found himself shielded from the blitz, the one road leading to the enemy position, absurdly, a safe conduit. The expression "fields of fire" popped into his head from the History Channel, but he had never really understood what it meant. Whatever fields of fire were, it suddenly became clear the Janjaweed hadn't prepared any. He was able to drive up the cavern along the road, completely hidden from the enemy.

A hundred meters later, at a tight turn to the left, he had to slow to a near stop. A figure in desert fatigues, face wrapped in an *immah*, darted from between two boulders and stood in front of the Rover. The man screamed, "Why you go? Bra'heem say no go!"

Sol laughed, sprang from the jeep, and hugged the man, who put one arm around Sol's shoulder hesitantly. "Ibrahim, I am so happy to see you. Listen, the helicopter belongs to me. No shoot. Do you understand?"

Ibrahim shook his head in confusion, so Sol physically turned him by the shoulders and pushed him back into the brush. He yelled, "Bring friends here."

A moment later, Ibrahim reemerged from the stone fissures, followed by DokDok and Ra'as. At first the dialog was vehemently angry, but it swiftly became exultant, and the meeting culminated with a wrathful chopping of hands into open palms.

Sol asked, "Are your men hurt?"

"Two, three." He pointed at the sky.

"I am sorry. But this is what we are going to do." Ibrahim translated, and Ra'as grunted as if offended, though Sol ignored him and continued in pidgin. He used hand signals to include DokDok. "You give me one radio. I in helicopter. I have big gun. I speak you where Janjaweed. You tell SLF soldier. If I see many Janjaweed, I shoot with grenade."

Sol stopped to allow Ibrahim to translate. The exchange was filled with bickering until DokDok growled something to Ibrahim, who ran into the bush and came out with a walkie-talkie. As Sol started to back out of the redoubt, he saw a figure in the rearview mirror waving madly, loping up the road toward them. Sol backed the jeep to meet him.

"Soli, I am not to stay back zere. I must do somesing."

"Okay. I'm happy you're here. Look, The Janjaweed saw our SLF friends and the helicopter firing on each other. So, they think it's coming with the money for them. They won't shoot at it. You stay on the ground and work the radio. When the helicopter goes back up, we'll have the SLF shoot behind it, pretend they're trying to shoot it down. The Janjaweed'll see the tracers and allow it to fly over, maybe even behind them. Crisanto can fake trying to find a place to land. Meanwhile, I'll be calling you with the Janjaweed's position. Ibrahim will understand you in person, but he'll never get it over the radio."

"So now we are ze mercenary advisor. From the 'ealer to ze slayer. Not so 'ard for ze change, *non*?"

"Yes, Dr. Guillotine. Look, I want her back. You want her back. I want Romeo back. What they've gone through. And I want those people from our camp freed. As of this minute, I don't personally give a rip what happens to me. You need to take care of yourself. Your decision."

"Soli, I was only sinking, sinking how easy for a man's life to change in ze instant. I want her back. I do anysing."

"You comfortable working with these men? They can be a pain in the ass."

"It is no problem." He smiled broadly. "I 'ave work wis you!"

Sol gave him a bump in the shoulder. "Good man. I'm leaving the jeep for you. When you get Lila and Romey, go back to the bus and fill the Rover from our jerry cans, then refill those cans from the fuel drum in the bus. Screw'em. It's our gas."

* * *

Sol dove into the jeep, stuffed what was left of the money into his pants, jumped out, hugged André hard, and whispered, "The happiest moment of my life will be when I see you and Lila together in Cairo." He shoved several thousand dollars into André's hand, turned to run, but looked back and shouted, "The Cairo Ramses Hilton. Next week. Leave word at the desk the instant you get there." He sprinted off the mountain into the desert.

At the helicopter, Crisanto rolled his eyes. "Doctor, so we have two armies who are killing each other and trying to kill us, and you pay for both. You are like the US Government." He laughed and put his hand on Sol's arm. "When this is over, Doctor, and I have a baby, he will be Sol."

Jati also laughed. "My son's name to be Suleiman. The same as Solomon. Maybe he will be a doctor."

Sol grabbed the grenade launcher and handed it to Jati, who showed him how to load and fire. Crisanto leaned back from his seat and warned, "Doctor, flat on floor. Stay inside until I tell you. Do *not* load until we are on station, and don't ever bring the muzzle into the ship if the gun's loaded. Muzzle is always out the door—never inside, and *never* let it point up toward the rotor, loaded or unloaded."

Sol nodded, and Crisanto called out the starting sequence. They lifted off, skimming the surface until reaching the first out-cropping of scarlet rock. As the ship climbed toward the Janjaweed encampment, the SLF dutifully fired at them, though some of the tracers crossed near the nose of the helicopter. Crisanto turned back to Sol, yelling at him to plug his earphones into the jack by the door, but he was on his stomach and did not hear. When the ship neared the bivouac area, Crisanto jinked a few times to inform the Janjaweed of his friendly intentions, then pretended to be avoiding the rifle fire so Sol could see the entire camp. Cages of metal fencing were filled with hundreds of black souls. They stood shoulder to shoulder, not a square inch to sit nor or a speck of shade from the burgeoning sun.

Sol came to his knees and crawled to the opposite door to count soldiers. He described to André the position of the enemy soldiers who had exposed themselves to fire down on the rebels.

Crisanto looked back toward Sol, who hollered, "Pretend to be landing." Then he called on the radio, "André, tell them to shoot in the air again."

There was static and an eventual, "I tell zem."

Sol came to his knees and crawled behind the pilots. "I have an idea. When our soldiers start to shoot again, lift up and pretend to run away, but first, fly real, real low and slow right over that main tent." He pointed. "Right there."

DokDok's men unleashed their weapons, and the helicopter inched across the Janjaweed camp. Sol pulled a handful of bills from his pants and dropped them out his door, letting the rotor wash blow the money directly onto the command tent. Dozens of Janjaweed appeared from the cracks in the earth they had exploited as bunkers. Their *jellabiyas* billowed, and their bodies twirled, hundreds of hands scraping the air to catch the windfall. It reminded Sol of the Dervish. A moment later, he laughed as a Janjaweed patrol nearing the SLF reversing its attack to sprint back up the hill.

The helicopter flew off the mountain again, settling onto the desert near the bus. Crisanto let the engine idle while he and Sol scripted the next distraction. They were too far from the mountain to raise André on the radio, the walkie-talkies limited, they had discovered, to a range of two or three hundred yards. So, they decided to come in from the opposite direction, drop more money, and count heads on the far side of the base camp. Sol pulled a dozen tens out of his pants and held them outside the door. When they got over the tent, twenty or so Janjaweed belched out into the sun, dancing about, their hands raised in Pavlovian anticipation. An angry man in Western-style fatigues and combat boots ran out of a bunker waving one fist above his head and firing an M-16 into the air with the other hand. The frenzy slowly stopped, and the foot soldiers walked, heads hung, back to their battle stations. Sol waited until the troops were inside their shallow foxholes to let the money drop, laughing as the men poured back out and trampled each other. A few bills fluttered near the commander—he dropped his rifle and leapt into the air.

Crisanto feigned an approach, but there was firing from the SLF, so they flew back to the bus. Sol took Crisanto aside, away from the howl of the jet engine. "That was the last recon, Crisanto. What if we drop your fifty-five-gallon drum of jet fuel out the door, and I shoot at it with the grenade launcher? You think that'll work?"

"Maybe, maybe not. It is JP-4. It might catch fire eventually, but it will not explode, not like gasoline."

Sol smiled and slapped his forehead. "I'm so dumb! We *got* gasoline." Crisanto shook his head in confusion. "There's a fifty-five-gallon drum on the bus. We'll load it on the helicopter. I'll push it out, it'll drop on them, and I'll shoot at it with a grenade. It'll end the war."

"Doctor, how are we going to load that much weight, just three of us, and how are you going to push it out by yourself?"

"How much can it weigh?"

"Three to four hundred pounds is how much." Crisanto thought for a moment. "Wait. If we can get it off the bus, we can sling it in the cargo net."

Sol answered. "Perfect. We can roll it out the back door of the bus and over the ground into the net. You hover, and I'll hook it up. When we get there, we can fly over the command tent. That's a good hundred yards from the hostages. I think it's gonna work."

At the bus, though, Crisanto stopped Sol. "The barrel is so corroded, it's going to split open before we get it out of the vehicle." He looked up at the sky and muttered, "Now, Singh is going to charge me for the net, and probably the helicopter." But he smiled and raised a perfect bird, aiming it into the sky toward El Fasher.

When the barrel tumbled from the back hatch of the bus, a small crack opened in a rusted patch. A bit of fuel dribbled out, so they moved quickly, but as the ship came up and the net gained purchase against the drum, the metal buckled, and the dribble became a stream. Sol yelled to Crisanto, who flew faster than on the other sorties. This time, they hovered over an area as far from the cages as they could get, and with money raining down in clumps, even the soldiers guarding the captives lunged toward headquarters, dropping to their knees, a hundred men crawling about like maddened rats.

Crisanto looked back to Sol, who nodded violently and gave the thumbs up. Crisanto pulled maximum power, and the ship vaulted straight up, leveling three hundred feet above the troops. Crisanto slammed the cargo release pedal so hard, Sol could feel the floor thump. As the barrel dropped away, Sol threw himself onto the deck of the aircraft, grenade launcher clutched to his chest, pockets stuffed with rounds.

When the crude bomb reached the ground, though, it landed in the single patch of trees in the entire base camp. Instead of rupturing, it rolled off the foliage and downhill toward a ledge of sharp rock directly over the SLF rebels. Sol tensed, realizing that if it went over the precipice, it would rupture at the first outcropping of the razor-sharp volcanic stone. The gasoline would shower down upon the rebels and André, though much of it would vaporize in the building heat before it hit the ground. Then the fuel would not just burn, it would explode with the equivalent of three thousand pounds of TNT, all of it just feet over the heads of a few dozen near-starving rebels. The Janjaweed would laugh as they tossed grenades over the side of the mountain. The fire and concussion waves from the atomized fuel would massacre DokDok and his band. No living creature would survive. Sol's gut seized. He realized he was about to end their lives, and André's as well, while the Janjaweed would be perfectly protected by the walls of stone.

But after the first bounce, the barrel rolled into the last obstacle between it and the edge, a Russian supply truck. The barrel broke open, and thirty or forty gallons of explosive fuel belched out. Sol watched it disperse into a lethal mist that suspended itself over the Janjaweed position.

He screamed, "Oh, my God!" and aimed the grenade launcher at the center of the saturated soldiers who were still foraging for the cash. As he placed his index finger on the trigger, he crossed himself, and recited the Lord's Prayer. The words, "…deliver us from evil…" hit him in the chest, and he suddenly grasped he was about to commit wholesale murder, not only the Janjaweed, but the captives as well, a hundred of the very people he had travelled so far to rescue.

Sol looked up when Crisanto screamed, "Fire now! Now, Doctor!"

He aimed again but was paralyzed with the notion that he would have to live for forty more years with what it would take less than a tenth of a second to do. He lost concentration, but with Crisanto's screams, he castigated himself for his weakness, and his finger slid back onto the trigger. And then he pictured the hapless souls along the road to Umm Balla, and the desperate nomads, and the boys in the *madrasa*. Were some of them Janjaweed, fighting for a few kilos of *durra* the monsters in Khartoum granted its mercenaries? But the vision of the women these very swine had mutilated in Umm Balla cleared his mind. He blew out a breath and aimed, but in the mist of the evaporating gasoline, a rainbow had formed, one of strange colors, unctuous hues, and, because he had delayed so long, the heat had lifted some of the gas to the altitude of the helicopter. He could smell the fumes. If he fired, the ship would be consumed as well. He turned to Crisanto and screamed at him to fly off a distance.

The Janjaweed commander, having just divined what was about to transpire, gesticulated wildly for the men to disperse, but one of the foot soldiers took it upon himself to punish the helicopter, and as the first round left the muzzle, a fireball of nuclear proportions lifted from the ground, carrying with it an inferno of orange-blazing *jellabiya*s.

The helicopter had flown just far enough to allow the air rushing through it to cleanse the cabin of atomized gasoline. The blast, though, was so intense, the stinking heat nearly caused the ship to overturn. Sol bounced against the bare metal walls of the helicopter until Crisanto regained control and flew back toward the bus. Sol's right arm began to throb, and he watched it swell before his eyes.

Sol forced himself to look back at the Janjaweed's position. A few of those sufficiently alive to move were staggering in circles. He tried to call André, but there was no response, and all he could see of the lower battlefield were SLF fighters standing in the open, firing at unarmed men stumbling down the road, many ablaze, all with hands high above their heads.

He called André again, and this time there was an answer, but when Sol told him to get the SLF to cease-fire, André screamed, "Zey no listen, no listen!"

The helicopter put down at the base of the mountain. Sol launched from the rear hatch and charged up the hill. He focused on the maddened SLF, who were picking off the frantic, burning enemy by twos and threes. He fired a grenade at a protruding wedge of rock, the unexpected recoil of the launcher nearly flattening him. The round burst between two boulders, concentrating the noise and fire into a deafening cylinder. It was so loud, the men of both sides froze in their tracks.

Ibrahim screeched at Sol, "SLF die devil Janjaweed." He was laughing and chopping at his hand. "*Al hum de ley la, al hum de ley la!*"

Sol ran past Ibrahim to DokDok and put his hand in front of the man's face. "No, you stop. Now, goddamnit." When the ancient man cocked his head in surprise, Sol sprinted back to Ibrahim and jammed the barrel of the unloaded M-79 into his chest. He bellowed, "You tell him stop. Now!"

Ibrahim began to tremble but gathered himself and yelled to DokDok, who fired a burst from his AK-47 into the air. He gabbled orders to Ra'as, who issued them to his men in a half-hearted grunt. For the most part, the firing stopped. One SLF, though, squatted behind a thick rock, waited until there was quiet, then bolted upright and screamed, "My wife and my son!" He dispatched a few more of the stragglers as they stumbled down the mountain.

Sol called to André, and the two met on the road. "We need to go up into the base camp and open the cages. Who the hell knows? We may have killed them, too."

Silently, they set off uphill, passing smoldering bodies, ignoring the calls of Ibrahim and DokDok to halt. A half mile up the road, they came to a set of bunkers, all abandoned, rifles lying about haphazardly. A seared, thin, oily, black patina of grease covered the red earth. They grabbed AKs and continued up another quarter of a mile to the next set of barricades. Scorched bodies lay about. Nothing moved. They pushed on, drawn by high-pitched screaming.

At the final plateau, the terrain was deeply blackened, but the fire had not reached the cages across the mesa. They sprinted the last several hundred yards, yanked open the gates, and were nearly trampled by the flood. Sol recognized some of the children from the village of Umm Balla. After the prisoners galloped away, both men realized neither Lila nor Romeo were amongst the captives. It was quiet now, aside from the occasional rifle shot at the base of the mountain. André fell to his knees. "All zis, for what, for what?"

* * *

At the rebels' position, the SLF were lugging the Janjaweed who had survived the burst, lining them up on the ground, spitting on them, and shooting those who had the temerity to beg for their lives. One man was urinating in the face of a soldier whose skin had peeled off. It made the victim appear white. Sol ripped the rifles from several men and ordered Ibrahim to tell them to move away from the prisoners.

Sol implored, "If you kill them, they cannot tell us where the woman and the pilot are. We need them alive."

"This Janjaweed. Die mother, father, baby. Not you mother, father, baby. Bra'heem mother, girl-brother. Now die Janjaweed."

"No, no, no. You want money, tell me where are *khawajii* woman and pilot. Ask them."

Ibrahim shook his head impatiently then yelled down to one of the cowering hostages, who whispered back tremulously that he had no idea what Ibrahim was talking about. Another of the SLF lowered what looked like a Civil War musket and discharged a round into the man's head. Ibrahim, with the slightest hint of a smirk, squared his shoulders and moved to the next prisoner in line, a grizzled old man whose face was covered in the brains, blood, and bone of his former companion. This one had more to say, and Sol leaned down to listen.

"Bra'heem tell *Doctori*. Woman go N'Djamena. That country Chad." He pointed west. "Sell Saudi man." He took his index finger and put it in his closed other fist, drawing it in and out, in and out.

The rebel with the AK aimed it at the old man's head, grinned openly as he charged the weapon, and looked to Ibrahim for a nod. But Sol grabbed the barrel, pulled it out of the man's hands, and flung it to the side. Ra'as spit on the ground and started to move furiously toward Sol, but Ibrahim put his hand in the man's gigantic face and spoke softly until Ra'as spun around and bridled back to DokDok.

"Ask him when they left," Sol commanded.

"Night," Ibrahim answered, searching for the word, pointing a finger over his shoulder.

Sol hissed, "What does that mean?"

Ibrahim made the motion again, and André intervened. "I think 'ee is say 'yesterday night.'"

"Yes, yes, yesterday night."

"What time?" Sol persisted.

Ibrahim asked, and the hostage pointed up at the sky to the east.

André declared, "Ah, when ze moon come up. Maybe nine. Zey knew we are coming. For sure. But 'ow zey know?"

"Ask him how fast the truck can go."

Ibrahim held up three, then five, fingers. André nodded, "Thirty to fifty kilometer in one hour."

Sol mumbled, "Okay, with a loaded truck, the best they can average is fifteen to twenty miles per hour until they get to a highway. Nah, they don't dare get on a public road, even in Chad. They're going to have to stay in the sand, out of sight of main roads. Ask him how many Janjaweed soldiers in the truck."

Three fingers.

"What kind of weapons do they have?"

The prisoner pointed to AKs.

"Do they have a radio?"

"Yes."

"How far can the radio talk?"

When the hostage turned his head away from Ibrahim, one of the SLF charged his assault rifle, took a step out of Sol's grabbing range, and lowered the muzzle toward the man's eyes. The Janjaweed soldier responded. Ibrahim translated, "Radio here, maybe," took a ten-dollar bill from his pocket, pointed at the number, and raised it three times.

"Truck left long before we got here. How the hell did they know we were coming? Ask him how they found out."

The man turned his face away again, the last volitional act of his life. Sol screamed at the executioner and appealed to DokDok, who ignored Sol and quietly took a pace sideways to stop at the head of the next man. That soldier said tremulously that a man who had worked for the whites had told them.

"Where is that man now?"

He pointed up the hill and added without emotion, "*Mat.*"

Sol turned to André. "So, what do we know? The truck left maybe three hours before we got here. That's five, six hours ago. They may have gone a couple of hundred kilometers by now, at the outside, but too far for us to catch them in the rover. But they probably don't know about the helicopter." Sol yelled at the prisoner. "What road?"

"A-43, A-5."

Sol turned to Crisanto. "That's, let's say, a hundred and twenty miles at the outside. Less than an hour-and-a-half flying if you don't have to look for them. Then about that, or a little more, to get back to El Fasher. Crisanto, do you have that much fuel with you?"

"We can get there if we use what we have left of the two barrels of fuel on board. But that isn't enough to come back with Lila and my father. We're already low."

"Can you burn diesel?"

"Not by itself. It has to be mixed with gasoline and benzene and some other stuff. But JP-4 is mostly diesel and gasoline. If we mix just those two, it might work for a while."

"Okay. Let's go back up and see what the Janjaweed have stockpiled. But we gotta move fast."

They found two barrels of diesel and one of gasoline half buried, but the metal was terribly oxidized, no different than the SLF's barrel. As they tried to pry them out of the ground, the rotted tops pulled off and handfuls of sand dribbled in.

Crisanto brought the helicopter up to the base camp, and they worked for an hour pulling fuel out of the barrels with cooking pots, straining it through death shroud, and mixing gasoline and diesel, gallon for gallon, until the ship's tanks were brimming. They refilled the two barrels aboard the helicopter and the jerry cans from the jeep with their mixture.

Crisanto had Jati wait outside the helicopter with a fire extinguisher pointed at the air intake as he started the engine, then set the power to one-hundred percent for six minutes. He waited for either an explosion or the engine to peter out in a whimper. He checked the temperature, and when it stayed in the green, albeit at the bottom, he lifted the collective, and the aircraft rose very slowly. He motioned with his head for the co-pilot to come aboard. This time they rose even more sluggishly, and Crisanto laughed sarcastically, "This stuff is like trying to fly on goddamn piss."

Jati grimaced. "Must you say this word?"

Jati pointed at Sol and André and motioned to the rear hatch. Sol directed Ibrahim to come aboard as well, but he approached the ship timidly, trying to hold down his fluttering *jellabiya*. "You need to come with us," Sol screamed over the engine noise, "you're very important to us. You're the translator."

"Bra'heem no go…" He poked his index finger into the air and wagged it wildly.

Sol began to argue but gave up quickly, jumped from the helicopter, and ran to DokDok, using hand signals and his infantile Arabic to convince the commander that there were more Janjaweed to kill, promising this time not to spare a single soul, and that even more money would be theirs if they got the girl and the old pilot back. He reached into his pants and pulled out a clump of bills, took a deep breath to calm himself, and offered them to DokDok with the hint of a bow.

DokDok barked to Ibrahim to climb aboard, and the young man did, trembling as violently as the prisoners from whom they had plied the intelligence. DokDok ordered three rebels to join Sol and Ibrahim. DokDok yelled to Ibrahim, "These are the best soldiers in Darfur. Bring them home to me."

Crisanto attempted a meager hover, but the ship only came light on the skids. "Two-hundred pounds too heavy," he called back over his shoulder. Sol and André looked at each other, and without a word, Sol jumped off.

"You get her, *mon ami*. It is your job. I will stay here and treat the wounded for a while, then I'll drive to El Fasher. If I don't see you there, do not forget, next week, Cairo Ramses Hilton. Check every day at the desk."

Sol lifted his thumb toward Crisanto. The ship barely rose but soon resettled. Crisanto tried again, this time tipping forward on the skids, not actually hovering, but ever so slowly starting a slide along the sand to pick up speed. Sol laughed to himself about the new sign he'd recommend Singh hang over the office:

CALCUTTA HELICOPTER—ZERO TO SIXTY IN A DAY OR SO
OUR PROMISE TO THE POOR OF THE WORLD.

As the velocity built, Crisanto pointed the nose into the building wind and the helicopter became airborne. He flew around the flank of Jebel Mara in sweeping circles, gaining altitude, before departing toward Chad. Sol wondered if the helicopter had the guts to fly high enough to see large swaths of the desert without being spotted and downed by troops on the ground. He shrugged, accepting that he would probably never find out, and likely never lay eyes on André, Lila, or Romey again.

He went to the wounded men; thirteen Janjaweed suffering burns and gunshot wounds were left, and the two SLF who had been hit with shrapnel from the grenades launched by Jati. He did what he could, stemming the bleeding and teaching the SLF where to apply pressure. He demanded they dribble water down the throats of their enemy. DokDok ordered the men up to the base camp to gather every single thread of matériel not burned beyond recognition, and some of that as well.

The men loaded two of the Russian trucks to the brim with ammunition, rifles, grenade launchers, two radios, uniforms, *jellabiya*s, *immah*s, sandals, and shoes stripped from the dead and wounded. There were cooking pots, kerosene stoves, plastic water bottles, paper, pencils, Korans, tents, prayer mats, tinned food, tea, *jabana*, salt, pepper, camel yogurt, a huge bottle of feta cheese floating in brine, rock-hard pita, and a box of Kit Kats, which the men ate with their tea when DokDok granted a break.

Sol took the medical equipment and sorted through it, but when he started to use it to treat one of the Janjaweed who was just minutes from meeting his maker, Ra'as's face flushed to the hue of a ripe grape, and he lunged forward, swiping the hemostat and suture material from Sol's hand. Sol went to the jeep, checked the fuel gauge, estimated twenty gallons, and decided it was enough to limp up to El Fasher.

* * *

As he drove away, he came to groups of refugees. They were no longer running, and many had to be helped to walk. One of the children called out "*Doctori*, jeep!" recognizing Sol from the day he'd let the boys drive. The gang howled in laughter, pointing to each other, then to the Rover, making motions as if steering. One of the boys came forward carrying a foot-long model of the Land Rover he'd fashioned from scraps of cardboard. The pieces had been sewn together by hand, the thread but wisps of nylon from the bags that had held milk powder and *durra*. The axels were crafted from twigs, and red plastic caps from the vegetable oil bottles served as headlights and wheels. Another tattered piece of nylon thread had been tied to the front to pull it along. He presented it silently to Sol, his eyes lowered. Sol lowered his eyes as well. That culled more howls of laughter. He gave the boy ten dollars, and the other children surrounded him to see what they could get for shredded tee shirts, pebbles, twigs, and torn flip flops.

Sol asked where the clan elder could be found, and several of the boys rushed off to find him. Sheik Muhammad, the man who had died several times at the hands of his stubborn friends, stumbled toward the jeep. The boys held his thin arms to keep him upright. Sol handed the old man a thousand dollars, but made him promise aloud, in Allah's name, he would feed all of the people, and not a grain extra for his own family. As Sol sped off, he yelled to the chief that he would send the UN to rescue them.

* * *

He reached El Fasher that night after having stopped four times to repair tires in hamlets along the way. The local boys beat the dried rubber with rock-headed sledge hammers until their gowns dripped with sweat. Sol left each child ten dollars. He called Mr. Chun from a hotel. The diplomat promised to go to the safe, collect the shoebox, and leave the remaining money and Sol's passport under a rock at the edge of town.

Chun also offered his advice. "Doctor, you must leave the Sudan four day ago. That is one day before you start war between India and Pakistan, and three day before you destroy detachment of Janjaweed their regional headquarter. And, please, Doctor," the Korean man laughed, "you never use Chun name. You never meet Chun."

Sol drove to the hostel, gave the mother superior two thousand dollars, and left a plastic bag in her hand with five thousand dollars for Bra'heem and the SLF. The nun assured Sol it would get to them, though she implored, "You never to tell any person or use name of this church."

Sol hugged her. She was startled for a moment but did not pull away. He shook his head in disbelief that he had embraced a nun then laughed aloud, "Orthodox Church, I mean they've got married priests, so it's probably okay. Just another deed for the confessional and Father Tony." He touched her hand as he walked off. She lowered her head.

He made his way to the airport, stopping first at Calcutta Helicopter to settle Crisanto's bill for fuel and engine time. He added two thousand to patch the bullet holes, an act that garnered not a thank you, but a mention of the loss of the first helicopter and the burial fees for the British co-pilot. He threw in another three thousand.

Sol drove to the Sunset Airways hangar at the far end of the field and traded the Rover and two thousand dollars for an eight-hundred-mile flight to N'Djamena, the capital of Chad. It was a major city, one large enough to hide for a day or so, then escape central Africa without having to go through Khartoum. He paid another thousand for a no-questions flight from N'Djamena to Tripoli, and fifteen-hundred more for the trip to Egypt in a World War Two DC-3, where he sat in the back on a rotting plywood floor.

CHAPTER TEN

In Cairo, he phoned Please Help the Children's office in London. They went on speakerphone. Not a single question was tendered about his sudden reappearance, or by the tales he spewed as fast as the phone line could carry them. When he was done, they did, however, query at length about how he was going to account for the money he'd squandered. Next, they reported they had not heard from Lila or André, or about the helicopter crew, but were in touch with the Sudanese officials in Khartoum, who had expelled Please Help the Children. Nigel, the CEO, ordered him to leave Cairo on the next flight and report to the home office in Great Britain, and it was to be no later than tomorrow.

He had been taught at his last clinic in the US that one should always smile on the phone, that that emotion would carry over the lines, softening anything said. So, he grinned, "Hey, Nigel, fuck you and the camel you rode in on." The smile broadened as the phone slammed down.

He left a letter at the desk of the Cairo Ramses Hilton, though the clerk asked if he was a guest. When he allowed he was staying elsewhere, the man apologized that they were not a postal service. When Sol offered up three tens, the man wrote on the envelope, using an exclusive code for favored, arriving guests. Sol waited in the lobby for hours, the clerk flashing him smiles and sending over cups of tea. At dusk Sol went back to his hotel.

The next morning, on his way to the Hilton, he stopped at a flower vendor on an ancient street, telling the owner in broken Arabic of his time in Sudan. The man plucked three dozen blood-red roses from his stock, took Sol's ten-dollar bill, and gave him nine in change. Sol tried to get him to take more, but the man pushed the money back each time.

In the street, Sol passed a woman covered from head to toe in rags, a municipal street sweeper. He handed her a rose and walked on. At the leather workshops, gangs of men stopped their labor of tanning hundreds and hundreds of hides to stare at him. Their hands and arms were stained as brown as the leather they worked. He sat with them on break and bought tea and cigarettes for the whole shift, another two dollars. He grinned to himself at the notation he would make on his expense report for Please Help the Children—tea and smokes for laborers who smell like leather.

He took a breakfast of falafel on soft, warm, spotless pita, and a glass of cold orange juice, then sat for an hour reading the International Herald Tribune. He drank strong coffee lightened with tablespoons of sweetened condensed milk. At the Hilton, he checked with the clerk, who waited expectantly for another ten. No one had asked for him. He wrote in his diary for a few hours in the ornate lobby, stunned by the striking health of the kids tagging behind gentle, beautifully attired Egyptians. He was soon sitting with the African families, discussing politics and refugee policy. The women, in particular, were informed and articulate. They were adamant that without secular education, famine and violence would remain the salient driving force of life in Africa for the next thousand years.

The men, on the other hand, wanted to know why Arabs had been blamed for 9-11. They flushed angrily as they informed Sol it was dynamite planted in the towers that brought the buildings down. Even a table of Egyptian university professors sipping tea in the lounge were convinced the attack on the World Trade Center had been carried out by the Israelis on the order of President Bush. When Sol asked how they could dispute the video of the planes smashing into the buildings, the men shot back angrily that the film had been Photoshopped.

By afternoon, Sol had grown restless and called Please Help the Children in London. He, again, ignored their fiscal inquiries, and asked abruptly if there had been word. He went to dinner at another hotel, one that served beer, and as he finished the second, he began to accept that he had returned to the real world, and that there were extradition laws, and his bravado notwithstanding, he would eventually have to pay back every penny he'd frittered. He stopped by the Hilton once again before midnight. The next day was indistinguishable from the one before.

On the fourth day, he started to put in a call to his lawyer in Whitaker to ask if the State Medical Abuse Commission had rendered a decision regarding his future as a doctor, but he understood the answer did not matter, and that it was simply time to go home. He hung up before the call went through.

He paid the clerk another twenty dollars to accept the call if his friends telephoned, but by seven there was no word, and he made his way back to the hostel to pack. He passed the closed British Airways office, though a light was burning, and a kind Egyptian woman opened the door. She listened to his story and booked a flight home through Frankfurt. It would have been cheaper and faster to leave from Paris or London, but he could not bear touching British or French soil.

He presented six of the roses to the travel agent. She gasped that she had never been given a bouquet, then reopened the computer and placed him in first class for the whole trip home to Whitaker. He touched her hand, as he had the nun in El Fasher, and left.

The next morning, he had the desk at his hostel call a cab. The driver was a gruff, toothless man. The taxi's windshield was so soiled, Sol could not fathom how the man could see the road. The inside stank of rancid breath and cigarettes, and the driver growled when Sol asked him to stop at the Hilton first and wait while he checked at the desk. There was no word. He exhaled deeply and went back to the foul vehicle.

As he was lowering himself into the backseat, another cab skidded to a stop at the front of the hotel. A man and a woman, both shabbily dressed, emerged unsteadily. Sol recognized neither, but when the woman turned toward him, he was struck by the architecture of her face, the flawless bone structure, the perfect nose, the dark and intense eyes. She seemed so small, though, and he ignored the mirage.

The man with her barely glanced at Sol's cab. When Sol noticed they were Caucasians, his heart leapt into his mouth, but he quickly calmed for they were so small, so insignificant, he thought they might be children. He turned away disinterestedly, nodding to the cabbie to start out, but before the driver could shift into gear, a dull spark burst from the interstices of Sol's subconscious and grew at light speed into a flare so bright, so intense, he hardly felt the clutch of his chest that really did stop his heart. With that came a stippling of the outside world, and it took him a moment to find the door handle.

By now, the cab was pulling into traffic, and Sol screamed, "Stop!" so loud, the flock of pedestrians outside the hotel startled and watched fearfully as Sol flew from inside the cab and ran toward them. André, alone, took a step forward, puffing his chest, a pit bull guarding Lila. Then André shrieked, and as he lunged toward Sol with open arms, the onlookers dispersed as if a bomb had landed in their midst. The two men hugged wildly, nearly falling into Lila. She stood frozen for a moment, expressionless, but began to tremble and wobbled toward Sol. The two embraced desperately, as if it were the last moments of their lives. The world had stopped for three of its minor souls.

Sol sensed nothing until five or six cabbies jumped from their vehicles to pull wildly at the three Westerners, separating them, screaming epithets in the most guttural of Arabic. The desk clerk came from the lobby, saw Sol, called back inside, and was joined by a gang of hotel employees. They hollered at the cabbies to leave, or they would never be given another fare from the Hilton. The clerk hissed to Sol. "Muslim Brotherhood. They say you must not touch a woman. They are crazy, yes, but also, very dangerous."

In the lobby, the three fell into the plush chairs on which Sol had spent days praying. "Oh, my God, André. This is what I wanted more than anything on Earth. You and Lila together. May it be forever. May I be the godfather of your children. A dozen of them. This is the answer to my prayers. I will want for nothing in life after this."

André shook his head in disbelief. "You still do not understand zis sing." He looked at Lila. "You are to tell 'im, or is it me? But I cannot wis out ze giggle."

Lila laughed openly. "Soli, we are *not* going to be married. No, André, you tell him. It's too funny. I simply can't do it."

"Okay. *Mon ami*, 'ow do I say zis? *Mais non*, first, I give you zis." He pulled a newspaper-wrapped packet from his bag. "Zis is from your pal, Bra'heem." Sol smiled and tore at the paper, exposing an *immah*. "It is 'is. 'Ee send it to you as ze gift from ze Liberation Force of ze Sudan."

Sol unwound the five-foot length of cloth as both Lila and André rolled their eyes at the fabric, stiff with dried saliva, sand, oil, burn marks, and reminiscence. Sol leaned back and clutched the gift tightly. André waited for another moment then took a deep breath. "Now, I tell you. Mademoiselle Lila is not my, what is it you say, my cup of tea. I prefer ze man." Sol's jaw dropped, and André went on. "Zat is unless you are ze interested one." André raised his eyes seductively. "All zis one talk about is ze American doctor who is so brave, so handsome, who free ze refugees, who jump out of ze 'elicopter so André may save 'er, because he sink I am ze one to marry 'er. On and on. Soli zis and Soli zat. I am tired of it by now."

Lila's eyes reddened, a few drops rolling onto her cheek. Sol whispered, "So this is how an angel cries." He leaned forward to wipe the tears away then leaned back again, his hand shaking.

André huffed, "You kiss 'er, or I will kiss you."

EPILOGUE

Dr. Solomon Forte appeared before the State Medical Abuse Commission's newly elected chairman the day after he arrived home. It was a private meeting. The two talked for nearly four hours. Sol agreed to write a paper on the use of pain medication in the dying.

The chairman ordered, "You will deliver, at the Commission's yearly meeting, a formal lecture based on your research, and it will be published in our journal. Make it good, and be sure you include the story of your patient, the one who landed you in my office. It's a lesson for all of us. And I trust that when you address our lofty council, you will include half-an-hour about the delivery of medical care in darkest Africa. God forbid, one of our colleagues might learn something."

When Sol arrived in London after his presentation to the State Medical Abuse Commission, Lila was at Heathrow Airport. She cried for an hour and refused to stop touching him. On the drive to her home in a chauffeured limousine, they sat holding hands in the back. They did not speak for a long time until she gasped, "Okay. Here it goes. I have something to tell you before you meet my family. Promise me you won't run away. Please, don't run away." Sol was too startled to answer. "I am, shall we say, of, oh, what the bloody hell, royal birth."

They married six months later at the castle, the one in which she had been born. Rachmaninoff's *Piano Concerto in C Minor, Opus 18* played before and after the ceremony.

The next day, Lila was informed that her graduate work had been sufficient to merit a PhD at Selwyn College, Cambridge. Two weeks later, while on their honeymoon in Scotland, she received another e-mail offering her a joint professorship, one in international relations at Selwyn, and the other in nursing at Addenbrooke's Hospital.

Though it took over a year to be licensed to practice in England, Solomon Forte accepted a position as a clinician in the City of Cambridge. In 2005, Lila gave birth to a boy. They named him André.

During the year he studied for his British medical examination, Sol began to write. He was admitted to his wife's college and eventually elected to a fellowship in sociology. He spent his free time writing novels about the human condition.

André Anseau graduated from medical school in Paris in 2004. He returned to Darfur in 2011 as a senior physician. He died there of AIDS a year later.

OTHER TITLES BY
WILLIAM S. GOULD, MD

William Stuart Gould, M.D.

AT YONAH MOUNTAIN

Brand new Second Lieutenant J.W. Weathersby is on orders to depart for a combat tour in Viet Nam. At a West Point wedding, though, he commits a very public faux pas and is thrust as punishment into a class of 160 select young officers who sweat and freeze through months of brutal training at the United States Army Ranger School.

J.W. joins an African American PhD candidate and a Rose Bud Sioux Harvard graduate, the three pushed together to trudge the mountains, forests, and deserts as Ranger buddies. As half the class is weeded out, they share their disparate lives and dreams. J.W. struggles to be cut from the program, and at the same time fights desperately to remain.

At Yonah Mountain is a coming of age adventure, an examination of race relations in the military, and an authentic tale of Army Ranger training.

CAPTAIN IRON MUSTACHE

Captain Iron Mustache takes place in 1968 and 1969. United States Army lieutenant, J.W. Weathersby, just out of Ranger School, volunteers for duty in Viet Nam. It is not long before he changes from naïve youngster to hardened soldier.

Something about rural Viet Nam, though, captivates him, and he convinces his commanding officer to allow him to live as the sole American in a remote rice-farming hamlet. His mission is to win the hearts and the minds of the peasants. J.W. forms a deep friendship with the village chief, and falls in love with the schoolteacher, Miss Lin.

During a mid-night battle, Miss Lin is arrested and tortured as a communist agent. At the same time, the chief is critically wounded, and disappears after being flown out of the village by an American medevac helicopter.

J.W. and the chief's wife spend the last month of his tour driving the deadly roads of Viet Nam searching hospital after hospital for the man.

Nearly half a century later, J.W. and his wife return to Viet Nam in a surreal effort to find the chief. He also wants to see Miss Lin, but the Vietnamese government is suspicious of his motives, and the days of his sojourn are fraught with struggle and frustration until a simple act of kindness changes his life.

William Stuart Gould, M.D.

IN BLACK GRANITE

In Black Granite is set in the decade after J.W. Weathersby returns from the war in Viet Nam. He eventually accepts the assessment of family, friends, and medical school deans that he will never become a doctor. He drifts without focus until the miracle of his first child's birth rekindles the craving to study medicine.

This is a narrative of his dogged struggle to beat the overwhelming odds against a man in his mid-thirties gaining admission to an American college of medicine. In Black Granite scrutinizes the ruthless battle for places in medical school, and how the psyches of the chosen are sieved as they are herded through the decade as students and residents. The strain of endless days and nights away from family, of sleepless months, and of pervasive arrogance, distort the souls of even the strongest. Some find the path more treacherous than surviving a war.

C.O.L.A.

The day his father died, Dr. Solomon Forte promised his mother he would honor the man's memory by dedicating his years as a doctor to the treatment of injured workers. It seemed so clear a decision—his patients would be like his dad, stoic, honest, working-class stiffs who sought nothing more from a doctor than an arm around the shoulder, a word of reassurance, and an ally in dealing with the state industrial insurance system.

His life at the Whitaker Hospital and Medical Center is, though, the antithesis of his dream. He can't tell which of the roadblocks is most daunting: that posed by his medical colleagues, the threats of S.M.A.C., the State Medical Abuse Commission, the bureaucracy at C.O.L.A., the state's Commission on Labor Affairs, or the duplicitous patients, some of whom spend every waking moment trying to dupe him out of drugs and government benefits.

Occasionally, a case is obvious—the worker really was devastated by an industrial accident. It seems to Sol, though, that those are the very patients C.O.L.A. torments. On the other hand, claimants skilled at ripping off the Commission run free for decades. C.O.L.A. also examines the specter of serious medical errors, and how they are so much easier to make on patients whose care is mired in the aggravation of government-sponsored insurance plans. Questions are also raised about the state-appointed morality commissions that determine which doctors relinquish their licenses for treating pain.

Finally, it is a disturbing look behind the scenes of a modern, multi-specialty medical clinic.

A HEART WIND FROM THE DESERT

Dr. Solomon Forte has lost everything. There is little left but to offer himself to the wretched in war-torn Sudan. Arriving in the desert, heart brimming with hope, it does not take long to recognize that the social and political beliefs that have spawned the war and famine are the very forces that prevent him from carrying out his dream of caring for the dispossessed.

At first, despite the warnings of the tiny European medical team left at the refugee camp in Darfur Province, he fights back with typical, strident, American resolve to save the entire population of refugees. The obstacles of life in Central African, however, soon draw the spirit from him, and he turns his efforts to preserving the lives of his Western companions.

He falls deeply for a gorgeous, but outwardly hardened, British nurse. When she disappears from camp, he spends what strength is left searching for her.

A Heart Wind from the Desert examines the need in all of us to accomplish something meaningful in the tiny fragment of time we are allotted, and the impossible hurdles faced when trying to change the way people have thought and behaved for the millennia.

It is a tale of beautiful, warm children, but also of the stark life in the sub-Saharan Sahel.

RAPHAEL'S BLANKET

Raphael Blumenkopf is born clandestinely at the Bergen Belsen Nazi death camp on the 14th of April, 1945. His birth is an unprecedented miracle, as is the liberation of the camp by British forces that very afternoon. He has only his mother and a few surviving villagers from their home in Checzonovska, Poland. While the majority of the refugees leave Central Europe for Israel and the West, his band travels across Russia to China. A relative has promised jobs in Shang Hai's old Jewish settlement.

The journey is fraught with threats from starving Russians, barbaric border guards, and destitute Chinese peasants. Just as the lives of the immigrants begin to normalize in China, the victory of Mao Zedong's communist army forces them to flee, this time to Hanoi.

Five years later, the communist movement in North Viet Nam topples the French government, and the Jews run again. They settle in Saigon until the unrest there compels them to emigrate to America. Raphael's years in the U.S. are colored indelibly by the poison that follows him from the Holocaust, and he formulates a plan to extract revenge from a federal judge with ties to the Nazis.

Who could have envisaged the price he'd pay?

LINCOLN FRIDAY

Lincoln Friday is born into nothing, an obscure, dirt farmer's son, destined to live dominated by the jagged edges of two wars. His early years are an endless series of losses, yet he struggles back after each blow, and slowly, a strongbox of dreams emerges from the fog of his hopelessness.

The harshest test of Lincoln's life, though, comes when the effects of his exposure to Agent Orange devastate both his and his daughter's lives. While the Fridays fight back passionately, the courts, Congress, and the VA turn their backs on them.

In the end, his deeds were neither profound nor dazzling, but he left his mark on disparate people in disparate lands. The world he touched chafed less for his quiet dignity.

SABRINA'S SUIT

Sabrina Friday, a gorgeous, young Doctor of Psychology, was born with a spinal defect as a result of her father, Lincoln Friday's exposure to Agent Orange in Viet Nam. Nonetheless, she leads a perfectly normal life until she becomes pregnant, and her care is botched. The complications change her life forever.

She and her husband finally bring suit against the doctor and hospital responsible for her tragedy. This is the narrative of that medical practice lawsuit, an anatomy of a case that lays forth the ends to which doctors and hospitals go to sidestep responsibility for shoddy care.

SASS

Reuben and Miriam Sassovitch emigrate from Romania to the promised land of the Bronx in the late 1970s. Crafting a new name and brimming with optimism, they enroll their only child, Elliott, in public school. Though a virtuoso in chemistry, his gifts do not extend beyond the lab doors.

His neuroses only deepen with time, nearly costing him his life in New York's drug underworld. Worse, though, they poison his bond with a blemished, but magical woman he pursues across the world.

For Elliott, life is one sharp-toothed puncture wound after another, until a flicker of light transforms him. It is a coming-of-age tale, but one that weaves an improbable path. It is also the saga of a love not destined to be that succeeds.

www.ingramcontent.com/pod-product-compliance
Lightning Source LLC
Chambersburg PA
CBHW070624260626
47161CB00007B/2578

* 9 7 8 0 9 9 7 9 8 0 4 2 4 *